D1611245

The Lumbar Intervertebral Disc

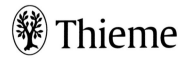

I dedicate this book to my family. To my parents, David and Shirley, whose unwavering love, support, and dedication have been an inspiration. They instilled in me a passion for knowledge and learning. To my wife, Denny: I cannot adequately express how much I value your being behind, alongside, and in front of me every step on this incredible journey. Thanks for all your sacrifices. I love you. Gina and Jay, you two are special people and make it all worthwhile.

–Frank M. Phillips

I dedicate this book to my family, for all time.

– Carl Lauryssen

Thieme Medical Publishers, Inc.
333 Seventh Ave.
New York, NY 10001

Editorial Director: Michael Wachinger
Executive Editor: Kay Conerly
Managing Editor: J. Owen Zurhellen IV
Vice President, Production and Electronic Publishing: Anne T. Vinnicombe
Production Editor: Grace R. Caputo, Dovetail Content Solutions
Medical Illustrator: Anthony M. Pazos
Cover illustration by Karl Wesker
Vice President, International Sales and Marketing: Cornelia Schulze
Chief Financial Officer: Peter van Woerden
President: Brian D. Scanlan
Compositor: Thomson Digital
Printer: Leo Paper Group

Library of Congress Cataloging-in-Publication Data

The lumbar intervertebral disc / editors, Frank M. Phillips and Carl
Lauryssen.
     p. ; cm.
  Includes bibliographical references.
  ISBN 978-1-60406-048-5
  1. Intervertebral disk—Diseases. 2. Lumbar vertebrae. I. Phillips, Frank
M. II. Lauryssen, Carl.
  [DNLM: 1. Intervertebral Disk. 2. Lumbosacral Region. 3. Spinal Diseases.
WE 750 L956607 2010]
  RD771.I6L855 2010
  617.5'6—dc22
                              2009012072

Important note: Medical knowledge is ever-changing. As new research and clinical experience broaden our knowledge, changes in treatment and drug therapy may be required. The authors and editors of the material herein have consulted sources believed to be reliable in their efforts to provide information that is complete and in accord with the standards accepted at the time of publication. However, in view of the possibility of human error by the authors, editors, or publisher of the work herein or changes in medical knowledge, neither the authors, editors, nor publisher, nor any other party who has been involved in the preparation of this work, warrants that the information contained herein is in every respect accurate or complete, and they are not responsible for any errors or omissions or for the results obtained from use of such information. Readers are encouraged to confirm the information contained herein with other sources. For example, readers are advised to check the product information sheet included in the package of each drug they plan to administer to be certain that the information contained in this publication is accurate and that changes have not been made in the recommended dose or in the contraindications for administration. This recommendation is of particular importance in connection with new or infrequently used drugs.

Some of the product names, patents, and registered designs referred to in this book are in fact registered trademarks or proprietary names even though specific reference to this fact is not always made in the text. Therefore, the appearance of a name without designation as proprietary is not to be construed as a representation by the publisher that it is in the public domain.

Printed in China

5 4 3 2 1

ISBN 978-1-60406-048-5

The Lumbar Intervertebral Disc

Frank M. Phillips, MD
Professor
Department of Orthopedic Surgery
Co-Director, Spine Fellowship
Rush University Medical Center
Chicago, Illinois

Carl Lauryssen, MD
Director, L.A. Center for Spine Care and Research
Olympia Medical Center
Associate Professor
Department of Neurosurgery
University of Southern California
Los Angeles, California

WITHDRAWN

Thieme
New York • Stuttgart

Contents

Foreword

The clinical, social, and economic implications of back pain are monumental. In the United States, health care expenditure related to back pain in 2005 was $86 billion, a figure similar to what the country spent on the treatment of diabetes. Forty million Americans with spinal or back pain will consult a doctor annually. In the United Kingdom, 13% of the working population will miss work because of back pain for a month or more. In terms of economy (national and individual), of employees who are off work for 6 months, only half return to work; of those off for 12 months, a quarter return. Two years of incapacitating back pain and the worker may never return to work.

There is thus an understandable pressure on the physician to "cure" the problem, an unachievable goal for many patients from the start considering the results reported in the literature and the comorbidities of pain in other sites and obesity in most back pain sufferers. The diametric treatment options of operation and no surgery are due to the less than universal success of the myriad of interventions and also the wide variety of somatic and psychological factors that can evince back pain. It requires a detailed clinical history to identify mechanical back pain; unfortunately, too many decisions to operate are based on magnetic resonance imaging, and the "black disc" is too often the scapegoat. In the United States, there is a 15-fold variation in the incidence of lumbar disc surgery across the country, and an industry has developed around failed back and revision surgery.

Controlled clinical trials of surgery have not given the hoped-for advantage of surgery versus a nonoperative approach for acute sciatica in The Netherlands or fusion for chronic back pain in the United Kingdom. The multicenter SPORT trial in the United States, which appeared to favor surgery, was confounded by the fact that the actual cost of the operation, implant, and reimbursement varied in the 13 trial centers, which interfered with the outcome calculations.

As health dollars become scarcer and a once-adoring public becomes more questioning, it is essential that physicians, surgeons, and health care workers understand much more deeply than before the causes, pathomechanics, and likely national history of a condition that causes much misery but very little mortality.

In this text, Frank Phillips and Carl Lauryssen—themselves expert clinicians, surgeons, and academics—have brought together a group of experts to look at the lumbar intervertebral disc, with considerable success. Natural aging and pathological changes are carefully presented in different chapters. The etiology of pain associated with acute disc injury as well as with a chronic degenerative condition is presented. The editors face up to the still-large gaps in our understanding of the condition and concede that "the mechanisms of discogenic pain is not well understood." But their authors provide the latest in the biology of degeneration and pain generation to stimulate the inquiring reader. In addition, the role of presurgical psychological screening, the importance of education, and the value of back schools and cognitive therapy are addressed. Conventional microsurgical techniques are described, as are new approaches, such as annular repair and barrier techniques and developments in arthoplasty. All the chapters are well researched and extensively referenced to allow the reader to pursue further individual lines of investigation.

The Lumbar Intervertebral Disc is important reading for those who wish to know the current thinking on this most difficult topic. I commend it, wholeheartedly.

Alan Crockard, DSc, FRCS, FRCS (Ed), FDS, RCS (Eng), FRCP
Emeritus Professor of Surgical Neurology
Victor Horsley Department of Neurosurgery
The National Hospital for Neurology and Neurosurgery
Queen Square, London
United Kingdom

Preface

Diseases of the intervertebral disc and associated degenerative disorders of the lumbar spine are a major focus of contemporary spinal care. These conditions are formidable clinical problems as well as a leading cause of suffering and disability, resulting in substantial health care costs. Disc degeneration may itself cause symptoms but is also an early event in the spinal degenerative cascade, ultimately leading to a variety of pathologies of the spine. This book, *The Lumbar Intervertebral Disc*, is devoted to the understanding and treatment of disorders of the disc. The editors' vision was to provide the reader with a text that comprehensively explores the latest knowledge pertaining to the lumbar intervertebral disc, with detailed information regarding the diagnosis and treatment of disc-related conditions, as well as the basic science of the disc, including anatomy, biology, pathophysiology, and biomechanics. We are very fortunate to have leaders in the field contributing chapters to this book.

In recent years, unprecedented advances in understanding of the biology and biomechanics of the disc in health and disease have led to developments in novel nonsurgical and surgical approaches to treatment of disc-related pain. Emerging over the past decade are less-invasive surgical strategies as well as motion-sparing surgical alternatives, and *The Lumbar Intervertebral Disc* explores these and other scientific frontiers relating to the disc, covering the breadth of pathologic syndromes and treatment options for the lumbar disc. Chapters are arranged logically, covering the herniated disc as well as degenerative disc disease. In each area, we describe the anatomy and biology, biomechanics and kinematics, pathophysiology and natural history, diagnostic workup, and surgical and nonoperative management of the condition. There is also focus on the patient as a whole, and the psychological aspects of disc disease are covered. We hope that the accurate surgical drawings will be helpful for surgical preparation.

Expert contributors in the field share their knowledge and expertise covering a wide variety of topics, and learning gems are numerous. Although specially intended for orthopedic and neurologic spinal surgeons (and advanced-level trainees including spine fellows and residents), the comprehensive and inclusive nature of *The Lumbar Intervertebral Disc* makes it of interest to pain specialists, scientists, physical therapists, chiropractors, and physiatrists — indeed, of anyone fascinated with the intricacies of the disc.

Frank M. Phillips
Carl Lauryssen

Acknowledgments

We thank our friends and colleagues who contributed to this book, for making time, in their incredibly busy lives, to share their thoughts and knowledge for the betterment of patients. Thanks to our teachers, mentors, and fellow surgeons who continually shape our professional and personal lives. Thanks to J. Owen Zurhellen and Kay D. Conerly at Thieme Publishers for all your guidance. You made this task relatively painless with your necessary and welcomed nudges. Also, thank you, Tony Pazos; your artistic contributions are greatly appreciated. To our industry friends — in this critical time, without you our patients would not benefit from the development of new technologies. We need each other and are grateful to have been part of great improvements in spinal care that have happened in such a short time. We have much to do still.

Dr. Phillips also wishes to acknowledge:

- Michael Simon, Larry Pottenger, and Henry Bohlman who mentored, trusted, and inspired me. I owe you all a great deal. To all my friends and colleagues who have supported me along the way, especially Carl, my co-editor and friend.

Dr. Lauryssen would also like to acknowledge:

- Professor Alan Crockard, Professor Mark Hadley, Professor Ralph Dacey, Professors Bruce Tranmer, Frank Leblanc, big bad Betty MacRae, Terry Myles, Mike Hunter, Marie Long, Ollie Dold, Harvey Thomas, Gary Dix, Celine Deaan (Deon Louw), Jerry Krcek, Owen Williams, Richard Brownlee, Sean McFadden, JB, Amgad, and Azzie: I have learned so much from all of you. Thank you.

- My office — Trysten, Pablo, Jessica, Jonathan, Alfonso, Jing, Jeannie, OMC nurses, OMC OR team (Big Julie), OMC 3 East caregivers, POM, and Dr Calderone, for getting things done; I am grateful to be surrounded by such outstanding individuals and team.

- Dad, Mom, Liezel, Craig, Jordan, Taylor, Emma, MIL, Charles, Evan, Mora, Taina, Noe, Carlos, Whitney, Jack, Erin, and Wiley, for being the best family in the world. I would like to acknowledge my co-editor Frank M. Phillips for his sincere friendship and his invitation to co-author this book.

- My wife, Alisa, for always encouraging me to pursue my passion for my profession. An enormous amount of gratitude goes to her for keeping Rex and Liv occupied at a time when she needed me more than I ever realized. Thank you; I love you.

Contributors

Michael A. Adams, BSc, PhD
Department of Anatomy
University of Bristol
Bristol, United Kingdom

Vijay Agarwal, BS
Department of Orthopaedic Surgery
Stanford University School of Medicine
Stanford, California

Todd F. Alamin, MD
Associate Professor
Department of Orthopaedic Surgery
Stanford University School of Medicine
Stanford Hospitals and Clinics
Stanford, California

Todd J. Albert, MD
Richard H. Rothman Professor and Chair
Department of Orthopaedics
Professor of Neurosurgery
Thomas Jefferson University and Hospital
The Rothman Institute
Philadelphia, Pennsylvania

Howard S. An, MD
The Morton International Professor
Department of Orthopedic Surgery
Rush Medical College
Rush University Medical Center
Chicago, Illinois

Neel Anand, MD
Institute for Spinal Disorders
Cedars-Sinai Medical Center
Los Angeles, California

Gunnar B.J. Andersson, MD, PhD
Professor and Chairman Emeritus
Department of Orthopedic Surgery
Rush University Medical Center
Chicago, Illinois

Qi-Bin Bao, PhD
Vice President
Advanced Spine
Marquette, Minesotta

Eli M. Baron, MD
Institute for Spinal Disorders
Cedars-Sinai Medical Center
Los Angeles, California

Maneesh Bawa, MD
Assistant Professor
Orthopaedic and Spine Center
Emory University School of Medicine
Atlanta, Georgia

Ashok Biyani, MD
Associate Professor
Department of Orthopaedic Surgery
University of Toledo Medical Center
Toledo, Ohio

Scott D. Boden, MD
Director, The Emory Spine Center
Department of Orthopaedic Surgery
Emory University School of Medicine
Staff Physician
Atlanta Veterans Administration Medical Center
Atlanta, Georgia

Pablo R. Pazmiño, MD
Director, Beverly Spine and Santa Monica Spine Institutes
Orthopaedic Spine Department
Olympia Medical Center
Cedars-Sinai Medical Center
Los Angeles, California

Mario L. Pereira, MD
Fellow, Texas Back Institute
Plano, Texas

Frank M. Phillips, MD
Professor
Department of Orthopedic Surgery
Co-Director, Spine Fellowship
Rush University Medical Center
Chicago, Illinois

Thomas J. Raley, MD
Director, Minimally Invasive Spine Institute
Department of Orthopaedics
Georgetown University
George Washington University
Washington, DC
Virginia Hospital Center
Arlington, Virginia

Thomas F. Roush, MD
Spine Surgeon
Southeastern Spine Institute
Mount Pleasant, South Carolina

Daphne R. Scott, DSc
Physical Therapist
Regional Manager, Athletico
Chicago, Illinois

Kern Singh, MD
Assistant Professor
Department of Orthopedic Surgery
Rush University Medical Center
Chicago, Illinois

Curtis W. Slipman, MD
Miami, Florida

Gwendolyn A. Sowa, MD, PhD
Assistant Professor
Department of Physical Medicine and Rehabilitation
Co-Director, Ferguson Laboratory for Orthopaedic and
    Spine Research
University of Pittsburgh Medical Center
Pittsburgh, Pennsylvania

Selvon St. Clair, MD, PhD
Chief Resident
Department of Orthopaedic Surgery
The Cleveland Clinic
Cleveland, Ohio

E. Andrew Stevens, MD
Resident
Department of Neurosurgery
Wake Forest University Health Sciences
North Carolina Baptist Medical Center
Medical Center Boulevard
Winston-Salem, North Carolina

William R. Taylor, MD
Professor
Department. of Neurosurgery
University of California, San Diego, School of
    Medicine
UCSD Medical Center
San Diego, California

Cary R. Templin, MD
Department of Orthopaedic Surgery
Hinsdale Orthopaedic Associates, SC
Hinsdale, South Carolina

Michael N. Tzermiadianos, MD

Alexander R. Vaccaro, MD
Professor
Departments of Orthopaedics and Neurosurgery
The Rothman Institute
Thomas Jefferson University
Philadelphia, Pennsylvania

Mark C. Valente, DO
Resident
Department of Orthopaedic Surgery
Michigan State University
Botsford Hospital
Farmington Hills, Michigan

Nam Vo, PhD
Research Assistant Professor
Department of Orthopaedic Surgery
Ferguson Laboratory for Orthopaedic
    and Spine Research
University of Pittsburgh Medical Center
Pittsburgh, Pennsylvania

Jeffrey C. Wang, MD
Professor
Department of Orthopaedic Surgery and Neurosurgery
UCLA School of Medicine
Chief, Orthopaedic Spine Service
UCLA Comprehensive Spine Center
UCLA Center for Health Sciences
Los Angeles, California

Andrew P. White, MD
Instructor
Department of Orthopaedic Surgery
Harvard Medical School
Carl J. Shapiro Department of Orthopaedic Surgery
Beth Israel Deaconess Medical Center
Boston, Massachusetts

Anthony T. Yeung, MD
Desert Institute for Spine Care
Phoenix, Arizona

Christopher A. Yeung, MD
Desert Institute for Spine Care
Phoenix, Arizona

Hansen A. Yuan, MD
Professor Emeritus
Department of Orthopaedic and Neurological Surgery
State University of New York, Upstate Medical University
Syracuse, New York

Basic Science

1 The Epidemiology and Economics of Intervertebral Disc Disease

Maneesh Bawa and Scott D. Boden

■ Epidemiology

Epidemiology refers to the study of occurrence rates and provides important insights into understanding intervertebral disc (IVD) disease. It provides information about the natural history of a disease so patient counseling about prognosis and appropriate treatment recommendations can be made. It also helps establish associations between a disease and individual or external factors, which allow risk factors to be identified. Finally, it provides information on the demand for social and medical resources, which is important for formulating public health policies.

Epidemiologic research on back disorders is difficult for several reasons. First, there is no standard definition of disc degeneration, so comparisons between studies are difficult because each study defines disc degeneration differently. Second, measures of disc degeneration often lack reliability and precision. Third, accurate measures of lifetime exposures, such as vibration or physical loading, are impossible. Finally, disc degeneration and back pain are not synonymous. Pain is a symptom, whereas the definition of disc degeneration varies with the method used to evaluate the disc; for example, radiographic versus biochemical. Disc degeneration is commonly thought to be associated with severe symptoms and is often targeted diagnostically and therapeutically, but most of the findings associated with disc degeneration, such as desiccation, osteophytes, and disc narrowing, have unclear mechanisms in pain production. Indeed, there is a large body of research into the mechanisms of pain production, but a clear understanding of how the disc causes pain has yet to be gained.

Recently, our views on the etiology of disc degeneration have been changing given our new understanding of genetic influences. Disc degeneration is the result of lifetime degradation and remodeling of both the vertebrae and the disc in response to physical loading and healing. This traditional view of disc degeneration was espoused by Frymoyer[1] in 1992, "Among the factors associated with its occurrence are age, gender, occupation, cigarette smoking, and exposure to vehicular vibration." Therefore, most attention has been given to environmental exposures as risk factors. Only recently have studies been conducted on the hereditary aspects of disc degeneration, and they are dramatically changing the earlier concepts. In one review of current scientific literature, the authors noted that environmental factors may explain only a small portion of disc degeneration and concluded that "genetic factors play an important role in disc pathology, and perhaps a major one."[2]

Defining Disc Degeneration

Definitions of disc degeneration have not been uniform because the process is not well understood. Usually, it is largely defined by the modality used to evaluate it. Radiographic data, autopsy results, surgical samples, biochemical analyses, and microscopic evaluation have all been used in different studies to try to define degeneration. Currently, the preferred method of evaluating the disc for large population samples is magnetic resonance imaging (MRI). There are various qualitative measures of disc degeneration, such as disc space narrowing, desiccation, bulging, and signal intensity loss, to name a few. There are various scales to try to quantify these qualitative changes, but comparisons between studies are often limited because of suboptimal reliability, imprecision, and lack of uniformity of assessments.

Thompson et al[3] provided the first grading scheme for gross morphology of the disc using 15 cadaveric specimens. Once MRI became more widely accepted, disc space narrowing was the most commonly used criterion. Severe narrowing is an obvious sign of degeneration, but early changes in the disc do not always cause narrowing.[4] If changes in the neighboring vertebrae are taken into account, including vertebral rim osteophytes and concavity of the endplates, disc height actually increases initially, and measurements of disc volume may be more important.[5] Other commonly evaluated findings on MRI include Schmorl's nodes, herniations, bulges, vertebral rim osteophytes, disc signal intensity, and high-intensity zones with annular tears. Many studies calculate a summary score to try to take all these findings into account, but this may mask specific effects and miss important correlations, especially genetic ones.[2]

Prevalence of Disc Degeneration

Battie et al[2] performed a thorough review of the scientific literature regarding MRI findings associated with disc degeneration. They identified 20 studies that included information on "asymptomatic" subjects and 10 studies that reported on populations that were symptomatic. As expected, the reported prevalences varied widely between studies. The reported prevalences for asymptomatic subjects were 10 to 81% for bulges, 3 to 63% for protrusion, 0 to 24% for extrusion, 20 to 83% for reduction in signal intensity, 3 to 56% for disc narrowing, 6 to 56% for high-intensity zones with annular tears, and 8 to 19% for Schmorl's nodes. The corresponding prevalences for the symptomatic population were 22 to 48% for bulges, 0 to 79% for protrusion, 1 to 55% for extrusion, 9 to 86% for reduction in signal intensity, 15 to 53% for disc narrowing, 15% for high-intensity zones with annular tears, and 6 to 79% for Schmorl's nodes. The authors concluded that there was no clear difference between the ranges reported for the two groups. Variations in the reported prevalence ranges could be due to age, exposure to known and unknown risk factors, or the disc levels included, but much of the variation is probably due to the different definitions of degenerative changes in the studies.

Many studies do not report prevalences by the specific level, but report summary scores that include the entire lumbar spine. This is problematic because large variations in prevalence have been reported based on the level of the lumbar spine, and the effect of risk factors could vary by level. Schmorl's nodes are most common in the upper levels (L1–L3), while degenerative changes are most common in the lower levels (L4–S1). Between L1 and L3, degenerative changes were uncommon (0 to 14%), whereas between L4 and S1, disc narrowing occurred 20 to 37%, disc bulges 5 to 33%, protrusions 10 to 32%, extrusions 3 to 47%, and annular tears 0 to 20%.[2] Disc herniations are most common at the thoracolumbar and lumbosacral junctions. Therefore, studies that summarize degenerative findings over the entire lumbar spine may miss important differences that are level specific.

Risk Factors

Age and Gender

The risk factor studied most intensely in relation to the degenerative process has been age. Numerous studies involving both autopsy specimens and radiographic evaluation have shown a clear association between increasing age and progressive disc degeneration.[6] In a study of 1000 consecutive autopsies, Heine[7] showed that disc degeneration increased linearly from 0% to 72% between the ages of 39 and 70 years. Another study based on histologic sections of the disc found annular tears in 30-year-olds and nuclear clefts in 40-year-olds.[8] More recent studies have shown that degenerative changes can occur in the younger years. Histopathologic results from autopsy and surgical samples revealed annular tears and endplate cartilage pathology in 3- to 10-year-old children. Although there were significant variations in all age groups, the increase in degenerative

scores was linear between 2 and 88 years of age.[9] In studies using MRI, disc signal intensity also decreases with increasing age.[2]

The relationship of sex to disc degeneration is more complicated. In a review article of 600 autopsy specimens, Miller et al[10] concluded that discs in men started to degenerate a decade earlier than discs in women and were more degenerated than age-matched discs in women. A recent article on sexual differences in degenerative disorders reported that although "degenerative changes are observed at similar rates in both sexes, women seem to be more susceptible to degenerative changes that lead to instability and malalignment."[11] Some biochemical metabolites such as insulin growth factor binding protein 1 and calcium hemostasis factors have been shown to be associated with decreased disc space loss in women.[12] Clearly other factors, including genetics, play a role in the sexual variability seen in disc degeneration.

Environmental and Behavioral Factors

Many have suspected that heavy physical loading, related to occupation or sport, contributes to disc degeneration, but not all studies have supported this hypothesis.[6,13-16] The inconsistency in this body of literature is common in epidemiologic studies. Interestingly, some physical activities are viewed as harmful in the occupational literature, but beneficial in the sports medicine literature. No dose-response relationship between physical loading and disc degeneration has been clearly demonstrated. For example, in a study on weightlifters, 26 years of weightlifting could only explain 10% of the variability in disc degeneration compared with shooters who reported minimal time weightlifting.[17] In addition, heavy physical loading in occupations may be related to lower socioeconomic status, youth, or lifestyle factors, further confounding the interpretation of this body of literature. The causal role of driving and whole-body vibration, previously accepted as a risk factor for disc degeneration,[6] has also been called into question.[14] In a series of studies on exposure-discordant monozygotic (MZ) twins (to reduce confounding variables), exposures suspected of accelerating disc degeneration, such as heavy physical loading, resistance training, and driving, were consistently shown to have minimal effects on degeneration.[13,14,18]

An association between cigarette smoking and back disorders, including degenerative discs, has been promulgated by many authors.[19-24] Some have even espoused a dose-response relationship.[23,24] For example, Kelsey et al[23] reported an increased risk of developing a herniated disc of 20% for each 10 cigarettes smoked per day in the previous year (odds ratio [OR] = 1.2), but not all studies have confirmed this association. Battie et al[20] assessed lumbar MRI scans in MZ twins highly discordant for lifetime smoking history (mean of 32 pack-years) and could only explain 2%

of the variance in disc degeneration. In another similar study, no significant association was found between smoking and disc degeneration.[13]

Genetic Factors

Previously, environmental factors were thought to play the primary role in disc degeneration and only recently has the importance of genetic factors been appreciated. In the Finnish twin cohort, environmental factors were thought to explain more than 80% of the etiology of sciatica.[25] In 1995, the first two studies of familial aggregation of disc degeneration in MZ twins were published.[13,26] The one study demonstrated similar degenerative findings according to spinal level compared with what would be expected by chance alone.[26] The other study evaluated MRI scans in 115 male MZ twins to determine the relative effects of age, familial aggregation, and common exposures that were thought to be risk factors for disc degeneration.[13] In the T12–L4 region, 61% of the variability in disc degeneration summary scores could be explained by familial aggregation, compared with 7% for physical loading and 9% for age. In the L4–S1 region, 34% of the variability in disc degeneration summary scores could be explained by familial aggregation, compared with 2% for physical loading and 7% for age. More of the variability in degeneration in the lower lumbar area remained unexplained. This, coupled with the fact that discs in the L4–S1 region are more degenerated than were those in the L1–L4 region, suggests that other unexplained variables have a disproportionate role in disc pathogenesis, affecting the lower lumbar levels more than the upper.

To distinguish between biologic and social sources of familial similarity, Sambrook et al[27] performed a classic study using MRI scans from 86 pairs of MZ twins and 154 pairs of dizygotic (DZ) twins. Heritability estimates for summary scores of degeneration in the lumbar spine were 74% (95% confidence interval [CI], 64 to 80%), after adjusting for age, weight, smoking, occupation, and physical activity. Disc bulging and disc height, not signal intensity, were the major determinants of the degenerative summary scores.

Disc degeneration is not synonymous with back pain or disc herniation. Some family and twin studies make a convincing case that disc herniations are influenced by familial factors, including genetics. In studies of juveniles with disc herniations, the risk of developing a disc herniation before the age of 21 was 4 to 6 times higher for patients with a positive family history.[28] Even adults undergoing surgery for disc herniations were 16.5 times more likely to have a family history of symptomatic disc herniations[29] and tended to have more severe disc degeneration on MRI.[30] Finally, in a classic study of 9000 Finnish twin pairs, the heritability estimate was 11% for hospitalization due to disc herniation.[25]

Although a substantial genetic influence on disc degeneration exists, the involved genes and pathophysiologic mechanisms have not been completely elucidated. Disc degeneration, like osteoarthritis, is best classified as a common, oligogenic, multifactorial disease. More than half a dozen gene loci have been associated with disc degeneration, mostly from chromosomes 2, 4, 6, 7, 11, 16, 19, and X, but those representing the most significant genetic susceptibility have yet to be identified.[2]

Most of the genes, except for the vitamin D receptor, associated with disc degeneration code for molecules that are involved in maintaining the structural integrity of the disc. Vitamin D receptor is a steroid nuclear receptor that is better known for its role in bone mineralization and calcium hemostasis. The *TaqI* and *FokI* polymorphisms have been associated with reduced disc signal intensity in lumbar and thoracic discs in a study of MZ Finnish twins.[31] This association has been confirmed in both the Japanese[32] and Chinese[33] populations. There is an age-dependent correlation with higher odds ratio in younger individuals.[32,33] Interestingly, the frequency of the risk t-allele is different among the different populations, 8% in Asians, 31% in Africans, and 43% in Caucasians.[34]

The only other genes, whose association with disc degeneration has been verified in different ethnic populations, are COL9A2 and COL9A3, which encode collagen IX. The tryptophan positive allele (*Trp2*) has been shown to be present in individuals with disc degeneration in both Finnish[35] and Chinese[36] populations. It is an age-dependent risk factor and is associated with structural changes, such as annular tears (OR = 2.4) and endplate herniations (OR = 4.0).[36] Another mutation, the *Trp3* allele, increases the risk of disc degeneration 3 times in the Finnish cohort,[37] but is absent in the Chinese.[36] This suggests that risk factors vary between different ethnic groups.

There are many other genes that have been studied but have less convincing data. In the Japanese population, more severe degeneration has been linked to shorter numbers of tandem repeats in the aggrecan gene,[38] to specific genotypes of the matrix metalloproteinase-3 gene,[39] and to mutations in the cartilage intermediate layer protein.[40] A recent Chinese study linked polymorphisms in the matrix metalloproteinase-2 gene to disc degeneration (OR = 3.08).[41] A study in the Dutch population showed that a collagen I gene (COL1A1) was also associated with disc degeneration, but the cohort was small.[42] In the Finnish population, interleukin-1 (IL-1) gene mutations were associated with disc bulges (OR = 3.0),[43] and further study showed that IL-1 modifies the effects of the COL9A3 polymorphism on disc degeneration.[44] The genes and genetic mechanisms involved in disc degeneration are incredibly complex; additional study is needed to clarify the contribution of genetics to the pathophysiology of disc degeneration.

■ Economics

Health care costs continue to rise at astronomical rates, and technological advances continue to outpace our ability to pay for them. In 2005, total national health expenditures in the United States were $2 trillion, which represents 16% of the gross domestic product, and are expected to rise to $4 trillion by 2015 (20% of gross domestic product).[45] There has been a 500% increase in spending in lumbar spine fusion surgery from 1992 to 2003 ($75 million to $482 million, respectively),[46] and the total costs of low back pain exceed $100 billion per year.[47] With the increased use of instrumentation and a broadening patient base, it is estimated that the spine market will compound at 22% annually.[48]

Determining the value of treatments and whether or not they improve the health of the population is the cornerstone of health economics. As costs rise and reimbursements fall, it is increasingly important that economic factors are included when evaluating treatment options. Unfortunately, there is a lack of well-designed and methodologically sound economic studies in the literature, and most surgeons are not familiar with basic health care economic principles. Currently, most studies address the economic impact of low back pain, which is too extensive to review here, and do not differentiate between the different diagnoses that can cause back pain.[49,50] Interpreting these studies is difficult because patients with different diagnoses, but similar procedures may have very different outcomes.

Luo et al[51] performed one of the only studies that correlated health expenditures to different diagnoses causing back pain. They used data from the 1998 Medical Expenditure Panel Survey, a national survey on health care utilization and expenditures. The most common diagnoses were unspecified back disorders (59.5%), back sprains and strains (16.2%), and IVD disorders (14.2%). Individuals with disc disorders had the highest per-capita total expenditures ($6010.70), while those with unspecified back disorders and back sprains were much lower ($3514 and $2494, respectively). For individuals with disc disorders, inpatient care expenditures per capita reached $2816, compared with only $634 for back sprains. Patients with disc disorders incurred much higher per-capita expenditures than individuals with other diagnoses.

For herniated discs, data from both the United States[52] and Sweden[53] have shown discectomy to be cost-effective, but the studies on lumbar fusion for degenerative disc disease are more controversial. Soegaard and Christensen[54] in a literature review from 1997 to 2004 determined that most studies had questionable methodologies, studied different populations, and used different outcome measures; thus, they could not draw any general conclusions about the cost-effectiveness of lumbar arthrodesis. Only the study by Fritzell et al[55] satisfied all of their methodological criteria and was limited to fusions for spondylosis. They determined that the spinal fusion group had better outcomes compared with the nonoperative group but higher costs, and therefore, lumbar fusion could be cost-effective depending upon the value put on the extra effect units gained by using surgery. In 2005, a randomized controlled trial in the United Kingdom concluded that spinal fusion was not a cost-effective use of scarce health care resources, but this could change if patients in the rehabilitation group required surgery in the future.[56] Unfortunately, this study included all patients with chronic back pain for more than 12 months and was not limited to just degenerative disc disease. The lack of adequate data to evaluate the economic benefit of lumbar fusion surgery for disc degeneration led Polly et al[57] to perform a cost-benefit analysis of lumbar fusion compared with other surgical interventions. They included patients with single-level degenerative disc disease that had participated in prospective multicenter trials conducted between 1995 and 2004 and concluded that "lumbar fusion cost per benefit achieved was very comparable to other well-accepted medical interventions (total hip replacement, total knee replacement, and coronary artery bypass surgery)." Even though this "thought experiment" included data from multiple other studies, it provided an important economic analysis, supporting lumbar fusion for degenerative disc disease.

In an environment with rising health care costs and diminishing resources, economic analyses are becoming increasingly important in assessing the utility of surgical procedures. In the future, study designs will need to include sound economic methodologies to help guide decisions regarding the most appropriate and efficient use of health care resources.

References

1. Frymoyer JW. Lumbar disk disease: epidemiology. Instr Course Lect 1992;41:217–223
2. Battie MC, Videman T, Parent E. Lumbar disc degeneration: epidemiology and genetic influences. Spine 2004;29(23):2679–2690
3. Thompson JP, Pearce RH, Schechter MT, Adams ME, Tsang IK, Bishop PB. Preliminary evaluation of a scheme for grading the gross morphology of the human intervertebral disc. Spine 1990;15(5):411–415
4. Frobin W, Brinckmann P, Kramer M, Hartwig E. Height of lumbar discs measured from radiographs compared with degeneration and height classified from MR images. Eur Radiol 2001;11(2):263–269
5. Shao Z, Rompe G, Schiltenwolf M. Radiographic changes in the lumbar intervertebral discs and lumbar vertebrae with age. Spine 2002;27(3):263–268

6. Andersson GB. The epidemiology of spinal disorders. In: Frymoyer JW, ed. The Adult Spine: Principles and Practice. 2nd ed. Philadelphia, PA: Lippincott-Raven; 1997:93–141

7. Heine J. Uber die Arthritis deformans. Virch Arch Pathol Anat 1926;260:521–663

8. Coventry MB, Ghormley RK, Kernohan JW. The intervertebral disc: its microscopic anatomy and pathology, II: Changes in the intervertebral disc concomitant with age. J Bone Joint Surg Am 1945;27:233–247

9. Boos N, Weissbach S, Rohrbach H, Weiler C, Spratt KF, Nerlich AG. 2002 Volvo Award in Basic Science. Classification of age-related changes in lumbar intervertebral discs. Spine 2002;27(23): 2631–2644

10. Miller JA, Schmatz C, Schultz AB. Lumbar disc degeneration: correlation with age, sex, and spine level in 600 autopsy specimens. Spine 1988;13(2):173–178

11. Manson NA, Goldberg EJ, Andersson GB. Sexual dimorphism in degenerative disorders of the spine. Orthop Clin North Am 2006; 37(4):549–553

12. Manek NJ, MacGregor AJ. Epidemiology of back disorders: prevalence, risk factors, and prognosis. Curr Opin Rheumatol 2005; 17(2):134–140

13. Battie MC, Videman T, Gibbons LE, Fisher LD, Manninen H, Gill K. 1995 Volvo Award in Clinical Sciences. Determinants of lumbar disc degeneration: a study relating lifetime exposures and magnetic resonance imaging findings in identical twins. Spine 1995;20(24):2601–2612

14. Battie MC, Videman T, Gibbons LE, et al. Occupational driving and lumbar disc degeneration: a case-control study. Lancet 2002; 360(9343):1369–1374

15. Frymoyer JW, Newberg A, Pope MH, Wilder DG, Clements J, MacPherson B. Spine radiographs in patients with low-back pain: an epidemiological study in men. J Bone Joint Surg Am 1984;66(7): 1048–1055

16. Savage RA, Whitehouse GH, Roberts N. The relationship between the magnetic resonance imaging appearance of the lumbar spine and low back pain, age and occupation in males. Eur Spine J 1997;6(2):106–114

17. Videman T, Sarna S, Battie MC, et al. The long-term effects of physical loading and exercise lifestyles on back-related symptoms, disability, and spinal pathology among men. Spine 1995;20(6):699–709

18. Videman T, Battie MC, Gibbons LE, et al. Lifetime exercise and disk degeneration: an MRI study of monozygotic twins. Med Sci Sports Exerc 1997;29(10):1350–1356

19. Battie MC, Bigos SJ, Fisher LD, et al. A prospective study of the role of cardiovascular risk factors and fitness in industrial back pain complaints. Spine 1989;14(2):141–147

20. Battie MC, Videman T, Gill K, et al. 1991 Volvo Award in Clinical Sciences. Smoking and lumbar intervertebral disc degeneration: an MRI study of identical twins. Spine 1991;16(9):1015–1021

21. Boshuizen HC, Verbeek JH, Broersen JP, Weel AN. Do smokers get more back pain? Spine 1993;18(1):35–40

22. Deyo RA, Bass JE. Lifestyle and low-back pain. The influence of smoking and obesity. Spine 1989;14(5):501–506

23. Kelsey JL, Githens PB, O'Conner T, et al. Acute prolapsed lumbar intervertebral disc. An epidemiologic study with special reference to driving automobiles and cigarette smoking. Spine 1984;9(6):608–613

24. Svensson HO, Vedin A, Wilhelmsson C, Andersson GB. Low-back pain in relation to other diseases and cardiovascular risk factors. Spine 1983;8(3):277–285

25. Heikkila JK, Koskenvuo M, Heliovaara M, et al. Genetic and environmental factors in sciatica: evidence from a nationwide panel of 9365 adult twin pairs. Ann Med 1989;21(5):393–398

26. Battie MC, Haynor DR, Fisher LD, Gill K, Gibbons LE, Videman T. Similarities in degenerative findings on magnetic resonance images of the lumbar spines of identical twins. J Bone Joint Surg Am 1995; 77(11):1662–1670

27. Sambrook PN, MacGregor AJ, Spector TD. Genetic influences on cervical and lumbar disc degeneration: a magnetic resonance imaging study in twins. Arthritis Rheum 1999;42(2):366–372

28. Varlotta GP, Brown MD, Kelsey JL, Golden AL. Familial predisposition for herniation of a lumbar disc in patients who are less than twenty-one years old. J Bone Joint Surg Am 1991;73(1):124–128

29. Richardson JK, Chung T, Schultz JS, Hurvitz E. A familial predisposition toward lumbar disc injury. Spine 1997;22(13):1487–1492 discussion 1493

30. Matsui H, Kanamori M, Ishihara H, Yudoh K, Naruse Y, Tsuji H. Familial predisposition for lumbar degenerative disc disease: a case-control study. Spine 1998;23(9):1029–1034

31. Videman T, Leppavuori J, Kaprio J, et al. Intragenic polymorphisms of the vitamin D receptor gene associated with intervertebral disc degeneration. Spine 1998;23(23):2477–2485

32. Kawaguchi Y, Kanamori M, Ishihara H, Ohmori K, Matsui H, Kimura T. The association of lumbar disc disease with vitamin-D receptor gene polymorphism. J Bone Joint Surg Am 2002;84-A(11):2022–2028

33. Cheung KM, Chan D, Karppinen J, et al. Association of the Taq I allele in vitamin D receptor with degenerative disc disease and disc bulge in a Chinese population. Spine 2006;31(10):1143–1148

34. Uitterlinden AG, Fang Y, Van Meurs JB, Pols HA, Van Leeuwen JP. Genetics and biology of vitamin D receptor polymorphisms. Gene 2004;338(2):143–156

35. Annunen S, Paassilta P, Lohiniva J, et al. An allele of COL9A2 associated with intervertebral disc disease. Science 1999;285(5426): 409–412

36. Jim JJ, Noponen-Hietala N, Cheung KM, et al. The TRP2 allele of COL9A2 is an age-dependent risk factor for the development and severity of intervertebral disc degeneration. Spine 2005;30(24): 2735–2742

37. Paassilta P, Lohiniva J, Goring HH, et al. Identification of a novel common genetic risk factor for lumbar disk disease. JAMA 2001; 285(14):1843–1849

38. Kawaguchi Y, Osada R, Kanamori M, et al. Association between an aggrecan gene polymorphism and lumbar disc degeneration. Spine 1999;24(23):2456–2460

39. Takahashi M, Haro H, Wakabayashi Y, Kawa-uchi T, Komori H, Shinomiya K. The association of degeneration of the intervertebral disc with 5a/6a polymorphism in the promoter of the human matrix metalloproteinase-3 gene. J Bone Joint Surg Br 2001;83(4):491–495

40. Seki S, Kawaguchi Y, Chiba K, et al. A functional SNP in CILP, encoding cartilage intermediate layer protein, is associated with susceptibility to lumbar disc disease. Nat Genet 2005;37(6):607–612

41. Dong DM, Yao M, Liu B, Sun CY, Jiang YQ, Wang YS. Association between the -1306C/T polymorphism of matrix metalloproteinase-2 gene and lumbar disc disease in Chinese young adults. Eur Spine J 2007;16(11):1958–1961

42. Pluijm SM, van Essen HW, Bravenboer N, et al. Collagen type I alpha1 Sp1 polymorphism, osteoporosis, and intervertebral disc degeneration in older men and women. Ann Rheum Dis 2004;63(1): 71–77

43. Solovieva S, Kouhia S, Leino-Arjas P, et al. Interleukin 1 polymorphisms and intervertebral disc degeneration. Epidemiology 2004; 15(5):626–633

44. Solovieva S, Lohiniva J, Leino-Arjas P, et al. Intervertebral disc degeneration in relation to the COL9A3 and the IL-1ss gene polymorphisms. Eur Spine J 2006;15(5):613–619

45. Health Insurance Cost. National Coalition on Health Care web site. Available at: www.nchc.org/facts/cost.shtml. Accessed August 23, 2007

46. Genuario JW, Mehta S, Nunley RM, The Washington Health Policy Fellows. Discrepancy in healthcare utilization: Is more better in orthopedic surgery? The American Academy of Orthopedic Surgeons web site. Available at: http://www.aaos.org/news/bulletin/jun07/reimbursement2.asp. Accessed August 23, 2007

47. Katz JN. Lumbar disc disorders and low-back pain: socioeconomic factors and consequences. J Bone Joint Surg Am 2006;88(Suppl 2): 21–24

48. Lieberman IH. Disc bulge bubble: spine economics 101. Spine J 2004;4(6):609–613

49. Pai S, Sundaram LJ. Low back pain: an economic assessment in the United States. Orthop Clin North Am 2004;35(1):1–5

50. van der Roer N, Goossens ME, Evers SM, van Tulder MW. What is the most cost-effective treatment for patients with low back pain? A systematic review. Best Pract Res Clin Rheumatol 2005;19(4):671–684

51. Luo X, Pietrobon R, Sun SX, Liu GG, Hey L. Estimates and patterns of direct health care expenditures among individuals with back pain in the United States. Spine 2004;29(1):79–86

52. Malter AD, Larson EB, Urban N, Deyo RA. Cost-effectiveness of lumbar discectomy for the treatment of herniated intervertebral disc. Spine 1996;21(9):1048–1054 discussion 1055

53. Hansson E, Hansson T. The cost-utility of lumbar disc herniation surgery. Eur Spine J 2007;16(3):329–337

54. Soegaard R, Christensen FB. Health economic evaluation in lumbar spinal fusion: a systematic literature review anno 2005. Eur Spine J 2006;15(8):1165–1173

55. Fritzell P, Hagg O, Jonsson D, Nordwall A. Cost-effectiveness of lumbar fusion and nonsurgical treatment for chronic low back pain in the Swedish Lumbar Spine Study: a multicenter, randomized, controlled trial from the Swedish Lumbar Spine Study Group. Spine 2004;29(4):421–434 discussion Z423

56. Rivero-Arias O, Campbell H, Gray A, Fairbank J, Frost H, Wilson-MacDonald J. Surgical stabilisation of the spine compared with a programme of intensive rehabilitation for the management of patients with chronic low back pain: cost utility analysis based on a randomised controlled trial. BMJ 2005;330(7502):1239

57. Polly DW Jr, Glassman SD, Schwender JD, et al. SF-36 PCS benefit-cost ratio of lumbar fusion comparison to other surgical interventions: a thought experiment. Spine 2007; 32(11, Suppl)S20–S26

2 Anatomy and Physiology of the Lumbar Intervertebral Disc and Endplates

Michael A. Adams

Intervertebral discs (IVDs) are pads of fibrocartilage that lie between the vertebral bodies of the spine. Their primary function is to confer some degree of flexibility to the spinal column, while at the same time distributing compressive loading evenly to the vertebral bodies, even when the spine is subjected to complex loading. Discs are generally too stiff and thin to be good shock absorbers, and leave most of this task to the body's natural shock absorbers—the tendons.[1]

In the first sections of this chapter, a detailed anatomy of IVDs, from the structure and composition of the extracellular matrix, to the characteristics of disc cells and their metabolite transport is given. Changes during growth and chronologic aging are then considered, to show progressive and inevitable changes in disc anatomy during the lifespan. This sets the scene for the final section on disc degeneration, which considers deleterious changes in structure and function, which occur in some discs but not in others. This discussion leads to a proposal for how disc degeneration should be defined, and a brief overview of causality.

■ Anatomy

The gross anatomy of a human lumbar IVD is illustrated in **Fig. 2.1**. The soft, pulpy nucleus pulposus is surrounded and constrained by the tough concentric layers (lamellae) of the anulus fibrosus (AF). High water content and low rigidity in the nucleus allow it to behave mechanically like a compressed fluid,[2] which generates a tensile "hoop stress" in the anulus when the spine is compressed. However, the mature anulus has sufficient rigidity to resist compressive loading directly,[2] as well as to resist nucleus pressure, so it is a complex mechanical structure. Overall disc dimensions vary with spinal level and increase with increasing body height.[3]

Anulus Fibrosus

Collagen fiber bundles of the anulus are oriented at ~30 degrees to the horizontal, with the direction alternating between adjacent lamellae (**Fig. 2.1**); 20 to 60 separate bundles are discernible in a vertical section.[4] Adjacent lamellae are of irregular thickness and often are discontinuous, especially in the posterolateral anulus.[4] Fibers of the outer anulus are strongly embedded in the adjacent vertebral bodies (forming Sharpey's fibers). In the inner anulus, they curve around the nucleus and blend in gradually with the hyaline cartilage of the endplate.

The collagen bundles of the anulus are mostly composed of coarse collagen type I fibers. They exhibit a planar zigzag "crimp" pattern when viewed under a polarizing microscope (**Fig. 2.2**). Crimp can be straightened out, allowing collagen type I fibers to be stretched ~4% with little resistance (as measured in tendon).[5] Stretching of the anulus also causes individual fibers to reorient and slide relative to each other.[6] Collagen fibers in the same lamella split and intertwine with each other laterally (**Fig. 2.2**) to form a cohesive planar structure.[7] Strong interactions between collagen fibers and other matrix constituents (collagen means "glue-maker") contribute toward structural integrity, even when collagen fibers are disrupted.[8] This makes the anulus very tough and difficult to pull apart. Approximately 20% of the collagen in the outer anulus is type II, which forms very fine "fibrils" rather than coarse type I fibers, and the proportion of collagen type II rises to 70% in the inner anulus.[9] Adjacent lamellae of the anulus are only weakly bonded together[10] probably by fine elastin[11] and collagen type II fibrils, with the former conferring the property of "elastic recoil," which is the ability to spring back into place after large deformations. Other constituents of the anulus include the water-binding proteoglycans, which compose ~10% of the dry weight of the outer anulus and 30% of the inner anulus.[9]

Excised samples of anulus can be stretched circumferentially by 40 to 60% before gross failure occurs, at a strain (elongation) of 40 to 64% and a stress (force per unit area) of 2 to 7 MPa.[12] The inner anulus is weaker and more deformable than the outer anulus[12,13]; the posterolateral anulus is particularly weak.[13]

Minor matrix components of both the anulus and nucleus include collagen types III and VI, which reinforce the pericellular matrix.[14] Fibronectin helps to bind cells to their matrix and is more abundant (often in fragments) in degenerated discs.[15]

Nucleus Pulposus

The nucleus is normally a soft and deformable proteoglycan gel, which is reinforced by fibrous proteins. Proteoglycans

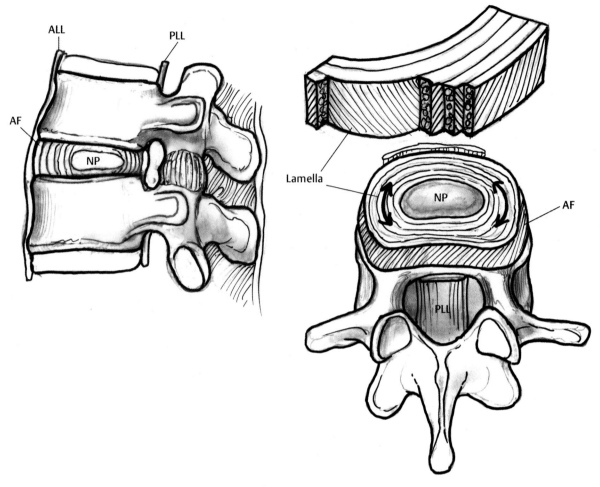

Fig. 2.1 An intervertebral disc lies between adjacent vertebral bodies of a spinal motion segment (left). The soft nucleus pulposus (NP) is surrounded by 15 to 25 lamellae (right, top) of the anulus fibrosus (AF). Spinal compression generates a hydrostatic pressure in the NP and a restraining tensile hoop stress in the anulus. The posterior longitudinal ligament (PLL) acts as a "nerve net" for the underlying disc. The anterior longitudinal ligament (ALL) helps to protect the disc from excessive backward bending.

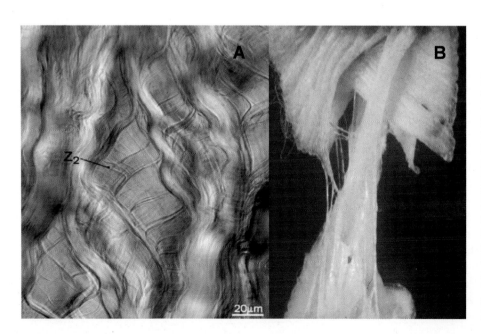

Fig. 2.2 **(A)** Phase-contrast microscopy of branching, crimped collagen fibers in bovine tail anulus fibrosus. **(B)** Sample of young adult human anulus pulled apart vertically in a tensile test in vitro: note the collagen fibers pulling out of the proteoglycan matrix, and the alternating fiber direction in adjacent lamellae. (**A,** From Pezowicz CA, Robertson PA, Broom ND. Intralamellar relationships within the collagenous architecture of the annulus fibrosus imaged in its fully hydrated state. J Anat 2005;207(4):299–312. Reprinted with permission. **B,** From Adams MA, Bogduk N, Burton K, Dolan P. The Biomechanics of Back Pain. 2nd ed. Edinburgh, UK: Churchill Livingstone; 2006. Reprinted with permission.)

are neutral molecules overall but are made up of glycosaminoglycan subunits, which have a preponderance of fixed negative charges on their exterior surface (balanced by positive charges internally). The fixed negative charges attract the positive charges found on either end of the polarized water molecule, thereby attracting water to the glycosaminoglycans. In young adults, proteoglycan molecules constitute 70% of nucleus dry weight,[9] and tissue water content can exceed 80%.[9] Proteoglycans aggregate with hyaluronic acid to form very large molecules that are trapped within the tissue by the loose network of collagen type II fibrils, which comprise more than 80% of collagen in the nucleus.[9] Elastin fibers appear to have a predominantly radial arrangement within the nucleus,[16] possibly serving to resist radial migration of nucleus tissue down radial fissures. Under high pressure, nucleus pulposus material can insinuate between collagen fibers of the inner anulus, causing microscopic disruption within and between lamellae.[17]

Cartilage Endplate

This thin layer of hyaline cartilage is only weakly bonded to the underlying bony endplate (**Fig. 2.3**). Like articular cartilage, it has a dense organized network of fine collagen II fibrils, which strongly maintain its structure and shape, prohibit swelling, and make it stiffer and denser than the adjacent nucleus. The cartilage endplate serves to maintain internal

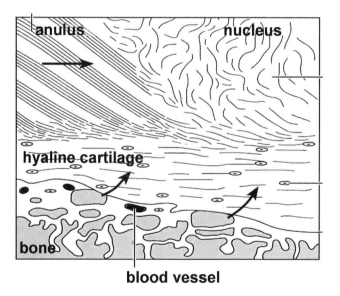

Fig. 2.3 Detail showing the hyaline cartilage endplate (center) bonded to the disc (top) and the bony endplate (bottom). Arrows show the two routes for metabolite transport into the center of the avascular disc: via the endplate route and via the peripheral anulus. Note how the coarse collagen fibers of the anulus blend in with the hyaline cartilage. (From Adams MA, Bogduk N, Burton K, Dolan P. The Biomechanics of Back Pain. 2nd ed. Edinburgh, UK: Churchill Livingstone; 2006. Reprinted with permission.)

pressurization of the disc by hindering the expulsion of water and proteoglycans from the disc through the bony endplate into the vertebral body. It also acts as a biological filter to restrict migration of cells and large solutes between nucleus and bone. The cells are rounded chondrocytes, similar to those in articular cartilage.

Bony Endplate

This is a thin sheet of bone, ~1 mm thick, which forms part of the cortex of the vertebral body. It contains a radiating anastomosing network of small marrow cavities, especially in the central regions,[18] which allow direct contact between bone marrow and hyaline cartilage endplate for ~5 to 10% of the central endplate area.[19] This facilitates the transfer of metabolites between blood vessels in the vertebral marrow and cells in the adjacent disc. Cranial endplates are 10 to 15% thinner[20] and weaker[21] than caudal endplates, and both are thinnest and weakest in their central region. Under normal levels of compressive loading, endplates bulge outward into their adjacent vertebral bodies, typically by 0.25 mm.[22] Not surprisingly, compressive fracture of the central region of the cranial endplate is common, both in vivo and in vitro.[20] The mechanical vulnerability of the bony endplate is probably a concession to the nutritional demands of the adjacent discs, and the relative vulnerability of the cranial endplate can be explained in terms of the extra loading applied to the caudal half of the vertebral body by muscles attached to the neural arch (and transmitted to the vertebral body at the level of the pedicle).

■ Physiology

Typical cells of the anulus are elongated fibroblasts, which tend to lie parallel to the lamellae of the matrix, although some anulus cells are more rounded.[23] They all appear to have long cytoplasmic extensions,[24] which can form gap junctions with extensions from neighboring cells,[6] suggesting that anulus cells are capable of forming a "nerve net" comparable to that created by osteocytes in bone. Anulus cells synthesize mostly collagen and proteoglycans.

Nucleus cells resemble the rounded chondrocytes found in articular cartilage, and their function is similar: to synthesize the proteoglycans and the fine, collagen type II fibrils of their matrix. Chondrocytes are not present in the nucleus from birth but replace the original notochordal cells during early childhood. Notochordal cells are larger and more active, form clusters, and appear to form gap junctions with each other.[25] Their demise after childhood may be attributable to increased mechanical loading, or to increasing difficulties in transporting metabolites into and out of the avascular disc as it grows larger. Probably for similar reasons, disc cell density decreases during growth, but then remains constant for most of adult life.[26] Mature nucleus cells retain sizeable cytoplasmic extensions.[24]

The relative isolation of nucleus cells from the general circulation suggests that autoimmune reactions will occur if nucleus cells escape from the center of the disc, as they do in disc herniation. Recent experiments on young pigs have shown that transplanted autologous nucleus pulposus tissue does indeed attract activated T and B cells to it,[27] but it remains to be seen if the same reaction occurs with nucleus cells from middle-aged humans.

Cell density in the adult human disc is maximal in the outer anulus,[23] close to the peripheral blood supply. It is noteworthy that only the outer anulus is capable of effective healing following injury.[28] In the absence of a nerve and blood supply, disc cells communicate by secreting and receiving low-molecular-weight chemical messengers (cytokines), which diffuse mostly to near-neighbor cells before being degraded. To suggest that cytokines (such as interleukin-1) are the "cause" of disc degeneration is rather like confusing the messenger with the message, although it is possible that malfunctioning of the cell-signaling apparatus could predispose a disc to degeneration.

Disc Metabolite Transport

In the first few years of life, blood vessels from the vertebral body penetrate the cartilage endplate and extend into the inner and outer anulus, but not into the nucleus.[29] These blood vessels are lost during infancy, presumably because weight-bearing causes hollow blood vessels to collapse within cartilage. High concentrations of proteoglycans may also play a role in inhibiting blood vessels from growing into central regions of a healthy disc.[30] Normal adolescent and adult discs are avascular, apart from a few capillaries penetrating the peripheral anulus, adjacent to the insertion of ligaments.[29]

In the absence of a blood supply, disc cells must receive their nutrients by the processes of diffusion and fluid flow. Diffusion involves flow down a concentration gradient, stimulated by random Brownian movements, and is an efficient system for the transport over short distances of small molecules such as glucose and oxygen. Large molecular weight solutes (such as the proteins, which control many cell activities) diffuse only very slowly in the disc and rely on being transported along with the bulk flow of fluid in response to changes in applied mechanical loading. Diurnal cycles of activity and rest cause 20% of disc water to be exchanged every day,[31] so fluid flow contributes substantially to metabolite transport,[32] especially in the anulus.[33] Rapid fluid "pumping" during locomotion probably has little effect, although alternating periods of rest and activity could possibly be beneficial. Disc cell metabolism is well adapted to an environment that is low in oxygen and yet high in the lactic acid that is an endproduct of anaerobic metabolism.[34]

Furthermore, cell density in the nucleus appears to reflect an adaptation to restricted metabolite transport.[35] Although viable, the resulting population of disc cells appears to be too small to effect major repairs,[28] or to overcome any disturbance in the already precarious supply of metabolites caused by heavy smoking[36] or endplate calcification.

Mechanical Influences on Disc Metabolism

Cells are most responsive to the type of loading they normally encounter, so nucleus cells respond to hydrostatic pressure, and outer anulus cells to stretch, but not vice versa. Inner anulus cells experience[2] (and respond to) hydrostatic pressure. Moderate mechanical stimuli cause both cell types to synthesize more matrix, whereas low and static stimuli cause them to synthesize less,[37] in accordance with the principles of "adaptive remodeling." High and static loading inhibits disc cell synthesis and can stimulate them to release and activate matrix metalloproteinases, enzymes that break down matrix macromolecules.[37,38] Sustained loading influences disc cell metabolism indirectly by increasing or decreasing the supply of metabolites, as discussed above. Furthermore, prolonged loading can greatly dehydrate disc tissue,[33] so that reduced pore size (and hence permeability) interferes with diffusion and fluid flow through the matrix.

Disc Innervation and Discogenic Pain

In normal adult human discs, both free and complex nerve endings are confined to the peripheral anulus, typically to the outermost 1 to 3 mm.[39] Anteriorly and laterally, the nerves are sympathetic, but in the posterior quadrant of the disc they originate from the mixed sinuvertebral nerve[40] and appear to be capable of nociception.[41] Pain provocation studies on sedated humans provide direct evidence that the posterior AF and the adhering posterior longitudinal ligament are the most common tissues of origin of severe and chronic back pain.[42] The same study supports the concept of "pain-sensitization" because it shows that patients' typical pain can be reproduced by relatively gentle mechanical probing of the posterior anulus. Animal experiments have confirmed that mere contact with the autologous nucleus pulposus can alter the morphology and conduction velocity of neurons[43] and produce pain-like behavior in rats, which is worsened if the nerve tissue is simultaneously stretched.[44]

Nerves believed to be capable of nociception can grow in toward the nucleus in severely degenerated discs, in both the anterior[45] and posterior[46] anulus. Nerves need to be close to blood vessels, and both structures appear to grow in together along the zone of granulation tissue within radial fissures.[46] Nerve ingrowth may be caused by revascularization, which itself is a consequence of reduced pressure and proteoglycan content in the degenerated nucleus. Nerve ingrowth may also be stimulated by neurotrophic factors released by disc cells[47] and by a loss of proteoglycans, which have an inhibitory effect on nerve growth.[48]

■ Effect of Aging on Anatomy and Physiology

Changes in the Extracellular Matrix

Microscopic changes including "mucoid degeneration" occur before the age of 2 years, and this is soon followed by decreased vascularization of the endplate and by decreased disc cellularity.[49] These changes may simply reflect necessary adaptations to weight-bearing and growth because they vary little with spinal level[49] and appear to have little effect on disc function.[2] Macroscopic disc changes before the age of 20 years have been characterized as "fibrous transformation,"[50] but their relationship to subsequent pain-related features such as radial fissures and disc prolapse (see below) is not clear because the latter do not normally appear for another 20 years.

After skeletal maturity, proteoglycan aggregates become increasingly fragmented, with the greatest changes occurring in the nucleus.[9] Some proteoglycan fragments are lost, so water content declines, especially in the nucleus, where tissue hydration falls from 87% to 74% between childhood and old age.[9]

The collagen network is affected rather differently. During growth, collagen fibers become stiffer and stronger as cross-links between adjacent collagen molecules become more stable.[51] From skeletal maturity onward, collagen cross-linking is supplemented by nonenzymatic (hence uncontrolled) cross-linking that involves sugar molecules. The biochemistry is complex, but the result of these adventitious chemical reactions is that the collagen network becomes excessively cross-linked, making the matrix stiffer (rather like a delicate woolen garment washed at a high temperature). **Figure 2.4** compares collagen fibers in young pig anulus and aging adult human anulus. Experiments on articular cartilage show that this phenomenon of nonenzymatic glycation makes cartilage more vulnerable to damage.[52] Nonenzymatic glycation occurs most in those tissues that do not turn over (i.e., replace) their collagen very quickly, so the avascular IVD, with a collagen turnover time of more than 100 years, is greatly affected with advancing age.[51] Nonenzymatic glycation causes collagenous tissue to develop the characteristic yellow-brown coloration typical of aging.

After the age of 60 years, less than 30% of the nucleus dry weight is collagen type II,[9] whereas the proportion of other matrix constituents, including collagen type I, increases. Overall, the proportion of denatured (damaged) collagen *molecules* rises from 3 to 12% in old age,[53] but extensive crosslinking ensures that most collagen fragments are retained within the tissue,[53] and the anulus becomes only slightly weaker.[12]

Changes in the Cells

Cell density does not normally decline after skeletal maturity,[26] and metabolic rates per cell are probably maintained with increasing age. However, an increasing proportion of aging disc cells become senescent in the sense that they lose the ability to divide, with up to 90% of cells being affected in the oldest and most degenerated discs.[54] Old discs appear to show increased levels of apoptosis (programmed cell death),[55] and this can be accelerated by trauma.[56] Matrix metalloproteinase production is elevated in old

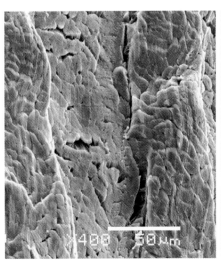

YOUNG (pig) **OLD (human)**

Fig. 2.4 Three adjacent lamellae of the anulus fibrosus of a young pig (left) and an elderly human (right) as imaged by environmental scanning electron microscopy. These images, which are reproduced to the same scale, show how lamellae and their individual collagen fiber bundles thicken with age. (Courtesy of Dr. Lee Neylon, Curtin University, Western Australia.)

discs, suggesting the presence of degenerative changes and/or repair.[9] With increasing age and number of cell divisions, oxidative stress can accumulate in disc cells, especially in the nucleus. This process is associated with internal damage created by reactive oxygen species, a phenomenon that can be likened to "rusting up" of the cell machinery. Oxidative stress is also associated with certain modifications of proteins in the pericellular matrix, especially in the nucleus pulposus.[57] Age-related changes in the biological activity of the cartilage endplate are similar to those in the adjacent nucleus pulposus.[58]

Structural Changes

The anulus becomes slightly thicker with disc aging,[59] and also starts to encroach on the nucleus (**Fig. 2.5B**). Osteoporotic bone loss from adjacent vertebrae can allow the

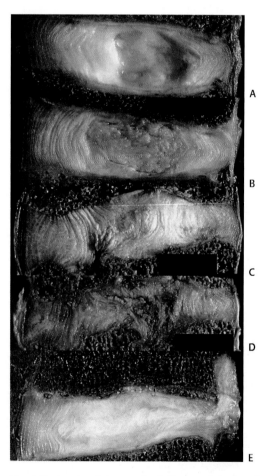

Fig. 2.5 Lumbar intervertebral discs sectioned in the midsagittal plane (anterior on left) illustrating grades of disc "degeneration." **(A)** Young adult disc, nondegenerated. **(B)** Middle-aged adult disc, nondegenerated. **(C)** Young adult disc, moderate degeneration. **(D)** Young adult disc, severe degeneration. **(E)** Middle-aged adult disc, prolapsed. (Adapted from color originals in Adams MA, Bogduk N, Burton K, Dolan P. The Biomechanics of Back Pain. 2nd ed. Edinburgh, UK: Churchill Livingstone; 2006. Reprinted with permission.)

endplates to bulge away from the nucleus, creating the "biconcave" deformity, typical of many elderly vertebrae,[59] which can give a misleading impression of a thick and healthy disc, even if its anulus is starting to collapse. Minor structural changes to the anulus and endplate appear during childhood,[50] but their relationship to gross structural defects (see below) is uncertain. With increasing age, fibrous accumulations occupy more space within the nucleus; they are separated by softer tissue, which accepts injected fluid, and this explains the typical "hamburger" discogram of discs of a middle-aged adult.[60]

Gross structural disruption is not inevitable in lumbar discs, but it does occur with increasing frequency after middle age, especially at the two lowest lumbar levels.[50] Changes include anulus tears, prolapse, endplate damage, anulus protrusion, internal disruption, and disc narrowing. Three types of anulus tear are conventionally recognized: radial fissures (**Fig. 2.5E**), circumferential tears, and rim lesions. Each is believed to form independently of the others.[61] Radial fissures usually extend to the posterior or posterolateral margins of the disc and can be created (in cadaveric experiments) by repetitive loading in bending and compression.[62,63] Circumferential tears are probably caused by interlaminar shear stresses[64] generated when the anulus is required to resist high concentrations of compressive stress (**Fig. 2.6**). Rim tears involve avulsions of the outer anulus fibers from bone and often occur in the anterolateral margins, suggesting an etiology involving torsional stresses. Radial bulging of the anulus occurs either outward or inward, and is facilitated by prior decompression of the nucleus[65] and by sustained bending of the disc.[66] Internal collapse ("internal disc disruption"[67]) is common, especially in the anterior anulus (**Fig. 2.5C**). Endplate fracture is the most common injury to occur after compressive overload. It causes an immediate decompression of the nucleus and is probably a potent cause of nucleus degeneration.[68,69] Disc prolapse involves relative movement between nucleus and anulus in such a manner that the outer surface of the disc is disturbed: typically, nucleus pulposus material is expressed into or through a radial fissure[70] as shown in **Fig. 2.5E**.

Functional Changes in the Disc

Old discs are capable of more or less normal function, with the fibrous nucleus still exhibiting hydrostatic behavior, albeit over a smaller central region.[2] The transition zone between nucleus and anulus changes from being a hydrostatic fluid to exhibiting solid behavior, and this may encourage cells in this region to produce coarse collagen type I fibers rather than fine type II fibrils. Water loss from the nucleus causes pressure within it to fall, so compressive load bearing is transferred increasingly to the anulus. This can result in concentrations of stress in the middle anulus, typically posterior to the nucleus,[2] and stress concentrations are intensified by water loss from the tissue.[71] The anulus becomes slightly weaker and less extensible.[12,13,72] Herniation of the nucleus pulposus can be reproduced most easily in the laboratory in specimens from adults aged 40 to 50 years (**Fig. 2.5E**), presumably because the anulus is weakening at a time when the nucleus still exhibits sufficient hydrostatic pressure to tension the anulus and burst through it.[73]

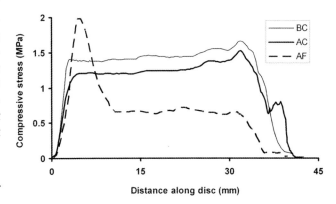

Fig. 2.6 Typical "stress profiles" recorded by pulling a miniature pressure transducer through a mature cadaveric lumbar intervertebral disc while it was subjected to a compressive force of 2 kN. Vertical compressive stress is plotted against position along the midsagittal diameter (posterior on left). BC = Disc fully hydrated (before creep). AC = After creep loading, which causes ~20% of tissue water to be lost, as in aging. AF = After fracture of the vertebral endplate during compressive overload. Damage decompresses the nucleus and generates a large concentration of compressive stress in the posterior anulus. (From Zhao F, Pollintine P, Hole BD, Dolan P, Adams MA. Discogenic origins of spinal instability. Spine 2005;30(23): 2621–2630. Reprinted with permission.)

■ Disc Degeneration

It is important to identify degenerative processes that differ from the inevitable age-related changes discussed above. A definition of disc degeneration is required to focus new research,[74] and to be useful, it must emphasize functional changes and pain. Various disc "degeneration" grading schemes have been proposed (for example, **Fig. 2.5A-D**), but they are merely exercises in pattern recognition, occasionally with some relevance to function.[60] They can be useful but do not explain the underlying processes.

Defining Disc Degeneration

Recently, we proposed that IVD degeneration should be defined as "an aberrant, cell-mediated response to progressive structural failure," and that the term *early degenerative changes* should be applied to accelerated age-related changes in a structurally intact disc.[75] Structural failure is important because it adversely affects the mechanical environment of disc cells (**Fig. 2.6**) so that cellular metabolism becomes abnormal.[9,76,77] Moreover, it does so permanently because adult discs have too few cells to repair their matrix. Structural failure of a disc or endplate is associated with dysfunction[2] and pain,[78,79] whereas age-related biochemical changes that manifest as dark discs on magnetic resonance imaging have little or no association with pain.[80] Some disrupted discs are not painful, but this may be because of variable processes such as pain sensitization[81] and stress shielding of a narrowed disc by the neural arch.[82] Structural disruption progresses, both mechanically and biologically, and animal models confirm that it always leads to typical degenerative changes[83] over a time span that increases with the size of the animal. Examples of mechanical progression are the propagation of fissures or cracks, and the buckling of already-collapsing lamellae in the anulus. Biological progression occurs because structural damage creates regions of high and low stress within the disc (**Fig. 2.6**), both of which impair disc cell metabolism.[37] Decreased proteoglycan synthesis in a decompressed nucleus would lead to a vicious circle as more load is transferred to the anulus so that the nucleus would be further decompressed. Disc cells are influenced mostly by their

immediate environment and are unaware of the "big picture": this is why they behave in an inappropriate or "aberrant" manner, and why the result is a degenerative process that can be likened to "frustrated healing" (**Fig. 2.7**) rather than adaptation or healing.

Causes of Disc Degeneration

The *underlying* cause of structural disruption is tissue weakness, arising from several causes. Genetic inheritance accounts for 30 to 50% of between-twin variability in disc degeneration, and the genes responsible appear to influence the strength of the extracellular matrix.[74] Genes influence

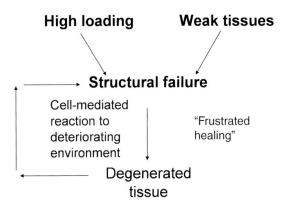

Fig. 2.7 Scheme summarizing the process of intervertebral disc degeneration.

"who gets" disc degeneration, whereas environmental factors probably determine which spinal levels are affected, and when. Aging also weakens discs, as discussed above, by making the matrix dehydrated and more brittle.[52] Nutritional compromise can limit the number of viable cells, leaving the discs incapable of effective repair.[84] However, nutritional compromise is probably not decisive because endplate fracture causes disc degeneration[69,85] even though it enhances disc metabolite transport.[86]

According to this scheme, the *precipitating* cause of disc degeneration is mechanical damage, but the forces involved need not be large if the disc is weak. For example, combined loading in bending and compression can cause radial fissures and disc prolapse, either as a sudden injury[73] (**Fig. 2.5E**) or by accumulating micro damage in the process of "fatigue failure."[62,63] There is direct evidence in humans that compressive injury to an endplate leads to disc degeneration.[69] The rate of progression of degeneration is very variable, but disc height loss averages 3% per year in middle-aged women,[87] increasing in those with physically demanding occupations.[88]

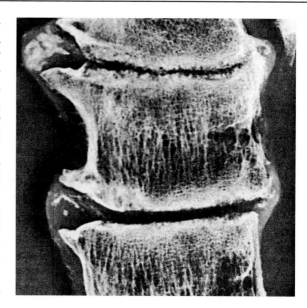

Fig. 2.8 Secondary changes to vertebrae following advanced disc degeneration and narrowing. Note the anterior osteophytes (on the left), sclerotic endplates, and thinning trabeculae.

Structural and Functional Changes following Disc Degeneration

Degenerated discs with disrupted structure exhibit highly abnormal "stress profiles" (**Fig. 2.6**). The nucleus is grossly decompressed, and high concentrations of compressive stress appear in the anulus. In animal models, experimental anulus damage increases endplate vascularity[19] and remodeling of underlying trabecular bone.[89] Nucleus decompression allows the anulus to bulge radially, like a flat tire,[65] and the resulting loss of disc height reduces tension in the outer anulus and intervertebral ligaments, allowing

the motion segment to "wobble" easily.[90] A combination of anulus bulge and segmental instability appears to stimulate the formation of osteophytes around the margins of the vertebral body,[91] especially in its anterolateral corners (**Fig. 2.8**)—these then restore stability in bending. Another long-term consequence of disc degeneration is osteoarthritis of the apophyseal joints.[92,93] Loss of disc height leads to high compressive load-bearing by the apophyseal joints[82] with much of the compressive force being concentrated on the rims of the inferior facets where they impinge on the lamina.[94,95]

References

1. Alexander RM. Elasticity in human and animal backs. In: Vleeming A, Mooney V, Dorman T, Snijders CJ, Stoeckart R, eds. Movement, Stability and Low Back Pain. Edinburgh, UK: Churchill Livingstone; 1997

2. Adams MA, McNally DS, Dolan P. "Stress" distributions inside intervertebral discs: the effects of age and degeneration. J Bone Joint Surg Br 1996;78(6):965–972

3. Pfirrmann CW, Metzdorf A, Elfering A, Hodler J, Boos N. Effect of aging and degeneration on disc volume and shape: a quantitative study in asymptomatic volunteers. J Orthop Res 2006;24(5):1086–1094

4. Marchand F, Ahmed AM. Investigation of the laminate structure of lumbar disc anulus fibrosus. Spine 1990;15(5):402–410

5. Screen HR, Lee DA, Bader DL, Shelton JC. An investigation into the effects of the hierarchical structure of tendon fascicles on micromechanical properties. Proc Inst Mech Eng [H] 2004;218(2):109–119

6. Duncan NA. Cell deformation and micromechanical environment in the intervertebral disc. J Bone Joint Surg Am 2006;88(Suppl 2): 47–51

7. Pezowicz CA, Robertson PA, Broom ND. Intralamellar relationships within the collagenous architecture of the annulus fibrosus imaged in its fully hydrated state. J Anat 2005;207(4): 299–312

8. Adams MA, Green TP. Tensile properties of the annulus fibrosus. Part I. The contribution of fibre-matrix interactions to tensile stiffness and strength. Eur Spine J 1993;2:203–208

9. Antoniou J, Steffen T, Nelson F, et al. The human lumbar intervertebral disc: evidence for changes in the biosynthesis and denaturation of the extracellular matrix with growth, maturation, ageing, and degeneration. J Clin Invest 1996;98(4):996–1003

10. Fujita Y, Duncan NA, Lotz JC. Radial tensile properties of the lumbar annulus fibrosus are site and degeneration dependent. J Orthop Res 1997;15(6):814–819

11. Yu J, Fairbank JC, Roberts S, Urban JP. The elastic fiber network of the anulus fibrosus of the normal and scoliotic human intervertebral disc. Spine 2005;30(16):1815–1820

12. Skrzypiec D, Tarala M, Pollintine P, Dolan P, Adams MA. When are intervertebral discs stronger than their adjacent vertebrae? Spine 2007;32(22):2455–2461

13. Ebara S, Iatridis JC, Setton LA, Foster RJ, Mow VC, Weidenbaum M. Tensile properties of nondegenerate human lumbar anulus fibrosus. Spine 1996;21(4):452–461

14. Roberts S, Menage J, Duance V, Wotton S, Ayad S. 1991 Volvo Award in Basic Sciences. Collagen types around the cells of the intervertebral disc and cartilage end plate: an immunolocalization study. Spine 1991;16(9):1030–1038

15. Oegema TR Jr, Johnson SL, Aguiar DJ, Ogilvie JW. Fibronectin and its fragments increase with degeneration in the human intervertebral disc. Spine 2000;25(21):2742–2747

16. Yu J, Winlove PC, Roberts S, Urban JP. Elastic fibre organization in the intervertebral discs of the bovine tail. J Anat 2002;201(6):465–475

17. Veres SP, Robertson PA, Broom ND. ISSLS prize winner. Microstructure and mechanical disruption of the lumbar disc annulus. Part II. How the annulus fails under hydrostatic pressure. Spine 2008;33: 2711–2720.

18. Francois RJ, Dhem A. Microradiographic study of the normal human vertebral body. Acta Anat (Basel) 1974;89(2):251–265

19. Moore RJ, Osti OL, Vernon-Roberts B, Fraser RD. Changes in endplate vascularity after an outer anulus tear in the sheep. Spine 1992;17(8):874–878

20. Zhao F, Pollintine P, Hole BD, Adams MA, Dolan P. Vertebral fractures usually affect the cranial endplate because it is thinner and supported by less-dense trabecular bone. Bone 2009;44(2): 372–379

21. Grant JP, Oxland TR, Dvorak MF. Mapping the structural properties of the lumbosacral vertebral endplates. Spine 2001;26(8):889–896

22. Brinckmann P, Frobin W, Hierholzer E, Horst M. Deformation of the vertebral end-plate under axial loading of the spine. Spine 1983; 8(8):851–856

23. Hastreiter D, Ozuna RM, Spector M. Regional variations in certain cellular characteristics in human lumbar intervertebral discs, including the presence of alpha-smooth muscle actin. J Orthop Res 2001;19(4):597–604

24. Errington RJ, Puustjarvi K, White IR, Roberts S, Urban JP. Characterisation of cytoplasm-filled processes in cells of the intervertebral disc. J Anat 1998;192(Pt 3):369–378

25. Hunter CJ, Matyas JR, Duncan NA. The functional significance of cell clusters in the notochordal nucleus pulposus: survival and signaling in the canine intervertebral disc. Spine 2004;29(10):1099–1104

26. Nerlich AG, Weiler C, Weissbach S, et al. Age-associated changes in the cell density of the human lumbar intervertebral disc. Washington, DC; Orthopaedic Research Society; 2005

27. Geiss A, Larsson K, Rydevik B, Takahashi I, Olmarker K. Autoimmune properties of nucleus pulposus: an experimental study in pigs. Spine 2007;32(2):168–173

28. Osti OL, Vernon-Roberts B, Fraser RD. 1990 Volvo Award in Experimental Studies. Anulus tears and intervertebral disc degeneration: an experimental study using an animal model. Spine 1990;15(8): 762–767

29. Nerlich AG, Schaaf R, Walchli B, Boos N. Temporo-spatial distribution of blood vessels in human lumbar intervertebral discs. Eur Spine J 2007;16(4):547–555

30. Johnson WE, Caterson B, Eisenstein SM, Roberts S. Human intervertebral disc aggrecan inhibits endothelial cell adhesion and cell migration in vitro. Spine 2005;30(10):1139–1147

31. Botsford DJ, Esses SI, Ogilvie-Harris DJ. In vivo diurnal variation in intervertebral disc volume and morphology. Spine 1994;19(8): 935–940

32. Ferguson SJ, Ito K, Nolte LP. Fluid flow and convective transport of solutes within the intervertebral disc. J Biomech 2004;37(2): 213–221

33. McMillan DW, Garbutt G, Adams MA. Effect of sustained loading on the water content of intervertebral discs: implications for disc metabolism. Ann Rheum Dis 1996;55(12):880–887

34. Bibby SR, Jones DA, Ripley RM, Urban JP. Metabolism of the intervertebral disc: effects of low levels of oxygen, glucose, and pH on rates of energy metabolism of bovine nucleus pulposus cells. Spine 2005;30(5):487–496

35. Horner HA, Urban JP. 2001 Volvo Award Winner in Basic Science. Effect of nutrient supply on the viability of cells from the nucleus pulposus of the intervertebral disc. Spine 2001;26(23):2543–2549

36. Battie MC, Videman T, Gill K, et al. 1991 Volvo Award in Clinical Sciences. Smoking and lumbar intervertebral disc degeneration: an MRI study of identical twins. Spine 1991;16(9):1015–1021

37. Ishihara H, McNally DS, Urban JP, Hall AC. Effects of hydrostatic pressure on matrix synthesis in different regions of the intervertebral disk. J Appl Physiol 1996;80(3):839–846

38. Neidlinger-Wilke C, Wurtz K, Urban JP, et al. Regulation of gene expression in intervertebral disc cells by low and high hydrostatic pressure. Eur Spine J 2006;15(Suppl 3):372–378

39. Palmgren T, Gronblad M, Virri J, Kaapa E, Karaharju E. An immunohistochemical study of nerve structures in the anulus fibrosus of human normal lumbar intervertebral discs. Spine 1999;24(20):2075–2079

40. Bogduk N. Clinical Anatomy of the Lumbar Spine. 3rd ed. Edinburgh, UK: Churchill Livingstone; 1997

41. Sekine M, Yamashita T, Takebayashi T, Sakamoto N, Minaki Y, Ishii S. Mechanosensitive afferent units in the lumbar posterior longitudinal ligament. Spine 2001;26(14):1516–1521

42. Kuslich SD, Ulstrom CL, Michael CJ. The tissue origin of low back pain and sciatica: a report of pain response to tissue stimulation during operations on the lumbar spine using local anesthesia. Orthop Clin North Am 1991;22(2):181–187

43. Olmarker K, Rydevik B, Nordborg C. Autologous nucleus pulposus induces neurophysiologic and histologic changes in porcine cauda equina nerve roots. Spine 1993;18(11):1425–1432

44. Onda A, Murata Y, Rydevik B, Larsson K, Kikuchi S, Olmarker K. Nerve growth factor content in dorsal root ganglion as related to changes in pain behavior in a rat model of experimental lumbar disc herniation. Spine 2005;30(2):188–193

45. Freemont AJ, Peacock TE, Goupille P, Hoyland JA, O'Brien J, Jayson MI. Nerve ingrowth into diseased intervertebral disc in chronic back pain. Lancet 1997;350(9072):178–181

46. Peng B, Wu W, Hou S, Li P, Zhang C, Yang Y. The pathogenesis of discogenic low back pain. J Bone Joint Surg Br 2005;87(1):62–67

47. Johnson WE, Sivan S, Wright KT, Eisenstein SM, Maroudas A, Roberts S. Human intervertebral disc cells promote nerve growth over substrata of human intervertebral disc aggrecan. Spine 2006;31(11):1187–1193

48. Johnson WE, Caterson B, Eisenstein SM, Hynds DL, Snow DM, Roberts S. Human intervertebral disc aggrecan inhibits nerve growth in vitro. Arthritis Rheum 2002;46(10):2658–2664

49. Boos N, Weissbach S, Rohrbach H, Weiler C, Spratt KF, Nerlich AG. 2002 Volvo Award in Basic Science. Classification of age-related changes in lumbar intervertebral discs. Spine 2002;27(23): 2631–2644

50. Haefeli M, Kalberer F, Saegesser D, Nerlich AG, Boos N, Paesold G. The course of macroscopic degeneration in the human lumbar intervertebral disc. Spine 2006;31(14):1522–1531

51. Duance VC, Crean JK, Sims TJ, et al. Changes in collagen cross-linking in degenerative disc disease and scoliosis. Spine 1998;23(23): 2545–2551

52. DeGroot J, Verzijl N, Wenting-Van Wijk MJ, et al. Accumulation of advanced glycation end products as a molecular mechanism for aging as a risk factor in osteoarthritis. Arthritis Rheum 2004;50(4): 1207–1215

53. Roughley PJ. Biology of intervertebral disc aging and degeneration: involvement of the extracellular matrix. Spine 2004;29(23): 2691–2699

54. Gruber HE, Ingram JA, Norton HJ, Hanley EN Jr. Senescence in cells of the aging and degenerating intervertebral disc: immunolocalization of senescence-associated beta-galactosidase in human and sand rat discs. Spine 2007;32(3):321–327

55. Gruber HE, Hanley EN Jr. Analysis of aging and degeneration of the human intervertebral disc: comparison of surgical specimens with normal controls. Spine 1998;23(7):751–757

56. Heyde CE, Tschoeke SK, Hellmuth M, Hostmann A, Ertel W, Oberholzer A. Trauma induces apoptosis in human thoracolumbar intervertebral discs. BMC Clin Pathol 2006;6:5

57. Nerlich AG, Bachmeier BE, Schleicher E, Rohrbach H, Paesold G, Boos N. Immunomorphological analysis of RAGE receptor expression and NF-kappaB activation in tissue samples from normal and degenerated intervertebral discs of various ages. Ann N Y Acad Sci 2007;1096:239–248

58. Antoniou J, Goudsouzian NM, Heathfield TF, et al. The human lumbar endplate. Evidence of changes in biosynthesis and denaturation of the extracellular matrix with growth, maturation, aging, and degeneration. Spine 1996;21(10):1153–1161

59. Shao Z, Rompe G, Schiltenwolf M. Radiographic changes in the lumbar intervertebral discs and lumbar vertebrae with age. Spine 2002;27(3):263–268

60. Adams MA, Dolan P, Hutton WC. The stages of disc degeneration as revealed by discograms. J Bone Joint Surg Br 1986;68(1):36–41

61. Vernon-Roberts B, Fazzalari NL, Manthey BA. Pathogenesis of tears of the anulus investigated by multiple-level transaxial analysis of the T12–L1 disc. Spine 1997;22(22):2641–2646

62. Adams MA, Hutton WC. Gradual disc prolapse. Spine 1985; 10(6):524–531

63. Gordon SJ, Yang KH, Mayer PJ, Mace AH Jr, Kish VL, Radin EL. Mechanism of disc rupture. A preliminary report. Spine 1991;16(4): 450–456

64. Goel VK, Monroe BT, Gilbertson LG, Brinckmann P. Interlaminar shear stresses and laminae separation in a disc: finite element analysis of the L3–L4 motion segment subjected to axial compressive loads. Spine 1995;20(6):689–698

65. Brinckmann P, Horst M. The influence of vertebral body fracture, intradiscal injection, and partial discectomy on the radial bulge and height of human lumbar discs. Spine 1985;10(2):138–145

66. Adams MA, Dolan P, Hutton WC. The lumbar spine in backward bending. Spine 1988;13(9):1019–1026

67. Crock HV. Internal disc disruption: a challenge to disc prolapse fifty years on. Spine 1986;11(6):650–653

68. Przybyla A, Pollintine P, Bedzinski R, Adams MA. Outer annulus tears have less effect than endplate fracture on stress distributions inside intervertebral discs: relevance to disc degeneration. Clin Biomech (Bristol, Avon) 2006;21(10):1013–1019

69. Kerttula LI, Serlo WS, Tervonen OA, Paakko EL, Vanharanta HV. Post-traumatic findings of the spine after earlier vertebral fracture in young patients: clinical and MRI study. Spine 2000;25(9):1104–1108

70. Moore RJ, Vernon-Roberts B, Fraser RD, Osti OL, Schembri M. The origin and fate of herniated lumbar intervertebral disc tissue. Spine 1996;21(18):2149–2155

71. Adams MA, McMillan DW, Green TP, Dolan P. Sustained loading generates stress concentrations in lumbar intervertebral discs. Spine 1996;21(4):434–438

72. Adams MA, Green TP, Dolan P. The strength in anterior bending of lumbar intervertebral discs. Spine 1994;19(19):2197–2203

73. Adams MA, Hutton WC. 1981 Volvo Award in Basic Science. Prolapsed intervertebral disc: a hyperflexion injury. Spine 1982;7(3): 184–191

74. Battie MC, Videman T, Levalahti E, Gill K, Kaprio J. Genetic and environmental effects on disc degeneration by phenotype and spinal level: a multivariate twin study. Spine 2008;33:2801–2808

75. Adams MA, Roughley PJ. What is intervertebral disc degeneration, and what causes it? Spine 2006;31(18):2151–2161

76. Weiler C, Nerlich AG, Zipperer J, Bachmeier BE, Boos N. 2002 SSE Award Competition in Basic Science. Expression of major matrix metalloproteinases is associated with intervertebral disc degradation and resorption. Eur Spine J 2002;11(4):308–320

77. Nerlich AG, Bachmeier BE, Boos N. Expression of fibronectin and TGF-beta1 mRNA and protein suggest altered regulation of extracellular matrix in degenerated disc tissue. Eur Spine J 2005;14(1):17–26

78. Weishaupt D, Zanetti M, Hodler J, et al. Painful lumbar disk derangement: relevance of endplate abnormalities at MR imaging. Radiology 2001;218(2):420–427

79. Videman T, Nurminen M. The occurrence of annular tears and their relation to lifetime back pain history: a cadaveric study using barium sulfate discography. Spine 2004;29(23):2668–2676

80. Boos N, Rieder R, Schade V, Spratt KF, Semmer N, Aebi M. 1995 Volvo Award in Clinical Sciences. The diagnostic accuracy of magnetic resonance imaging, work perception, and psychosocial factors in identifying symptomatic disc herniations. Spine 1995;20(24): 2613–2625

81. Olmarker K, Nutu M, Storkson R. Changes in spontaneous behavior in rats exposed to experimental disc herniation are blocked by selective TNF-alpha inhibition. Spine 2003;28(15):1635–1641 discussion 1642

82. Pollintine P, Przybyla AS, Dolan P, Adams MA. Neural arch load-bearing in old and degenerated spines. J Biomech 2004;37(2):197–204

83. Lotz JC. Animal models of intervertebral disc degeneration: lessons learned. Spine 2004;29(23):2742–2750

84. Urban JP, Smith S, Fairbank JC. Nutrition of the intervertebral disc. Spine 2004;29(23):2700–2709

85. Holm S, Holm AK, Ekstrom L, Karladani A, Hansson T. Experimental disc degeneration due to endplate injury. J Spinal Disord Tech 2004;17(1):64–71

86. Rajasekaran S, Babu JN, Arun R, Armstrong BR, Shetty AP, Murugan S. ISSLS Prize Winner. A study of diffusion in human lumbar discs: a serial magnetic resonance imaging study documenting the influence of the endplate on diffusion in normal and degenerate discs. Spine 2004;29(23):2654–2667

87. Hassett G, Hart DJ, Manek NJ, Doyle DV, Spector TD. Risk factors for progression of lumbar spine disc degeneration: the Chingford Study. Arthritis Rheum 2003;48(11):3112–3117

88. Videman T, Battie MC, Ripatti S, Gill K, Manninen H, Kaprio J. Determinants of the progression in lumbar degeneration: a 5-year

follow-up study of adult male monozygotic twins. Spine 2006; 31(6):671–678

89. Moore RJ, Vernon-Roberts B, Osti OL, Fraser RD. Remodeling of vertebral bone after outer annular injury in sheep. Spine 1996;21(8): 936–940

90. Zhao F, Pollintine P, Hole BD, Dolan P, Adams MA. Discogenic origins of spinal instability. Spine 2005;30(23):2621–2630

91. Lipson SJ, Muir H. Vertebral osteophyte formation in experimental disc degeneration: morphologic and proteoglycan changes over time. Arthritis Rheum 1980;23(3):319–324

92. Tischer T, Aktas T, Milz S, Putz RV. Detailed pathological changes of human lumbar facet joints L1–L5 in elderly individuals. Eur Spine J 2006;15(3):308–315

93. Moore RJ, Crotti TN, Osti OL, Fraser RD, Vernon-Roberts B. Osteoarthrosis of the facet joints resulting from annular rim lesions in sheep lumbar discs. Spine 1999;24(6):519–525

94. Dunlop RB, Adams MA, Hutton WC. Disc space narrowing and the lumbar facet joints. J Bone Joint Surg Br 1984;66(5):706–710

95. Adams MA, Bogduk N, Burton K, Dolan P. The Biomechanics of Back Pain. 2nd ed. Edinburgh, UK: Churchill Livingstone; 2006

3 Biology of the Lumbar Intervertebral Disc

Ashok Biyani, Philip D. Nowicki, and Howard S. An

A daily accretion in the knowledge of intervertebral disc (IVD) biology and biochemistry is advancing rapidly due, in part, to the advent of newer biochemical techniques and more precise disc models. New discoveries regarding the form and function of the IVD extracellular matrix as well as the complex interaction and balance of growth factors, proteinases, and proteinase inhibitors have opened the door for new and exciting options for clinical therapeutics of IVD degeneration. Though currently in their infancy, such therapies may one day become routine in preventing disc degradation and providing pain relief to patients with degenerative disc disease. In this chapter, we will discuss the important biological processes that characterize the intervertebral disc in both health and disease.

■ Biology of the Normal Lumbar Intervertebral Disc

Development

To understand the biology of the healthy IVD, a review of the normal development and embryology of the disc is in order. The notochord is derived from embryologic mesoderm that becomes the predecessor for multiple tissues that ultimately form the spine and its various elements. The first tissue is the neural tube, which creates the formation of the floor plate.[1] The second tissue is that of the ventral somites, which ultimately develop into the sclerotomes and subsequent skeletal elements of the ribs and vertebral column.[1,2] Portions of this ventral somite tissue remain in an axial position and ultimately form the anulus fibrosus and the vertebral bodies through chondrification.[2,3] The notochord itself degrades and disappears where the vertebral bodies condense, but is maintained in the areas between the bodies, giving rise to the nucleus pulposus (NP).[1,4,5] Type II collagen has been recognized as important in this differentiation.[1] A cascade of events occurs as the fetus grows, establishing the distinct spinal levels and anteroposterior polarity of the spinal column. Various transcription factors are imperative to this development and include *Sox9, Pax1, Pax9, Shh*, and *Bapx1.*[2] The primitive notochord cells remain within the pulposus until approximately

12 years of age, when they develop into mature tissue.[6] These cells are replaced by infiltrating chondrocyte-like cells that form a fibrocartilaginous matrix rich with chemical markers responsible for cell migration, extracellular matrix digestion, and cell proliferation.[5]

The gradual change of cell populations from notochordal cells to chondrocytic cells occurs at different ages in different species.[7] In the human IVD, notochordal cells to predominate in the very young nucleus and are present in a limited number until the age of 12 years. Although the precise mechanism of transition from notochordal cells to chondrocytic cells in the nucleus is not known, there is evidence in rabbits and rats that chondrocytes from cartilaginous endplates migrate toward the NP region as notochordal cells undergo apoptosis.[8,9] The mechanism of apoptosis of the notochordal cells is by way of either an autocrine or a paracrine Fas-mediated mitochondrial caspase-9 pathway.[9] The migration of chondrocytes from cartilage endplates into the NP is accompanied by the expression of membrane-type I matrix metalloproteinase (a marker of cell migration and extracellular matrix digestion), K_i-67 protein (a cell proliferation marker), and type II collagen (a marker for cartilaginous matrix).

Structure and Function

There are a multitude of biochemicals in the anulus fibrosus (AF) and NP. These include specific collagens, proteoglycans, growth factors, and cytokines. Each tissue type is unique in its composition, which gives each tissue distinct properties employed in their distinct structure and function. **Figure 3.1** illustrates the anatomy of the anulus fibrosus and the NP in association with the spinal segment and surrounding structures.

The anulus fibrosus consists primarily of highly ordered arrangements of type I collagen. This lamellar structure provides the tensile strength of the IVD.[2,4–6,10–12] Approximately 70% of the dry weight of the anulus is composed of collagen molecules.[4] The anulus is divided into inner and outer portions. The outer portion is composed of cells that are ellipsoidal in shape and fibroblast-like in nature. The cells are aligned in a radial fashion to the collagen fibers within individual lamellae that take and distribute loads from the NP during various types of exercise.[4,5,10] The outer

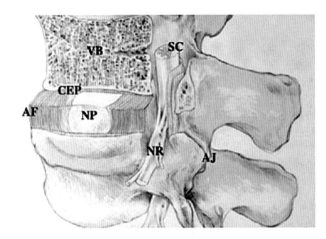

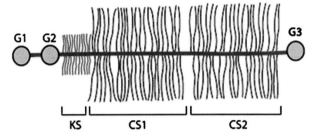

Fig. 3.1 Schematic view of a spinal segment and the intervertebral disc. The figure shows the organization of the disc with the nucleus pulposus (NP) surrounded by the lamellae of the anulus fibrosus (AF) and separated from the vertebral bodies (VB) by the cartilaginous endplate (CEP). The figure also shows the relationship between the intervertebral disc and the spinal cord (SC), the nerve root (NR), and the apophyseal joints (AJ). (From Urban JP, Roberts S. Degeneration of the intervertebral disc. Arthritis Res Ther 2003;5:120–130. Reprinted with permission.)

Fig. 3.2 The structure of human aggrecan. Aggrecan is a central core protein with keratan sulfate (KS) and chondroitin sulfate (CS) side chains. The core protein possesses three globular domains (G1, G2, and G3), with the G2 and G3 domains being separated by a KS-rich domain and two CS-rich domains (CS1 and CS2). (From Roughley PJ, Melching LI, Heathfield TF, Pearce RH, Mort JS. The structure and degradation of aggrecan in human intervertebral disc. Eur Spine J 2006;15(suppl 3): S326–332. Reprinted with permission.)

portion anchors the anulus and disc itself directly to the vertebral body at the endplate.[4] The inner layer of the anulus is less structured and more fibrocartilaginous in nature, with an increasingly higher concentration of type II collagen and other collagen types (i.e., types V and XI). These additional collagens allow for cross-bridging of other collagen molecules and form the fibrillar collagen network to add to the strength of the anulus.[4,5,10] Type VI collagen plays a unique role in the anulus, contributing along with the fibrillar collagen network to establish the major strength to tensile loads by way of fibrillar sliding.[4,10,13] The inner layer of the anulus is less cellular and is composed of a pericellular matrix that extends into the NP. This inner anulus tissue helps to modify the local environment at the annular–nucleus interface.[5] Included in this pericellular matrix are the proteoglycans decorin and biglycan, which are thought to help regulate fibroblast and matrix synthesis.[12]

The NP is derived from primitive interconnected notochord cells that gradually disappear and leave behind a collection of sparse chondrocytes, which comprise ~1% of the total disc material.[4,14] Despite this diminutive population, chondrocytes are the predominant cell type in the nucleus, decreasing in number in the central disc portions.[15] Water constitutes 70 to 80% of the nucleus. Up to 50% of the dry weight of the NP is made up of various proteoglycans and collagens. Aggrecan is the predominant proteoglycan type, and type II collagen is the predominant collagen type found in the nucleus.[4] The proteoglycans themselves are part of the highly organized extracellular matrix found in the nucleus. The unique and inherent chemical properties of the proteoglycans

to retain water give the nucleus its main function to resist compression loads.[11,12,16] This hydration ability grants the nucleus unique biologic responses to mechanical stimuli (**Fig. 3.2**). At low frequencies and moderate compressive forces, the nucleus is in a relative state of anabolism. With higher loading frequencies and magnitudes, higher rates of apoptosis and increased protease expression are found.[17,18] This response is thought to occur from biomechanically induced secondary messengers activating intracellular calcium gradients and cytoskeletal remodeling that effects downstream gene expression and posttranslational biosynthesis.[5]

The Extracellular Matrix

The extracellular matrix of the intervertebral disc has been the focus of more recent research. Through its distinct biochemical properties, this matrix is important in the absorption of shear and rotational stresses disseminated on the annular lamellae. The presence of an extensive communication array in the anulus allows for biologic and mechanical adjustments to occur between lamellae.[13] Other molecules of importance in the extracellular matrix include aggrecan, a family of proteoglycans known as leucine-rich repeat proteins, type VI collagen, and cartilage oligomeric matrix protein, among others (**Fig. 3.3**).

Aggrecan is the most important and abundant proteoglycan found in the extracellular matrix of the nucleus. It is bound centrally to chains of chondroitin and keratin sulfate, which bond to water and maintain hydration. A collection of aggrecan molecules attach to hyaluronan at their N-terminus ends.[10] At the opposite C-terminus, aggrecan can bind to other molecules of the extracellular matrix as well as to collagen and the fibrillar collagen network (**Fig. 3.4**).[10] This creates an extensive net of crosslinked molecules that support nucleus structure and function. Trivalent pyridinoline crosslinks have been found to be important in maintaining nucleus tissue

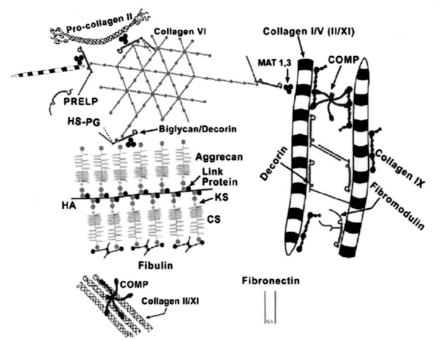

Fig. 3.3 Schematic illustration of assemblies of matrix proteins into structures in the intervertebral disc. COMP, cartilage oligomeric matrix protein; CS, chondroitin sulfate; H4, hyaluronan; HS-PG, heparin sulfate proteoglycan; KS, keratan sulfate; MAT, matrilin; PRELP, praline arginine-rich end leucine-rich repeat protein. (From Feng H, Danfelter M, Stromqvist B, Heinegard D. Extracellular matrix in disc degeneration. J Bone Joint Surg Am 2006;88A(suppl 2):25–29. Reprinted with permission.)

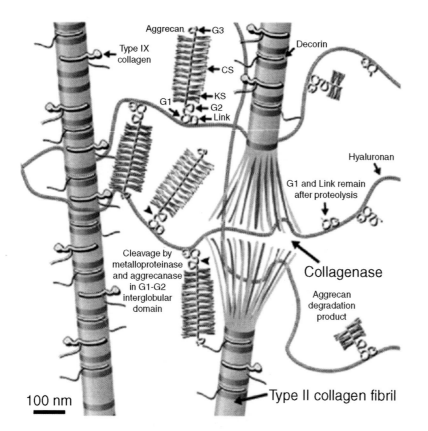

Fig. 3.4 Structure of collagen and the proteoglycan aggrecan. Sites of attack by collagenases and other proteinases (arrowheads). CS, chondroitin sulfate; G1-G3, globular domains; KS, keratan sulfate. (From Recklies AD, Poole AR, Banerjee S, et al. Pathophysiologic aspects of inflammation in diarthrodial joints. In: Buckwalter JA, Einhorn TA, Simon SR, eds. Orthopaedic Basic Science: Biology and Biomechanics of the Musculoskeletal System. 2nd ed. Rosemont, IL: American Academy of Orthopaedic Surgeons; 2000:489–530. Reprinted with permission.)

cohesiveness. With age, these crosslinks decrease and become replaced with pentosidine, a sign of advanced glycosylation.[19] This substitution alters the biochemistry of the extracellular matrix and leads to degeneration.

The leucine-rich repeat proteins (LRRPs) are a family of proteoglycans granting additional structural and functional properties to the extracellular matrix of the IVD. The most studied molecules in this group include fibromodulin, decorin, lumican, and versican. These proteins contain a central portion of 10 or 11 specific repeats that maintain leucine residues at conserved locations.[10] This biochemical structure enables direct interaction with collagen and aids in collagen crosslinking. Decorin and lumican have been found to play an important organizational role in assembly, transport, and incorporation of collagen fibrils into the extracellular matrix.[10,12] Versican is thought to attach adjacent annular lamellae to one another by way of elastic fibers, enhancing cellular adhesion as well as proliferation.[12,20] These LRRPs can bind to growth factors, with a predilection for binding to transforming growth factor-β, and thus may play a role in the development of the nucleus.[10] The LRRPs are expressed at various times within the life cycle of the IVD, reflecting the phenotypic differences of cell populations in different regions and at different times in the life of the disc.[12]

In addition to proteoglycans, the extracellular matrix is also composed of a variety of other molecules. Cartilage oligomeric matrix protein (COMP) is a pentameric extracellular matrix protein that is abundantly expressed in many tissues in the body, with the highest levels manifested in weight-bearing tissues.[21] It is a molecule important for the development of cartilage and cartilage growth, as mutations in the COMP gene lead to skeletal dysplasia, pseudoachondroplasia, and multiple epiphyseal dysplasia.[22,23] COMP is heavily bound to collagen and can concomitantly bind to other matrix molecules, especially in the anulus. COMP therefore may play a role in maintaining the structural stiffness of the normal IVD.[21] This multimolecular binding capacity of COMP allows for the rapid and efficient regulation of collagen fibril assembly into well-defined collagen fibers and maintains the stability of the fibrillar collagen network.[10]

Type VI collagen is secreted into a filamentous and beaded network that binds to LRRPs, which then bind to aggrecan and other collagen types, resulting in organization of the territorial matrix.[24] Type VI collagen is thought to be involved in remodeling of the pericellular microenvironment.[25] NG2 is a transmembrane proteoglycan that has been found to be closely associated with type VI collagen and the pericellular matrix.[26–28] Because of this association, NG2 is thought to be involved in cell-matrix interactions and transmembrane signaling pathways.[27] Specifically, NG2 binds to growth factors such as platelet-derived growth factor and basic fibroblast growth factor.[29,30] This binding potential likely makes NG2 important in cellular proliferation and migration.[27] The function of cartilage intermediate layer protein in the nucleus has yet to be elucidated, but it has been shown to be involved with degeneration of lumbar discs.[31]

Cellular Biology

The health of the IVD is dependent upon a balance between anabolic and catabolic factors as well as cellular demand and transportation limits.[6,11,32,33] There are numerous factors important in this balance, including blood supply, cellular metabolism, cytokines, growth factors, proteinases, proteinase inhibitors, and mechanical stimuli.

The IVD is almost completely avascular. Blood vessels are limited to the periphery of the AF. There is minimal penetration into the inner disc layers, leaving the central portion of the NP without direct nutritional supply (**Fig. 3.5**).[4,15,33] The metabolism of the disc is therefore highly dependent upon diffusion and glycolysis.[33,34] The vertebral endplates, which are composed of hyaline cartilage, are porous in structure and directly abut the blood

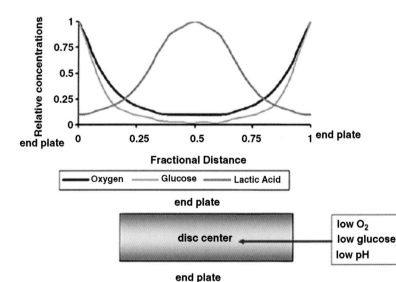

Fig. 3.5 Schematic showing the concentrations of oxygen, glucose, and pH levels across the disc from endplate to endplate. (From Grunhagen T, Wilde G, Mokhbi Soukane D, Shirazi-adl SA, Urban JP. Nutrient supply and intervertebral disc metabolism. J Bone Joint Surg Am 2006;88A(suppl 2):30–35. Reprinted with permission.)

vessels of adjacent vertebral bodies to allow for nutrient diffusion to occur.[15] Oxygen tension, pH, and glucose concentrations are the main determinants of cellular biology in the IVD. Their levels are closely maintained within specific narrow limits to allow optimal metabolism and matrix synthesis.[33] The osmotic pressure gradient is also important for disc metabolism. This gradient is affected by mechanical forces within the disc that help to regulate disc height and hydration, as well as intracellular signaling responsible for cell death or survival.[5] If the cellular environment of the disc strays too far from optimal concentration gradients, apoptosis and degradation ensue.

Growth Factors

IVD anabolism is regulated by insulin growth factor (IGF), transforming growth factor-β (TGF-β), and the bone morphogenetic protein (BMP) family. These molecules are involved in extracellular matrix production and regulation.[11,35] IGF has been shown to stimulate prostaglandin synthesis in the NP of bovine cells,[36] but gradually with time this response by IVD cells diminishes.[37] TGF-β has demonstrated similar effects on prostaglandin synthesis but also has shown the ability to stimulate disc regeneration.[38] Contrary to these findings, some authors have found that high TGF-β concentrations may actually be toxic to disc cells and in fact inhibit prostaglandin synthesis.[39]

BMP-2 appears to increase cell proliferation, prostaglandin synthesis, expression of type II collagen messenger ribonucleic acid (mRNA), aggrecan, and osteocalcin production in the AF.[40,41] BMP-2 is inhibited in the NP by nicotine.[41] BMP-2 also seems to be important in maintaining disc height, as direct injection into discs has been shown to reverse early height loss.[42] When utilized in conjunction with TGF-β and IGF-1, BMP-2 is especially beneficial in stimulating prostaglandin synthesis.[43]

Osteogenic protein 1 (OP-1), also known as BMP-7, stimulates and retains proteoglycan and collagen metabolism, doing so in fetal, adult, and old bovine annular and nuclear cells.[44–46] OP-1 has a role in repair of the degenerated nuclear extracellular matrix and the anulus.[47,48] OP-1 may play a role in maintaining, restoring, and regenerating intervertebral disc height as evidenced in multiple disc injection studies.[49–51] Annular and nuclear cells respond to OP-1 by dividing as well as enhancing their synthesis of aggrecan and collagen.[35]

Growth and differentiation factor-5 (GDF-5) is a member of the BMP family. Its absence has been implicated as a causative factor in multiple skeletal dysplasias.[52,53] It is also necessary for normal joint development as it is thought to play a crucial role in stimulating the formation and proliferation of chondrogenic cells.[52,53] In IVDs void of GDF-5, total glycosaminoglycan concentration is decreased, but total collagen is not altered; there is also a downregulation of type II collagen and aggrecan genes.[53] When rhGDF-5 was injected into degenerated IVDs, a dramatic restoration in disc height was observed.[52] The NP maintained its hydrophilic properties on magnetic resonance imaging (MRI) and chondrocytic cell concentration increased in the nucleus and anulus.[52] Injection of OP-1 (BMP-7) and GDF-5 into degenerated discs was found to have similar results, but the responses by the disc cells differed. OP-1 was found to have more of an effect on proteoglycan synthesis,[54] whereas GDF-5 was found to stimulate proteoglycan and collagen synthesis in a similar manner.[52]

■ Biology of the Diseased Lumbar Intervertebral Disc

The biology of the healthy IVD is invariably dependent upon the balance between anabolic and catabolic factors (**Fig. 3.6**). Disc degeneration is complex and involves alterations in local biomechanical forces and loads, cell loss, disc nutrition and metabolism, and quantitative and qualitative changes in matrix production. **Figure 3.7** illustrates the gross appearances and differences between healthy and degenerated discs. The inciting factor for the beginning of the disc degeneration cascade continues to elude researchers. Any one of these factors or multiple simultaneous factors may be responsible for initiating disc degeneration, and not necessarily one over another in sequence (**Fig. 3.8**).

The health of the IVD is dependent on its ability to retain water. As water content decreases, not only does the local biologic environment change but the biomechanical environment changes as well. With diminished water content, the disc becomes more susceptible to damage produced by abnormal forces. Bending and compressive loads can lead to disc bulging, endplate deformation, and volumetric changes within the nucleus, whereas torque loads deform the anulus. These changes in biomechanical loading can lead to accelerated deformation and degeneration and will be discussed in more detail in a later chapter.

Cellular Changes

Cell numbers within the IVD diminish with age and result in higher levels of apoptosis, especially in the anulus.[55,56] These cells are not necessarily biologically inactive, but instead produce inappropriate matrix molecules such as matrix metalloproteinases (MMPs).[56] Altered gene expression, altered posttranslational modifications, and altered transcription factors all contribute to this cellular senescence. These cell changes ultimately lead to a decreased ability for intact cells within the anulus and nucleus to recover from deforming forces.[15]

Intrinsic and extrinsic factors that decrease the vascular supply to the disc increase the risk for degeneration. Examples

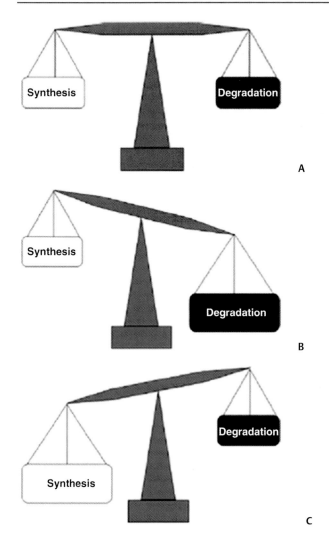

Fig. 3.6 Disc-matrix metabolism: balance of synthesis and degradation. **(A)** In the homeostatic state, the disc undergoes matrix synthesis and degradation in a balanced manner. **(B)** As the disc matrix undergoes a turnover during the course of an individual's lifetime, any small imbalance between synthesis and degradation can lead to significant changes in overall disc-matrix content. **(C)** One of the major goals of molecular therapy of the disc involves modulating this metabolic balance to the more favorable anabolic state. This can be accomplished by increasing the synthesis or decreasing the catabolism. (From Yoon ST, Patel NM. Molecular therapy of the intervertebral disc. Eur Spine J 2006;15(suppl 3):S379–S388.)

of such factors include sickle cell anemia, atherosclerosis, vibrational forces, trauma, cigarette smoking, scoliosis, and genetic predisposition.[11,33,57] The presence of any one or more of these factors may lead to endplate calcification between the vertebral bodies and the IVDs. Endplate calcification affects cellular metabolism by diminishing the diffusion capacity of the disc and leads to inappropriate changes in vital metabolic gradients. If the microenvironment pH rises due to lactate formation from decreased oxygen tension, glycolysis diminishes and leads to the inhibition of

cellular metabolism and the activation of apoptosis.[33] Extracellular matrix synthesis and degradation are directly dependent upon disc metabolism. If the diffusion concentration of glucose falls below critical levels, apoptosis rapidly accelerates.[33] If cell metabolism decreases, the cell phenotype changes and leads to decreased matrix synthesis and degeneration of the remaining matrix.[33] Disc degeneration occurs from inside of the nucleus toward the outer nucleus as cells in the internal portion have the smallest concentrations of vital metabolic gradients (**Fig. 3.5**).[58] Changes in cell phenotype activate new genes that activate the apoptotic cascade, the inflammatory response, and production of proteases. Specific enzymes and molecules involved in these degrading processes include the family of MMPs, aggrecanases, and proinflammatory cytokines.

Proteinases

The most widely studied family of enzymes in the IVD is the MMPs. These proteins are a family of zinc-dependent enzymes that degrade extracellular and basement membrane components, produced by the chondrocytes found within the IVD.[14] Individual MMPs have specific substrates enabling complete degradation of all components of the extracellular matrix.[59,60] The MMP family is divided into four major groups: (1) collagenases, (2) gelatinases, (3) stromelysins, and (4) membrane-type MMPs.[32,61] Collagenases cleave intact interstitial collagen molecules. Gelatinases work by metabolizing denatured collagen and basement membrane collagen. Stromelysins degrade noncollagenous matrix proteins. Membrane-type MMPs play a secondary role in matrix degradation. Their main activity is thought to be activation of other MMPs. The cells of the nucleus and inner anulus predominantly produce MMPs 1, 3, 13, and aggrecanase-1; the blood vessels, infiltrating cells, and cells of the outer anulus do not produce an appreciable amount of these particular enzymes.[61]

The MMPs are involved in the normal biological balance of the healthy IVD.[15,62] Their main purpose in healthy IVDs is matrix remodeling and recycling. With changes in nutrient supply and biomechanical stimuli, the genes encoding the MMPs and other catabolic factors become upregulated. This results in the transformation of cellular phenotypes and leads to an imbalance of anabolic and catabolic factors within the disc.[6,32] Radiographic evidence has confirmed that elevated levels of MMPs are directly associated with degenerative disc changes.[63]

Specifically, MMP-1 and MMP-3 have been implicated in the pathogenesis of disc herniation.[64] MMP-1 is the most abundant metalloproteinase in IVDs, found in both normal as well as diseased discs.[65] MMP-1 preferentially degrades type III collagen, but also collagen types I and II.[66,67] As degeneration occurs, a greater proportion of IVD cells produce MMP-1, which degrades type III collagen predominantly found in the inner anulus.[68,69] MMP-3 broadly binds and degrades many of

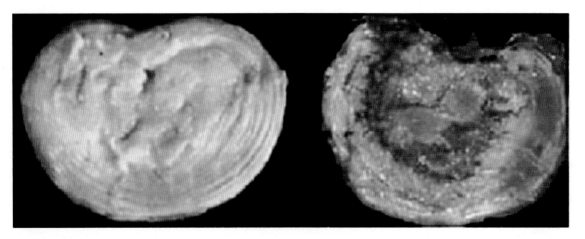

Fig. 3.7 The normal and degenerate lumbar intervertebral disc. The figure shows a normal intervertebral disc on the left. The anulus lamellae surrounding the softer nucleus pulposus are clearly visible. In the highly degenerate disc on the right, the nucleus is desiccated and the anulus is disorganized. (From Urban JP, Roberts S. Degeneration of the intervertebral disc. Arthritis Res Ther 2003;5:120–130. Reprinted with permission.)

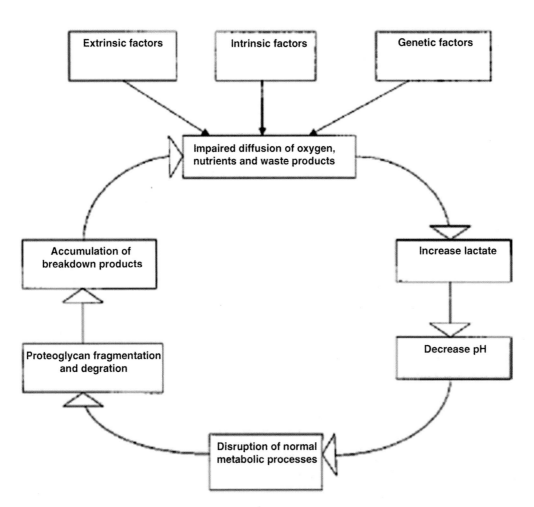

Fig. 3.8 The cycle of degenerative disc disease. The critical step in this process is the disruption of the normal diffusion of oxygen, nutrients, and waste products through the avascular disc. (From Guiot BH, Fessler RG. Molecular biology of degenerative disc disease. Neurosurgery 2000;47:1034–1040. Reprinted with permission.)

the molecules found in the extracellular matrix, as well as activates other MMP activity.[70] MMP-13 is the most potent binder of type II collagen of all the MMPs.[66] Not only does it efficiently cleave type II collagen, it also further degrades the initial cleavage products of various collagenases.[66] Although the activity of MMP-2 is yet to be fully elucidated, it has been found to have a substantial substrate list for degradation and is an activator of further MMP activity.[71]

As the MMPs become activated and the ratio of their concentrations to their inhibitors becomes altered, the biomechanical properties of the disc change and lead to inhibition of diffusion and cell metabolism. Partially degraded collagen molecules and glycolytic products that are produced from MMP activity stimulate the release of proinflammatory cytokines such as interleukin 1 (IL-1) and tumor necrosis factor alpha (TNF-α).[65] Proforms of MMPs secreted by IVDs may also become activated by cytokines.[72] These phenomena can occur at any time in a patient's life, with alterations in some patients occurring as early as adolescence.

In addition to the breakdown of collagen, MMPs and aggrecanases also degrade the chondroitin and keratin sulfate side chains of aggrecan (**Fig. 3.9**). The cleavage site for

aggrecanases and MMPs on aggrecan have been found to be distinct from one another.[73,74] Séguin et al demonstrated that with short-term exposure to TNF-α, proteoglycan degradation was more a result of induced aggrecanase activity rather than MMP-mediated catabolism.[75] Aggrecanase-1, found in the normal IVD, is thought to play a role in matrix remodeling.[61] With disc degeneration, the concentration of aggrecanase-1 increases from an increased production of nucleus cells, suggesting a strong role for matrix degradation.[61] Aggrecanase-2 is thought to be the major aggrecanase in the IVD.[75] Both aggrecanase-1 and -2 are not constitutively expressed in IVDs but become significantly upregulated with activation by the presence of TNF-α.[75] Such changes ultimately affect the disc's ability to maintain appropriate hydration and directly affect the biomechanical weight-bearing properties of the IVD and initiates the apoptotic cascade.[12,65]

Cytokines

Release of proinflammatory cytokines such as IL-1 and TNF-α in aged and diseased IVDs greatly enhances proteinase

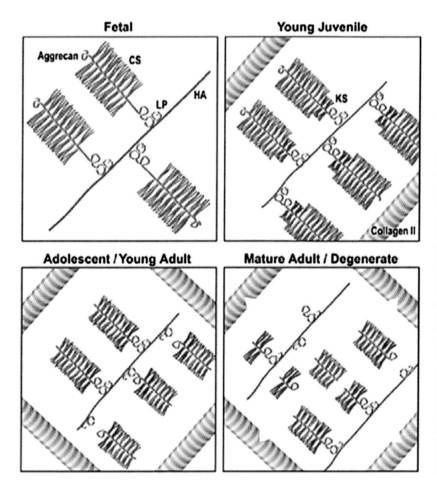

Fig. 3.9 Variation in composition of the human nucleus pulposus with age. The figure depicts the collagen fibrils and aggrecan-derived proteoglycans in the nucleus pulposus of fetal, young juvenile, adolescent/young adult, and mature adult/degenerate intervertebral discs. In the fetus, there is little collagen and the aggrecan is rich in chondroitin sulfate. In the young juvenile, the collagen fibril content is increased, the aggrecan contains both chondroitin sulfate and keratan sulfate, and proteolytic processing of the proteoglycan aggregates is evident. In the young adult, collagen content is maximal, the aggrecan and link proteins have undergone proteolytic processing, aggrecan is present as both proteoglycan aggregates and nonaggregated fragments, and the chondroitin sulfate chains of aggrecan are of decreased size, whereas its keratan sulfate chains are of increased size. In the mature adult, the collagen fibrils show evidence of enhanced proteolytic processing, the aggrecan and link protein have undergone extensive proteolytic processing, the proportion of aggrecan in a nonaggregated form is increased, and the hyaluronan content is increased. (From Roughley PJ. Biology of intervertebral disc aging and degeneration: involvement of the extracellular matrix. Spine 2004;29:2691–2699. Reprinted with permission.)

production.[6,35,76] They do so by upregulating cell production of these enzymes.[57] IL-1 in particular has been found to impede disc repair by inhibiting collagen and proteoglycan synthesis as well as stimulating production of MMPs.[57,75,77] If IL-1 is antagonistically blocked, apoptosis and production of degenerative disc markers are markedly reduced.[78] OP-1 has been shown to repair cellular tissue once IL-1 has begun to degrade disc tissue.[79] In particular, IL-1 has been found to induce a specific cleavage at the N-terminus of fibromodulin. This cleavage causes fibromodulin to lose its tyrosine sulfate-rich domain and its ability to maintain the integrity of the collagen network, which can lead to mechanical instability.[80,81] This change is most obvious in the anulus, where such instability could lead to annular wall weakness and subsequent herniation of the NP. Fibromodulin cleavage has also been shown to activate the classic complement cascade and a direct inflammatory response that may lead to pain and nerve root irritation.[82] TNF-α administration has been shown in vitro to decrease expression of aggrecan and type II collagen genes; decrease accumulation and synthesis of aggrecan and type II collagen; increase the expression of MMP-1, MMP-3, MMP-13, aggrecanase-1, aggrecanase-2; and induce aggrecanase-dependent proteoglycan degeneration.[75]

Proteinase Inhibitors

The metalloproteinases are not allowed to act uninhibited within the IVD. To balance the effects of the MMPs, chondrocytes in the disc also produce a family of enzymes known as tissue inhibitors of metalloproteinases (TIMPs). These proteins are the main inhibitors of the MMPs as well as the aggrecanases.[14,73,83,84] In normal discs, TIMPS and MMPs act together to balance extracellular matrix production and breakdown as a normal response for recovery. In diseased discs, an imbalance between the activity levels of the MMPs and the TIMPs occurs and has been implicated in disc resorption and degeneration.[63,85] Diseased discs have been found to contain not only higher levels of MMP production but also TIMP production, which demonstrates the disc's attempt to repair itself. The greater ratio of MMPs to TIMPs is what separates healthy discs from diseased discs.[86]

TIMP-1 has been found to specifically inhibit MMP-3 activity.[65] Delivery of TIMP-1 via adenoviral delivery to degenerated discs demonstrated an increase in extracellular matrix production, thought to be due to MMP inhibition.[86] TIMP-2 has been found to selectively bind to MMP-2 to inhibit its activity.[14] TIMP-2 also binds to the proform of MMP-2, and this collective complex has been demonstrated to inhibit other MMPs such as MMP-1, MMP-8, and MMP-9 through ternary complex binding.[87] In degenerated discs, TIMP-1 concentrations have been shown to increase, whereas TIMP-2 levels remain unchanged.[63,65]

As a result of increased catabolic processes by increased expression of proinflammatory cytokines and MMPs with aging and disc degeneration, IVD cells produce less proteoglycans and collagens in both the nucleus and the anulus. AF cells found in the early stages of disc degeneration synthesize proteoglycans and collagens at higher levels than annular cells from normal tissue, most likely representing a repair mechanism.[88] With advanced disc degeneration, the majority of matrix molecule levels are diminished, with the exception of biglycan and fibronectin.[88] In healthy discs, a balance is maintained between anabolic factors (such as endogenous BMPs and growth factors) and catabolic factors (such as proinflammatory cytokines and MMPs). With disc degeneration, this balance is lost as catabolic factor concentrations increase with advancing degeneration. Accordingly, therapeutic treatment strategies for human disc degeneration have been designed to block catabolic cascades and/or increase the levels of anabolic cascade growth factors (**Fig. 3.6**).

■ Potential Therapies

With our ever-increasing knowledge of IVD biology, potential therapies for disc disease have arisen. The focus of such therapies is to treat the underlying causative factors of disc degeneration rather than simply covering up the effects of degradation, which current conservative treatments do. The various pathways that have been discussed in this chapter have all been or are currently a focus of investigations for potential treatment.

Gene therapy is very young in its advent. Injecting deficient genes before patient symptoms or disc pathology begins into a diseased disc or the disc of patients who lack key molecules involved in normal disc biology seems logical and straightforward in regard to treatment. Current problems with this type of therapy include difficulties in the mechanism for transduction of the genes (transduction efficiency), maintaining the gene in the chosen tissue once implanted (duration of effect), and maintaining the benefit of these genes once delivered (proper regulation of gene expression). Our current understanding of gene transduction and transfer has shown success in animal models, but in vivo studies have failed to demonstrate beneficial efficacy to date. Furthermore, the safety of gene therapy has not been established, particularly the virus-mediated transduction methods. Nonviral transfection methods are generally safer, but efficiency and duration of effect are generally inferior to virus-mediated methods. Prior to human application, further research is needed to assess safety and efficacy of gene therapy that has shown promising results in preclinical experiments.

Currently, protein therapy appears to be the most promising therapy and treatment. Multiple studies have demonstrated the regeneration of disc height in early degeneration with direct disc injection of various growth factors including BMP-2, OP-1, GDF-5, and TGF-β as well as cytokine antagonists to IL-1 and TNF-α. More recent studies have demonstrated that an amalgamated mixture of two or more of these factors may prove superior in overall therapeutic potential.[35] Current treatments are in clinical trials and represent great promise for patients with degenerative disc disease.

■ Conclusion

The biology of healthy and diseased IVDs is a complex array of molecules, proteins, chemical gradients, and biomechanical stimuli that can be signified as being in or out of balance. Healthy discs maintain an appropriate balance between growth factors and degradative enzymes, whereas aged and diseased discs do not and therefore are prone to degeneration. A multitude of growth factors have been studied and shown to prevent and reverse degenerative

changes, establishing them as important candidates for future therapies in disc disease. Inflammatory and proteinase inhibition have also become important targets for potential therapies. Although a large gap remains in our understanding of the complexity of IVD biology, daily discoveries continue to be encouraging to the development of future noninvasive treatments for degenerative disc disease of the spine. Biologic treatment has the potential to prevent and reverse early degenerative changes, but it will probably not be effective in patients with more advanced changes such as significant disc space narrowing and spondylosis. For patients with advanced degeneration, biologic treatment combined with a biomechanical restoring posterior dynamic stabilization technique might be considered in the future. Finally, it should be stressed that there is poor correlation between pain and disc degeneration severity, and more research is needed to investigate the etiology of pain in chronic low-back pain patients.

References

1. Aszódi A, Chan D, Hunziker E, Bateman JF, Fässler R. Collagen II is essential for the removal of the notochord and the formation of intervertebral discs. J Cell Biol 1998;143:1399–1412
2. Behrens A, Haigh J, Mechta-Grigoriou F, Nagy A, Yaniv M, Wagner EF. Impaired intervertebral disc formation in the absence of *Jun*. Development 2003;130:103–109
3. Patwardhan AG, Gaitanis IN, Voronov LI, Biomechanics of the spine. In: Spivak JM, Connolly PJ, eds. Orthopaedic Knowledge Update 3: Spine. Rosemont, IL: American Academy of Orthopaedic Surgeons; 2006:25–34
4. Buckwalter JA, Mow VC, Boden SD, Eyre DR, Weidenbaum M. Intervertebral disk structure, composition, and mechanical function. In: Buckwalter JA, Einhorn TA, Simon SR, ed. Orthopaedic Basic Sciences: Biology and Biomechanics of the Musculoskeletal System. 2nd ed. Chicago: American Academy of Orthopaedic Surgeons; 2000:547–556
5. Setton LA, Chen J. Mechanobiology of the intervertebral disc and relevance to disc degeneration. J Bone Joint Surg Am 2006;88(supp 2): 52–57
6. An H, Masuda K. Relevance of in vitro and in vivo models for intervertebral disc degeneration. J Bone Joint Surg Am 2006;88(supp 2): 88–94
7. Hunter CJ, Matyas JR, Duncan NA. Cytomorphology of notochordal and chondrocytic cells from the nucleus pulposus: a species comparison. J Anat 2004;205:357–362
8. Kim KW, Lim TH, Kim JG, Jeong ST, Masuda K, An HS. The origin of chondrocytes in the nucleus pulposus and histologic findings associated with the transition of a notochordal nucleus pulposus to a fibrocartilaginous nucleus pulposus in intact rabbit intervertebral discs. Spine 2003;28:982–990
9. Kim KW, Kim YS, Ha KY, et al. An autocrine or paracrine Fas-mediated counterattack: a potential mechanism for apoptosis of notochordal cells in intact rat nucleus pulposus. Spine 2005;30: 1247–1251
10. Feng H, Danfelter M, Strömqvist B, Heinegård D. Extracellular matrix in disc degeneration. J Bone Joint Surg Am 2006;88(supp 2): 25–29
11. An H, Masuda K, Inoue N. Intervertebral disc degeneration: biological and biomechanical factors. J Orthop Sci 2006;11:541–552
12. Melrose J, Ghosh P, Taylor T. A comparative analysis of the differential spatial and temporal distributions of the large (aggrecan, versican) and small (decorin, biglycan, fibromodulin) proteoglycans of the intervertebral disc. J Anat 2001;198:3–15
13. Duncan NA. Cell deformation and micromechanical environment in the intervertebral disc. J Bone Joint Surg Am 2006;88(supp 2): 47–51
14. Kozaci LD, Guner A, Oktay G, Guner G. Alterations in biochemical components of extracellular matrix in intervertebral disc herniation: role of MMP-2 and TIMP-2 in type II collagen loss. Cell Biochem Funct 2006;24:431–436
15. Biyani A, Andersson G. Low back pain: pathophysiology and management. J Am Acad Orthop Surg 2004;12:106–115
16. Hukins D. Disc structure and function. In: Golsh P, ed. The Biology of the Intervertebral Disc. Boca Raton, FL: CRC Press; 1988:1–37
17. Maclean JJ, Lee CR, Alini M, Iatridis JC. Anabolic and catabolic mRNA levels of the intervertebral disc vary with the magnitude and frequency of in vivo dynamic compression. J Orthop Res 2004;22:1193–1200
18. Walsh AJ, Lotz JC. Biological response of the intervertebral disc to dynamic loading. J Biomech 2004;37:329–337
19. Pokharna HK, Phillips FM. Collagen cross-links in human lumbar intervertebral disc aging. Spine 1998;23:1645–1648
20. Yang BL, Yang BB, Erwin M, Ang LC, Finkelstein J, Yee AJ. Versican G3 domain enhances cellular adhesion and proliferation of bovine intervertebral disc cells cultured in vitro. Life Sci 2003;73: 3399–3413
21. Ishii Y, Thomas AO, Guo XA, Hung CT, Chen FH. Localization and distribution of cartilage oligomeric matrix protein in the rat intervertebral disc. Spine 2006;31:1539–1546

22. Hecht JT, Nelson LD, Crowder E, et al. Mutations in exon 17B of cartilage oligomeric matrix protein (COMP) cause pseudoachondroplasia. Nat Genet 1995;10:325–329

23. Briggs MD, Hoffman SM, King LM, et al. Pseudoachondroplasia and multiple epiphyseal dysplasia due to mutations in the cartilage oligomeric matrix protein gene. Nat Genet 1995;10:330–336

24. Wiberg C, Klatt AR, Wagener R, et al. Complexes of matrilin-1 and biglycan or decorin connect collagen VI microfibrils to both collagen II and aggrecan. J Biol Chem 2003;278:37698–37704

25. Chang J, Poole CA. Sequestration of type VI collagen in the pericellular microenvironment of adult chondrocytes cultured in agarose. Osteoarthritis Cartilage 1996;4:275–285

26. Midwood KS, Salter DM. NG2/HMPG modulation of human articular chondrocyte adhesion to type VI collagen is lost in osteoarthritis. J Pathol 2001;195:631–635

27. Akeda K, An HS, Pichika R, et al. The expression of NG2 proteoglycan in the human intervertebral disc. Spine 2007;32:306–314

28. Akeda K, An HS, Pichika R, et al. The expression of NG-2 proteoglycan in the human intervertebral disc. Spine 2007;32:306–314

29. Nishiyama A, Lin XH, Giese N, et al. Co-localization of NG2 proteoglycan and PDGF alpha-receptor on O2A progenitor cells in the developing rat brain. J Neurosci Res 1996;43:299–314

30. Goretzki L, Burg MA, Grako KA, et al. High-affinity binding of basic fibroblast growth factor and platelet-derived growth factor-AA to the core protein of the NG2 proteoglycan. J Biol Chem 1999;274:16831–16837

31. Seki S, Kawaguchi Y, Chiba K, et al. A functional SNP in CILP, encoding cartilage intermediate layer protein, is associated with susceptibility to lumbar disc disease. Nat Genet 2005;37:607–612

32. Weiler C, Nerlich AG, Zipperer J, Bachmeier BE, Boos N. Expression of major matrix metalloproteinase is associated with intervertebral disc degradation and resorption. Eur Spine J 2002;11:308–320

33. Grunhagen T, Wilde G, Soukane DM, Ahirazi-Adl SA, Urban JP. Nutrient supply and intervertebral disc metabolism. J Bone Joint Surg Am 2006;88(supp 2):30–35

34. Urban JP, Holm S, Maroudas A, Nachemson A. Nutrition of the intervertebral disk: an in vivo study of solute transport. Clin Orthop Relat Res 1977;129:101–114

35. Evans C. Potential biologic therapies for the intervertebral disc. J Bone Joint Surg Am 2006;88(supp 2):95–98

36. Osada R, Ohshima H, Ishihara H, et al. Autocrine/paracrine mechanism of insulin-like growth factor-1 secretion, and the effect of insulin-like growth factor-1 on proteoglycan synthesis in bovine intervertebral discs. J Orthop Res 1996;14:690–699

37. Okuda S, Myoui A, Ariga K, Nakase T, Yonenobu K, Yoshikawa H. Mechanisms of age-related decline in insulin-like growth factor-1 dependent proteoglycan synthesis in rat intervertebral disc cells. Spine 2001;26:2421–2426

38. Walsh AJ, Bradford DS, Lotz JC. In vivo growth factor treatment of degenerated intervertebral discs. Spine 2004;29:156–163

39. Wallach CJ, Latterman C, Gilbertson L, Kang J. Transduction of TGF-β_1 inhibits proteoglycan synthesis in intervertebral disc cells in a three dimensional culture. North American Spine Society. Spine J 2002;2:67S

40. Ahn S-H, Teng P-N, Niyibizi C, Gilbertson L, Kang J. The effects of BMP-12 and BMP-2 on proteoglycan and collagen synthesis in nucleus pulposus cells from human degenerated discs. Paper presented at 29th Annual Meeting of the International Society for the Study of the Lumbar Spine; May 14–18, 2002; Cleveland, OH

41. Tim Yoon S, Su Kim K, Li J, et al. The effect of bone morphogenetic protein-2 on rat intervertebral disc cells in vitro. Spine 2003;28:1773–1780

42. Larson JW III, Levicoff EA, Gilbertson LG, Kang JD. Biologic modification of animal models of intervertebral disc degeneration. J Bone Joint Surg Am 2006;88(supp 2):83–87

43. Sobajima S, Kim JS, Gilbertson LG, Kang JD. Gene therapy for degenerative disc disease. Gene Ther 2004;11:390–401

44. Masuda K, Takegami K, An H, et al. Recombinant osteogenic protein-1 upregulates extracellular matrix metabolism by rabbit annulus fibrosus and nucleus pulposus cells cultured in alginate beads. J Orthop Res 2003;21:922–930

45. Matsumoto T, An H, Thonar E, Andersson G, Masuda K. Effect of osteogenic protein-1 on the metabolism of proteoglycan of intervertebral disc cells in aging. Trans Orthop Res Soc 2002;27:826

46. Matsumoto T, Masuda K, Chen S, et al. Transfer of osteogenic protein-1 gene by gene gun system promotes matrix synthesis in bovine intervertebral disc and articular cartilage cells. Orthop Res Soc Trans 2001;26:30

47. Takegami K, An H, Kumano F, et al. Osteogenic protein-1 is most effective in stimulating nucleus pulposus and annulus fibrosus cells to repair their matrix after chondroitinase ABC-induced in vitro chemonucleolysis. Spine J 2005;5:231–238

48. Gruber HE, Norton HJ, Hanley EN Jr. Anti-apoptotic effects of IGF-1 and PDGF on human intervertebral disc cells in vitro. Spine 2000;25:2153–2157

49. An HS, Takegami K, Kamada H, et al. Intradiscal administration of osteogenic protein-1 increases intervertebral disc height and proteoglycan content in the nucleus pulposus in normal adolescent rabbits. Spine 2005;30:25–31

50. Masuda K, Aota Y, Muehleman C, et al. A novel rabbit model of mild, reproducible disc degeneration by an annulus needle puncture: correlation between the degree of disc injury and radiological and histological appearances of disc degeneration. Spine 2005; 30:5–14

51. Masuda K, Imai Y, Okuma M, et al. Osteogenic protein-1 (OP-1) injection into a degenerated disc induces the restoration of disc height and structural changes in the rabbit annular puncture model. Spine 2006;31:742–754

52. Chujo T, An HS, Akeda K, et al. Effects of growth differentiation factor-5 on the intervertebral disc: in vitro bovine study and in vivo rabbit disc degeneration model study. Spine 2006;31:2909–2917

53. Li X, Leo BM, Beck G, Balian G, Anderson DG. Collagen and proteoglycan abnormalities in the GDF-5-deficient mice and molecular changes when treating disk cells with recombinant growth factor. Spine 2004;29:2229–2234

54. Masuda K, Imai Y, Okuma M, et al. Injection of OP-1 induces the recovery of disc height after chondroitinase ABC-induced intervertebral disc degeneration in the rabbit. Spine J 2003;3:71S

55. Buckwalter JA. Aging and degeneration of the human intervertebral disc. Spine 1995;20:1307–1314

56. Gruber HE, Hanley EN Jr. Analysis of aging and degeneration of the human intervertebral disc: comparison of surgical specimens with normal controls. Spine 1998;23:751–757

57. Solovieva S, Lohiniva J, Leino-Arjas P, et al. Intervertebral disc degeneration in relation to the *COL9A3* and the *IL-1β* gene polymorphisms. Eur Spine J 2006;15:613–619

58. Holm S, Maroudas A, Urban JP, Selsatm G, Nachemson A. Nutrition of the intervertebral disc: solute transport and metabolism. Connect Tissue Res 1981;8:101–119

59. Nagase H, Woessner JF Jr. Matrix metalloproteinases. J Biol Chem 1999;274:21491–21494
60. Brinckerhoff CE, Matrisian LM. Matrix metalloproteinases: a tail of a frog that became a prince. Nat Rev Mol Cell Biol 2002;3:207–214
61. LeMaitre CL, Freemont AJ, Hoyland JA. Localization of degradative enzymes and their inhibitors in the degenerate human intervertebral disc. J Pathol 2004;204:47–54
62. Buckwalter JA, Mow VC, Boden SD, Eyre DR, Weidenbaum M. Intervertebral disc structure, composition, and mechanical function. In: Buckwalter JA, Einhorn TA, Simon SR, eds. Orthopaedic Basic Science: Biology and Biomechanics of the Musculoskeletal System. 2nd ed. Chicago: American Academy of Orthopaedic Surgeons; 2000:557–566
63. Kanemoto M, Hukuda S, Komiya Y, Katsuura A, Nishioka J. Immunohistochemical study of matrix metalloproteinase-3 and tissue inhibitor of metalloproteinase-1 in human intervertebral discs. Spine 1996;21:1–8
64. Nemoto O, Yamagishi M, Yamada H, Kikuchi T, Takaishi H. Matrix metalloproteinase-3 production by human degenerated intervertebral disc. J Spinal Disord 1997;10:493–498
65. Robert S, Caterson B, Menage J, Evans EH, Jaffray DC, Eisenstein SM. Matrix metalloproteinases and aggrecanase: their role in disorders of the human intervertebral disc. Spine 2000;23:3005–3013
66. Goupille P, Jayson MI, Valat JP, Freemont AJ. Matrix metalloproteinases: the clue to intervertebral disc degeneration? Spine 1998;23:1612–1626
67. Shingleton WD, Ellis AJ, Rowan AD, Cawston TE. Retinoic acid combines with interleukin-1 to promote the degradation of collagen from bovine nasal cartilage: matrix metalloproteinases-1 and -13 are involved in cartilage collagen breakdown. J Cell Biochem 2000;79:519–531
68. Nerlich AG, Schleicher ED, Boos N. 1997 Volvo Award Winner in Basic Science Studies. Immunohistologic markers for age-related changes of human lumbar intervertebral discs. Spine 1997;22:2781–2795
69. Nerlich AG, Boos N, Wiest I, Aebi M. Immunolocalization of major interstitial collagen types in human lumbar intervertebral discs of various ages. Virchows Arch 1998;432:67–76
70. Murphy G, Cockett MI, Stephens PE, Smith BJ, Docherty AJ. Stromelysin is an activator of procollagenase a study with natural and recombinant enzymes. Biochem J 1987;248:265–268
71. Sedowofia K, Tomlinson I, Weiss J, Hilton R, Jayson M. Collagenolytic enzyme systems in human intervertebral disc: their control, mechanism, and their possible role in the initiation of biochemical failure. Spine 1982;7:213–222
72. Kang JD, Georgescu HI, McIntyre-Larkin L, Stefanovic-Racic M, Donalson WF III, Evans CH. Herniated lumbar intervertebral discs spontaneously produce matrix metalloproteinases, nitric oxide, interleukin-6, and prostaglandin-E2. Spine 1996;21:271–277
73. Arner EC, Pratta MA, Trzaskos JM, et al. Generation and characterization of aggrecanase: a soluble, cartilage-derived aggrecan-degrading activity. J Biol Chem 1999;274:6594–6601
74. Tortorella MD, Burn TC, Pratta MA, et al. Purification and cloning of aggrecanase-1: a member of the ADAMTS family of proteins. Science 1999;284:1664–1666
75. Séguin CA, Pilliar RM, Roughley PJ, Kandel RA. Tumor necrosis factor-α modulates matrix production and catabolism in nucleus pulposus tissue. Spine 2005;30:1940–1948
76. Sequin CA, Bojarski OM, Pilliar RM, Roughley PJ, Kandel RA. Differential regulation of matrix degrading enzymes in a TNF-alpha induced model of nucleus pulposus tissue degeneration. Matrix Biol 2006;25:409–418
77. Pattison S, Melrose J, Ghosh P, Taylor T. Regulation of gelatinase-A (MMP-2) production by ovine intervertebral disc nucleus pulposus cells grown in alginate bead culture by transforming growth factor-1. Cell Biol Int 2001;25:679–689
78. Wehling P. Antiapoptotic and antidegenerative effect of an autologous IL-1ra/IGF-1/PDGF combination on human intervertebral disc cells in vivo. Paper presented at 29th Annual Meeting of the International Society for the Study of the Lumbar Spine; May 14–18, 2002; Cleveland, OH, 2002
79. Takegami K, Thonar EJ, An HS, Kemada H, Masuda K. Osteogenic protein-1 enhances matrix replenishment by intervertebral disc cells previously exposed to interleukin-1. Spine 2002;27:1318–1325
80. Heathfield TF, Önnerfjord P, Dahlberg L. Heinegård D. Cleavage of fibromodulin in cartilage explants involves removal of the N-terminal tyrosine sulfate-rich region by proteolysis at a site that is sensitive to matrix metalloproteinase-13. J Biol Chem 2004;279:6286–6295
81. Heinegård D, Aspberg A, Franzén A, Lorenzo P. Glycosylated matrix proteins. In: Royce PM, Steinmann B, eds. Connective Tissue and Its Heritable Disorders: Molecular, Genetic, and Medical Aspects. 2nd ed. New York: Wiley-Liss; 2002:271–291
82. Sjöberg A, Önnerfjord P, Mörgelin M, Heinegård D, Blom AM. The extracellular matrix and inflammation: fibromodulin activates the classical pathway of complement by directly binding C1q. J Biol Chem 2005;280:32301–32308
83. Guner A, Oktay G, Jerman M, Guner G. Immunoglobulins and alpha-1-proteinase-1 proteinase inhibitor in human intervertebral disc material. Biochem Soc Trans 1995;23:212S
84. Hashimoto G, Aoki T, Nakamura H, et al. Inhibition of ADAMTS4 (aggrecanase-1) by tissue inhibitors of metalloproteinases (TIMP-1, 2, 3, and 4). FEBS Lett 2001;494:192–195
85. Doita M, Kanatani T, Ozaki T, Matsui N, Kurosaka M, Yoshiya S. Influence of macrophage infiltration of herniated disc tissue on the production of matrix metalloproteinases leading to disc resorption. Spine 2001;26:1522–1527
86. Wallach CJ, Sobajima S, Watanabe Y, et al. Gene transfer of the catabolic inhibitor TIMP-1 increases measured proteoglycans in cells from degenerated human intervertebral discs. Spine 2003;28:2331–2337
87. Fujimoto N, Ward R, Shinya T, Iwata K, Yamashita K, Hayakawa T. Interaction between tissue inhibitor of metalloproteinase-2 and progelatinase A: immunoreactivity. Biochem J 1996;313:827–833
88. Cs-Szabo G, Ragasa-San Juan D, Turumella V, Masuda K, Thonar E, An HS. Changes in message and protein levels of proteoglycans of the annulus fibrosus and nucleus pulposus during interverterbal disc degeneration. Spine 2002;27:2212–2219

4 Biomechanics of the Lumbar Intervertebral Disc

Michael N. Tzermiadianos and Avinash G. Patwardhan

A disc comprises three distinct parts: the nucleus pulposus (NP), the anulus fibrosus (AF), and the cartilaginous endplates. The nucleus is composed of a loose network of fibrous strands that lie in a translucent mucoprotein gel containing various mucopolysaccharides. In a healthy young disc, the water content of the nucleus ranges from 70 to 90%. The water gives the tissue very low rigidity so that it can deform easily in any direction and equalize the stress applied to it.[1] The nucleus fills 30 to 50% of the total disc cross sectional area, and is located more posterior than central. The anulus gradually becomes differentiated from the periphery of the nucleus and forms the outer boundary of the disc. The anulus is made up of a series of 15 to 25 concentric lamellae.[2] The fibers within each lamina are arranged in a helicoid manner angled at 30 degrees with respect to the endplate.[2] The fibers of adjacent lamellae have similar arrangements, but run in opposite directions with the fibers of one layer angled to the right and the fibers of another layer angled to the left. The anulus is well suited to resisting torsion due to the characteristic orientation of the fibers in each layer. Because of this opposite orientation, torsional movements generate tension in half of the collagen fibers in the anulus, whereas the other fibers tend to become slack.[3] Fiber strains rarely exceed 6% under physiologic flexion and extension moments and 8.5% under physiologic axial rotation. The intervertebral disc (IVD) alone provides most of the compressive stiffness of the motion segment, whereas ligaments and facets contribute significantly to resisting bending moments and axial torsion.

The annular fibers are attached to the cartilaginous endplate in the inner zone, whereas in the outer zone they are attached directly to the osseous endplates. This attachment to the bone through Sharpey's fibers is significantly stronger than the other more central attachments to the cartilaginous endplates. The anulus contains the nucleus, surrounding it like a strong thick membrane. When the disc is compressed, the pressure inside the nucleus increases, generating a tensile hoop stress in the restraining anulus, thus maintaining the IVD height. Hoop stress decreases from the inner lamellae of the anulus to the outer lamellae. Cadaveric experiments have shown that a compressive force of 2000 N stretches the collagen fibers on the outer anulus by less than 2% and causes the anulus to bulge radially by 0.4 to 1.0 mm.[4] As the preload increases from 250 N to 4500 N, the height of a motion segment is reduced by 0.9 mm. Approximately half of the height reduction can be attributed to the endplates bulging into the vertebral bodies.[5,6] The anulus also resists compression directly; therefore, compressive stresses are distributed almost evenly throughout the entire disc area in a young, nondegenerated disc.[7]

■ Biomechanics of the Normal Lumbar Intervertebral Disc

Kinematic Properties

The natural human disc has 6 degrees of freedom, allowing independent angular motion about, and independent translation along each of the three anatomic axes.[8] Being a fibrocartilaginous joint, the disc offers resistance to both angular and translational motions. The kinematic properties of the disc, and those of the whole motion segment, can be assessed by measuring the range of motion (ROM) and the parameters that assess quality of motion.

ROM refers to the total amount of motion between the motion endpoints. The average ROM in the flexion–extension in healthy young men, measured using stereo radiographs was ~14 degrees at most spinal levels.[9,10] ROM was ~4 degrees in lateral bending, and 1.5 degrees in axial rotation. The L5–S1 segment showed significantly lower in vivo ROM compared with the other segments.

The term quality of motion refers to the characteristic kinematic signature of the disc (or a spinal segment), and characterizes the pattern of motion as opposed to its magnitude. When a spinal segment is subjected to flexion and extension moments, the load-displacement curve has a characteristic sigmoidal shape, with concavity toward the load axis (**Fig. 4.1**). Such a curve implies that the disc and the surrounding ligamentous structures provide little resistance (i.e., low stiffness) at low loads, but at higher magnitudes of load the stiffness is increased. Thus, it provides flexibility at low loads and stability at higher loads. Two commonly used parameters to characterize this curve pattern are neutral zone and stiffness in the high flexibility

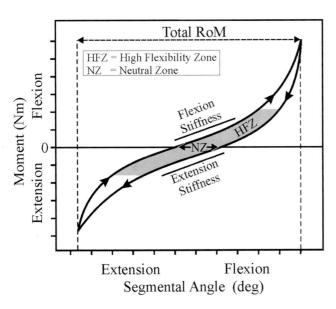

Fig. 4.1 Load versus displacement curve of a lumbar segment in flexion–extension.

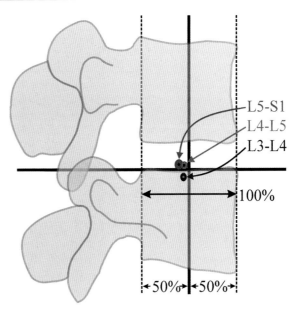

Fig. 4.2 Locations of flexion–extension centers of rotation for healthy lumbar segments.

zone. Neutral zone, expressed in degrees, is calculated as the difference in the segmental angle between the loading and unloading curves at 0 Nm bending moment.[11] The high flexibility zone is the region around the neutral posture in which the osteoligamentous spine can move with negligible resistance. The stiffness in the high flexibility zone is calculated using slopes of the linear portion of the load-displacement curve around the neutral posture.[12] These concepts of neutral zone and stiffness also apply to the discussion of quality of motion in lateral bending and axial rotation. The characteristic shape of the load-displacement curve, and therefore the values of neutral zone and stiffness are affected by compressive preload and disc degeneration.

Another measure of the quality of motion of a spinal segment is the location and orientation of the helical axis of motion (HAM) as the segment undergoes motion in response to physiologic loads. The quality of segmental motion in the sagittal plane can be assessed by the location of the center of rotation (COR), which is the intersection of the HAM with the midsagittal plane.[13–15] The COR location can be compared between healthy and degenerated segments to assess the difference in the quality of flexion–extension motion.

In a recent in vitro study,[16] the COR in flexion–extension for healthy L3–L4 and L4–L5 segments calculated using the flexion and extension endpoints was located close to or slightly posterior to the midpoint of the superior endplate of the inferior vertebra. In contrast, in the L5–S1 disc space, the COR was located ~4–5 mm posterior to the midpoint of the S1 endplate (**Fig. 4.2**). The instantaneous centers of rotation (ICR) calculated for incremental motions during flexion–extension in the relatively healthy segments tended to remain stationary as the segments moved through the

ROM.[16] These experimental results of COR in intact cadaveric specimens match closely with the in vivo results reported by Pearcy and Bogduk[17] and Schneider, Pearcy, and Bogduk.[13] In all three studies,[13,16,17] the COR was located close to the superior endplate of the inferior vertebra of the L4–L5 and L5–S1 segments, unlike the in vitro results of Zhao et al,[18] who reported the location of the COR in cadaveric specimens to be 30 mm caudal to the midpoint of the disc. Zhao et al's measurement puts the COR near the inferior endplate of the inferior vertebra, a location too distal when compared with the results reported in vivo. It should be noted that the location of the COR depends on the loads used in creating the motion. A combination of flexion moment and anterior shear would result in a COR that is located more distal than that for motions created by pure moments.

Load Transfer

Loads on the human spine are shared by the osteoligamentous tissues and muscles of the spine. Tensile forces in the paraspinal muscles, which exert a compressive load on the spine, balance the moments created by gravitational and external forces. Because these muscles have a small moment arm from the spinal segment, they amplify the compressive load on the osteoligamentous spine. The preload, produced by muscles, can be considered an "external" compressive load that acts on the spinal segments in vivo during different activities of daily living. The mechanical response of healthy, degenerated, or injured spinal segments will be influenced by this preload.

The internal compressive forces on the ligamentous spine have been estimated for different physical tasks using intradiscal pressure and electromyographic data in conjunction with three-dimensional biomechanical models. The compressive force on the human lumbar spine is estimated to range from 150–300 N during supine and recumbent postures to 1400 N during relaxed standing with the trunk flexed 30 degrees. The compressive force may be substantially larger when holding a weight in the hands in the static standing posture, and even more so during dynamic lifting. In healthy individuals, the spine sustains these loads without injury or instability.[19–21]

The IVD is the major load-bearing element in axial compression and flexion. In the young healthy spine, the disc transfers ~80% of the compressive load applied to the motion segment.[22] As load is applied to the healthy disc, forces are distributed equally in all directions from within the nucleus, placing the anulus fibers in tension. The collagen fibers of the anulus are well suited to resisting tension. The pressure in the nucleus causes the lamellae of the anulus to bulge outward, stretching the fibers in the anulus. Resistance of the fibers to tensile loading then allows the anulus to contribute to compressive load sharing. Measurements in young, healthy discs using stress profilometry show that most of the disc is under uniform load and because the stress is equal in the vertical and horizontal directions (isotropic), the nucleus behaves as a fluid.[23]

Experimental and finite element studies have shown that a compressive load applied to a healthy disc is shared by both the NP and the AF.[24] Adams et al[25] showed that when discs are subjected to compressive loading in the neutral posture they generally exhibit a small peak of compressive stress in the posterior anulus and a fairly even compressive stress throughout the nucleus and anterior anulus. In extension, the size of the peak in the posterior anulus increases, whereas moderately flexed postures usually distribute stresses evenly across the disc. In full flexion, stress peaks appear in the anterior anulus but are rarely as high as those in the posterior anulus are in full extension.[25] Posture also affects the hydrostatic pressure in the nucleus. Under compressive preload of 500 N, the nucleus pressure is 40% less in 4 degrees of extension than in the neutral posture, reflecting the increased load sharing by the facets in extension.[25] Nucleus pressure rises by 100% in full flexion because flexion stretches the ligaments of the neural arch, creating tension that compresses the disc. If the neural arch is removed, the ligamentous tension decreases, and the nucleus pressure increases only by 38% in flexion and by 8% in extension.[25]

Loading effects on the lumbar spine not only depend upon load magnitude but also upon loading rate and duration.[26,27] This dependency occurs because of the viscoelastic behavior of the IVD.[22] Viscoelasticity is defined as the time-dependent response of a material to rate of loading or deformation and is linked to the absorption of energy by the disc. Viscoelastic materials exhibit hysteresis, which is a measure of the loss of energy when a structure is subjected to repetitive load and unload cycles. Hysteresis can be thought of as a protective mechanism as this mechanism is mainly responsible for the discs absorbing the shock energy from the sacrum to the skull when a person lands on his or her feet. Hysteresis may vary according to the load applied as well as the spinal level and degree of degeneration. Hysteresis is also decreased when the same disc is loaded a second time, reaching a steady state after a few cycles.[28]

Viscoelastic behavior of the disc comes from two sources: the inherent viscoelasticity of collagen fibers and their interaction with the proteoglycan matrix, and the fluid flow within the disc under load. The outflow of interstitial fluid under loading causes approximately a 20% reduction in height and the volume of the disc.[29] Intradiscal pressure has been shown to decrease with creep loading,[30] rendering the tissue less resistant to bending.[26] When loading is removed, the disc reabsorbs water and recovers from the deformation.

As compared with compression, the lumbar discs appear less well suited to resist prolonged loading and low-frequency cyclic loading in shear. Biomechanical studies have reported that load transfer in compression occurs via the production of high disc pressures; whereas in shear, the mechanism appears to be via the AF without the development of significant disc pressure.[31,32,] Thus, the stiffness in shear under static and dynamic loads is significantly smaller than the values in compression.[33] The stress relaxation in shear is also significantly smaller than the values in compression.[33] This implies that under prolonged shear loading, the disc will retain a higher proportion of the applied shear load as compared with the proportion of the compressive load retained by the disc when loaded in pure compression. Conversely, under a low-frequency cyclic loading environment, the ability of lumbar discs to dissipate the dynamic energy (hysteresis) is significantly smaller in shear than in compression.[33] These findings suggest that the disc is susceptible to injury when loaded in shear.

■ Biomechanics of the Diseased Lumbar Intervertebral Disc

Disc Degeneration

Disc degeneration is associated with biochemical, morphologic, and material changes. A loss of proteoglycans, and hence loss of hydration, particularly in the nucleus is considered the principal biochemical sign of degeneration.[34] The loss of water content from the nucleus results in a loss of disc height. The nucleus becomes progressively more fibrous and opaque, with increased pigmentation. The demarcation between the anulus and the nucleus becomes less distinct, and delamination (separation of adjacent laminae) of the anulus occurs. Delamination leads to the development of concentric tears in the AF.[35] These annular tears increase in size and coalesce to form radial fissures. The radial fissures then expand and extend into the NP, disrupting the disc structure. Radial fissures and cracks in the anulus can form cavities within the disc.[36] In a cadaveric study, Krismer et al[37] reported that reduced disc height was consistently associated with the presence of fissures in the anulus. With disc dehydration and narrowing of the disc space, the nucleus is no longer able to exert a hydrostatic pressure on the anulus, meaning the annular fibers of the disc are no longer subjected to the same tensile stresses, as they would be in a healthy disc with a hydrated nucleus. Instead, the anulus in a degenerated disc under compression is more likely to directly bear the axial load from the vertebra above, resulting in an inward bulging of the inner anulus and accelerated delamination.[38]

Mechanical, chemical, age-related, autoimmune, and genetic factors have been implicated in the pathomechanisms of disc degeneration.[39] Considering the limited repair capacity of the IVD, accumulative structural damage is believed to contribute to disc degeneration. Experimental studies have shown that compressive load generally leads to failure of the endplate or the vertebral body but cannot produce disc herniation. The disc bulges circumferentially after compressive loading with no propensity for posterolateral protrusion.[40] Axial rotation is likely a more important injury-causing load as proposed by Farfan et al.[41] The IVD provides ~40 to 50% of the torsional strength, whereas the remaining strength is attributed to the posterior elements and the interspinous ligaments.[41] Axial rotation, especially in combination with flexion when the facet joints open and offer less constraint to rotation,[22] can lead to delamination and annular tears that can initiate the disc degeneration process. Depressurization of the nucleus reduces the intervertebral space height, subjects the anulus to more compressive load and allows more rotational flexibility because of the collapsed annular fibers and the capsular laxity of the facets that follows facet subluxation. Repeated loading in flexion has also been implicated in disc degeneration.[42] Other mechanical encumbrances implicated in disc degeneration include acute hyperflexion injury,[43] repetitive hyperextension injuries,[44] and vibration.[45] However, it must be noted that establishing a cause and effect relation in disc degeneration is difficult. Structural disruption is accompanied by cell-mediated changes, and progressive biochemical changes alter the structural integrity. Therefore, it is unclear whether mechanical disturbances or biochemical changes initiate the degenerative cascade.

As narrowing of the disc space occurs, the zygapophyseal joints undergo subluxation until the tips of the inferior facets impinge on the inferior lamina. This causes an increase in the load transmission by the facets. Increased peak pressures caused by the increased loads within the facet joint may give rise to degeneration of the joint cartilage. Thinning of the cartilage may cause capsular ligament laxity and allow abnormal motion or hypermobility of the facet joints. Cartilage degeneration seems to further increase the segmental movements that already were increased with disc degeneration. As degeneration progresses, the abnormal pressure and focal degeneration of the facets give rise to bony hypertrophy and osteophytes with a subsequent decrease in segmental mobility.

Altered Kinematics

The effect of disc degeneration on segmental ROM depends on the degree of disc degeneration. According to the degenerative cascade proposed by Kirkaldy-Willis and Farfan,[46] as degeneration increases the spinal segment progress from the dysfunction to the instability phase, and finally to the restabilization phase. Cadaveric studies have confirmed that segmental motion tends to increase with increasing severity of disc degeneration. However, a decrease in segmental motion has been found at the highest grade of degeneration.[47,48]

Flexion–extension radiographs have been traditionally used to diagnose spinal instability in vivo; however, the results have been inconsistent. Morgan and King[49] observed the presence of incomplete radial posterior tears in the lower lumbar discs and of anterior concentric fissures in the upper lumbar discs, and drew attention to the association between annular tears, radiographic signs of instability, and low back pain. Other clinical studies showed reduction of disc height to be significantly associated with reduced flexion–extension ROM,[50] a finding that has also been reported in cadaveric studies.[37,47] Mimura et al[47] reported that ROM in flexion–extension showed a tendency to decrease, whereas lateral bending showed a significant decrease with degeneration. On the contrary, Krismer et al[37] did not find a significant decrease in the lateral bending ROM with increasing degeneration. The differences between reports might be due to different specimen selection and inclusion of specimens with lateral osteophytes in some of the studies.

Increased axial rotation with higher degrees of disc degeneration has been more consistently reported among different investigators.[37,47,48,51] Kirkaldy-Willis and Farfan[46] focused on anteroposterior lateral bending radiographs from which rotational deformity and lateral translation were interpreted as indicators of instability. Cadaveric studies have confirmed the importance of torsional instability in disc degeneration. Krismer et al[37] reported that the ROM in axial rotation is increased in cases of severe degeneration. Furthermore they reported that in disc degeneration axial rotation is coupled with same-side lateral translation, a combination that was negligible in healthy segments. The authors also noted that reduced disc height in radiographs was associated with fissure formation in the disc. Schmidt et al[52] also reported that the presence of a high-intensity zone in the IVD, a radiologic sign of radial tears, is associated with reduced stiffness of motion segments, especially in axial rotation. Other studies have reported that the change in axial rotation motion caused by disc degeneration is greater than the change in flexion–extension and lateral bending.[47,48] These findings are in accordance with studies showing that the IVD plays a significant role in restricting rotation,[7,51] although there is some controversy about whether torsion of the lumbar spine is restricted primarily by the apophyseal joints.[51]

ROM is not an accurate measure of instability caused by degeneration. A patient with a painful degenerated spine may have decreased motion, whereas a ballet dancer with extensive motion may not have any clinical symptoms of instability. Furthermore, the ROM measurement is affected by voluntary effort and thus motion limitation because of pain. In a biomechanical sense, instability is quantified in terms of a loss of stiffness or an increase in flexibility of a functional spinal unit. Panjabi[53] postulated that increased laxity around the neutral posture would put increased demand on the spinal musculature to provide the stability needed during activities of daily living. In turn, increased muscle forces would increase the stresses in the spinal components and may contribute to pain.[53] Furthermore, increased joint laxity may be associated with insufficient tension in the spinal ligaments and anulus fibers, both of which contain nerve endings that allow them to act as proprioceptive transducers. Lack of sufficient tension in the anulus fibers and ligaments may delay detection of sensory information needed to regulate muscle tension, thus contributing to dysfunction of the active stabilization system of the spine.[54]

The neutral zone and stiffness around the neutral posture (**Fig. 4.1**) are important measures of the stability of the spine. In vitro studies have shown that neutral zone increases with disc degeneration, particularly in axial rotation and anteroposterior shear motions. Therefore, the neutral zone is considered to be a more sensitive parameter than ROM in relation to disc degeneration or spinal injury.[55] The neutral zone ratio, a quotient of the neutral zone and the ROM, increases in value with greater joint laxity. Mimura et al[47] reported that although disc degeneration decreased ROM in flexion–extension and lateral bending, degeneration increased the intervertebral joint laxity around the neutral position as demonstrated by an increase in the neutral zone ratio. The neutral zone and stiffness in the high flexibility zone offer excellent in vitro tools to assess the effects of disc degeneration or injury; however, their value in the in vivo assessment in patients is yet to be demonstrated.

The behavior of COR has also been used to assess the effect of degeneration on the quality of motion of a spinal segment. Although the instantaneous COR of the intact segments with mild degeneration tends to remain relatively stationary as the segments move through the ROM, discs with moderate to severe degeneration show substantially larger anterior and superior migrations.[13,18,56–58] This shift of the COR is a reflection of the mechanical instability of these segments.

Abnormal Load Transmission

Disc degeneration can significantly alter the normal load sharing between the components of a functional spinal unit. In vitro studies have shown that in a degenerative disc the nucleus becomes depressurized as a result of the reduction of water content and increased fibrosis.[59] This has been confirmed by in vivo studies that showed that the intradiscal pressure was significantly reduced in a degenerated disc,[60] and the decrease was in accordance with the degree of disc degeneration as estimated by magnetic resonance imaging (MRI).[19] Nucleus depressurization results in an increasingly larger load transmission through the anulus, especially in the posterior portion.[59] Furthermore, the principal area of load transmission is highly dependent on posture, with a more prominent increase of stress concentrations in the posterior anulus when the segment is extended.[60,61] With disc degeneration, the posterolateral anulus is no longer acting in its role of a nucleus-retaining membrane, but rather as a region transmitting compressive stress. This is associated with inward bulging of the inner lamellae.[62] In more advanced stages of degeneration with disc space narrowing, it is possible for the neural arch to stress shield the posterior anulus in extension, so that much of the compressive load is transmitted through the neural arch and the anterior anulus.[61] The facet joints in a healthy spine normally bear ~20% of the load, but when there is a loss of disc height due to degenerative changes facet load bearing can be as high as 70%.[22]

In the degenerated disc, the structure of the nucleus changes to a nonhomogeneous mixture of fragmented and condensed collagen, areas of fluid, and on occasion, areas of gas. Isolated fragments of the anulus or the cartilaginous endplate may add to the loose fragments in the disc.[63] Disc pressure profilometry studies in cadavers have demonstrated irregular areas of abnormal spot loading.[59] Similarly, in vivo studies have shown occasional stress concentrations in the nucleus and multiple stress concentrations in the posterolateral anulus.[60] The multiple stress concentrations in the posterolateral anulus probably correspond to annular fissures or radial tears. Extensive variability of stress distribution has been shown even in discs showing the same degree of radiographic degeneration.[60] This variability demonstrates that the radiographic or MRI appearance of a disc is not a direct indicator of its mechanical competence.

Abnormal pressure profiles measured by in vivo stress profilometry have been shown to correlate with abnormal discograms. Increase in pressure in the degenerated disc is related to pain provocation.[60] However, McNally et al[60] demonstrated that pain is not associated with simple overloading of the disc. Evidence from in vivo stress profilometry suggests that it is the pattern of loading rather than its absolute magnitude that causes pain. Abnormal loading of the posterolateral anulus was a predicting factor for pain on provocative discography. Shear stress generated between areas of low load and areas of high load may also cause acceleration of degeneration and painful loading of the endplate. Similarly, the focal loading of the nucleus observed in a smaller percentage of investigated levels may also lead to pain. In this manner, pain provoked by discography may result from overloading particular areas by the injection of the discographic dye.[60] The pain may be generated by pain-sensitive nerve fibers in the peripheral anulus, or by the abnormal loading of the vertebral endplate, which is highly innervated.[64]

Disc degeneration has also been associated with abnormal viscoelastic response.[30] Water loss from the nucleus after creep loading reduces the hydrostatic pressure in the nucleus, resulting in a transfer of load from nucleus to anulus.[30] Degenerated discs exhibit decreased compressive and shear stiffness under static and dynamic loads, greater initial deformation, and approach equilibrium at a more rapid rate compared with nondegenerated discs.[33,65–68]

■ Conclusion

The complex structure of the IVD allows mobility while offering resistance to angular and translational motions. The disc along with the surrounding ligamentous structures provides flexibility at low bending moments while offering stability at higher moments. In cadaveric studies, segmental ROM tends to increase with increasing severity of disc degeneration, with a decrease in segmental ROM at the highest grade of degeneration. On the contrary, in most in vivo studies disc degeneration is associated with a reduced flexion–extension ROM. Therefore, ROM may not be an accurate measure of instability caused by degeneration, which is better quantified in terms of an increase in the neutral zone or a decrease in the stiffness around the neutral posture as shown by in vitro studies. Increased laxity around the neutral posture theoretically puts increased demand on the spinal musculature to provide the stability needed during daily activities, thus increasing stresses in the spinal components. Increased joint laxity may also be associated with insufficient tension in the spinal ligaments and anulus fibers that may result in a delayed detection of sensory information from proprioceptive transducers, thus contributing to dysfunction of the active-neuromuscular stabilization system of the spine. Another reflection of the instability of degenerated lumbar segment is the substantially larger migration of the center of rotation as the segment moves through the ROM compared with nondegenerated or mildly degenerated segments where it tends to remain stationary. The biomechanical changes responsible for symptomatic disc degeneration are not clearly understood. In addition to the instability with the consequent abnormal muscle activation, altered load sharing between the components of a functional spinal unit, and abnormal spot loading and stress concentration in the nucleus and the posterolateral anulus have been hypothesized as factors contributing to pain.

References

1. Adams MA, McNally DS, Dolan P. Stress distributions inside intervertebral discs: the effects of age and degeneration. J Bone Joint Surg Br 1996;78:965–972
2. Marchand F, Ahmed AM. Investigation of the laminate structure of lumbar disc annulus fibrosus. Spine 1990;15:402–410
3. Krismer M, Haid C, Rabl W. The contribution of annulus fibers to torque resistance. Spine 1996;21:2551–2557
4. Stokes IA. Surface strain on human intervertebral discs. J Orthop Res 1987;5:348–355
5. Brinckmann P, Frobin W, Hierholzer E, et al. Deformation of the vertebral endplate under axial loading of the spine. Spine 1983;8:851–856
6. Holmes AD, Hukins DW, Freemont AJ. Endplate displacement during compression of lumbar vertebra-disc vertebra segments and the mechanisms of failure. Spine 1993;18:128–135
7. Adams MA, Dolan P, Hutton WC. The stages of disc degeneration as revealed by discograms. J Bone Joint Surg Br 1986;68:36–41
8. Panjabi MM, Krag MH, Goel VK. A technique for measurement and description of three-dimensional six degrees-of-freedom motion of a body joint with an application to the human spine. J Biomech 1981;14:447–460
9. Pearcy MJ, Tibrewal SB. Axial rotation and lateral bending in the normal lumbar spine measured by three-dimensional radiography. Spine 1894;9:582–587
10. Pearcy M, Portek I, Shepherd J. Three-dimensional x-ray analysis of normal movement in the lumbar spine. Spine 1984;9:294–297
11. Wilke HJ, Wolf S, Claes LE, Arand M, Wiesend A. Stability increase of the lumbar spine with different muscle groups. Spine 1995;20:192–198
12. Patwardhan AG, Havey RM, Carandang G, et al. Effect of compressive follower preload on the flexion–extension response of the human lumbar spine. J Orthop Res 2003;21:540–546
13. Schneider G, Pearcy MJ, Bogduk N. Abnormal motion in spondylolytic spondylolisthesis. Spine 2005;30:1159–1164
14. Dimnet J, Pasquet A, Krag MH, et al. Cervical spine motion in the sagittal plane: kinematic and geometric parameters. J Biomech 1982;15:959–969

15. Panjabi MM, Krag MH, Dimnet JC, et al. Thoracic spine centers of rotation in the sagittal plane. J Orthop Res 1984;1:387–394

16. Patwardhan A, Wharton N, Havey R, et al. Instantaneous centers of rotation of the intact lumbar spine and total disc replacement. Paper presented at International Society for the Study of the Lumbar Spine; June 13–17, 2006; Bergen, Norway

17. Pearcy MJ, Bogduk N. Instantaneous axes of rotation of the lumbar intervertebral joints. Spine 1988;13(9):1033–1041

18. Zhao PP, Hole BD, Dolan P, Adams MA. Discogenic origins of spinal instability. Spine 2005;30(23):2621–2630

19. Sato K, Kikuchi S, Yonezawa T. In vivo intradiscal pressure measurement in healthy individuals and in patients with ongoing back problems. Spine 1999;24(23):2468–2474

20. Nachemson AL. Disc pressure measurements. Spine 1981;6(1):93–97

21. Schultz A. Loads in the lumbar spine. In: Jayson MVI, ed. The Lumbar Spine and Back Pain. Edinburgh, UK: Churchill Livingstone; 1987:204–214

22. Adams MA, Hutton WC. The mechanical function of the lumbar apophyseal joints. Spine 1983;8(3):327–330

23. McNally DS, Adams MA, Goodship AE. Development and validation of a new transducer for intradiscal pressure measurement. J Biomed Eng 1992;14:495–498

24. Goel VK, Weinstein JN, Patwardhan A. Biomechanics of the intact ligamentous spine. In: Goel, VK, Weinstein, JN, eds. Biomechanics of the Spine: Clinical and Surgical Perspective. Boca Raton, FL: CRC Press; 1990:97–156

25. Adams MA, McNally DS, Chinn H, et al. Posture and the compressive strength of the lumbar spine. Clin Biomech (Bristol, Avon) 1994;9:5–14

26. Adams MA, Dolan P. Time-dependent changes in the lumbar spine's resistance to bending. Clin Biomech (Bristol, Avon) 1996;11:194–200

27. Hutton WC, Adams MA. Can the lumbar spine be crushed in heavy lifting? Spine 1982;7:586–590

28. Virgin WJ. Experimental investigations into physical properties of the intervertebral disc. J Bone Joint Surg Br 1951;33:607–611

29. Botsford DJ, Esses SI, Ogilvie-Harris DJ. In vivo diurnal variation in intervertebral disc volume and morphology. Spine 1994;19:935–940

30. Adams MA, McMillan DW, Green TP, et al. Sustained loading generates stress concentrations in lumbar intervertebral discs. Spine 1996;21:434–438

31. Frei H, Oxland TR, Nolte LP. Thoracolumbar spine mechanics contrasted under compression and shear loading. J Orthop Res 2002;20:1333–1338

32. Tencer AF, Ahmed AM, Burke DL. Some static mechanical properties of the lumbar intervertebral joint, intact and injured. J Biomech Eng 1982;104:193–201

33. Bunag J. Viscoelastic properties of lumbar spine segments in shear and compression [master's thesis]. Chicago, IL: Department of Mechanical Engineering, University of Illinois at Chicago; 1995

34. McDevitt CA. Proteoglycans of the intervertebral disc. In: Ghosh P, ed. The Biology of the Intervertebral Disc. Boca Raton, FL: CRC Press; 1988:151–170

35. Vernon-Roberts B, Fazzalari NL, Manthey BA. Pathogenesis of tears of the anulus investigated by multiple-level transaxial analysis of the T12-L1 disc. Spine 1997;22(22):2641–2646

36. Gruber HE, Hanley EN Jr. Ultrastructure of the human intervertebral disc during aging and degeneration: comparison of surgical and control specimens. Spine 2002;27(8):798–805

37. Krismer M, Haid C, Behensky H, Kapfinger P, Landauer F, Rachbauer F. Motion in lumbar functional spine units during side bending and axial rotation moments depending on the degree of degeneration. Spine 2000;25(16):2020–2027

38. Gunzburg R, Parkinson R, Moore R, et al. A cadaveric study comparing discography, magnetic resonance imaging, histology, and mechanical behavior of the human lumbar disc. Spine 1992;17(4):417–426

39. Hadjipavlou AG, Simmons JW, Pope MH, Necessary JT, Goel VK. Pathomechanics and clinical relevance of disc degeneration and annular tear: a point-of-view review. Am J Orthop 1999;28(10):561–571

40. Lin HS, Liu YK, Adams KH. Mechanical response of the lumbar intervertebral joint under physiological (complex) loading. J Bone Joint Surg Am 1978;60(1):41–55

41. Farfan HF, Cossette JW, Robertson GH, Wells RV, Kraus H. The effects of torsion on the lumbar intervertebral joints: the role of torsion in the production of disc degeneration. J Bone Joint Surg Am 1970;52(3):468–497

42. Adams MA, Hutton WC. Gradual disc prolapse. Spine 1985;10(6):524–531

43. Adams MA, Hutton WC. 1981 Volvo Award in Basic Science. Prolapsed intervertebral disc: a hyperflexion injury. Spine 1982;7(3):184–191

44. Granhed H, Morelli B. Low back pain among retired wrestlers and heavyweight lifters. Am J Sports Med 1988;16:530–533

45. Pope MH, Hansson TH. Vibration of the spine and low back pain. Clin Orthop Relat Res 1992;(279):49–59

46. Kirkaldy-Willis WH, Farfan HF. Instability of the lumbar spine. Clin Orthop Relat Res 1982;(165):110–123

47. Mimura M, Panjabi M, Oxland TR, Crisco JJ, Yamamoto I, Vasavada A. Disc degeneration affects the multidirectional flexibility of the lumbar spine. Spine 1994;19:1371–1380

48. Fujiwara A, Lim TH, An HS, et al. The effect of disc degeneration and facet joint osteoarthritis on the segmental flexibility of the lumbar spine. Spine 2000;25(23):3036–3044

49. Morgan FP, King T. Primary instability of lumbar vertebrae as a common cause of low back pain. J Bone Joint Surg Br 1957;39-B(1):6–22

50. Burton AK, Battie MC, Gibbons L, Videman T, Tillotson KM. Lumbar disc degeneration and sagittal flexibility. J Spinal Disord 1996;9(5):418–424

51. Adams MA, Hutton WC. The relevance of torsion to the mechanical derangement of the lumbar spine. Spine 1981;6:241–248

52. Schmidt TA, An HS, Lim TH, Nowicki BH, Haughton VM. The stiffness of lumbar spinal motion segments with a high-intensity zone in the annulus fibrosus. Spine 1998;23(20):2167–2173

53. Panjabi MM. The stabilizing system of the spine. Part II. Neutral zone and instability hypothesis. J Spinal Disord 1992;5(4):390–396

54. Panjabi MM. A hypothesis of chronic back pain: ligament subfailure injuries lead to muscle control dysfunction. Spine J 2006;15:668–676

55. Oxland TR, Panjabi MM. The onset and progression of spinal injury: a demonstration of neutral zone sensitivity. J Biomech 1992;25(10):1165–1172

56. Gertzbein SD, Seligman J, Holtby R, et al. Centrode patterns and segmental instability in degenerative disc disease. Spine 1985;10:257–261

57. Gertzbein SD, Seligman J, Holtby R, et al. Centrode characteristics of the lumbar spine as a function of segmental instability. Clin Orthop Relat Res 1986;208:48–51

58. Ogston NG, King GJ, Getzbein SD, et al. Centrode patterns in the lumbar spine. Baseline studies in normal subjects. Spine 1986; 11:591–595

59. McNally DS, Adams MA. Internal intervertebral disc mechanics as revealed by stress profilometry. Spine 1992;17(1):66–73

60. McNally DS, Shackleford IM, Goodship AE, Mulholland RC. In vivo stress measurements can predict pain on discography. Spine 1996;21(22):2580–2587

61. Adams MA, May S, Freeman BJ, Morrison HP, Dolan P. Effects of backward bending on lumbar intervertebral discs: relevance to physical therapy treatments for low back pain. Spine 2000;25(4):431–438

62. McNally DS. The objectives of the biomechanical evaluation of spinal instrumentation have changed. Eur Spine J 2002;11(Suppl 2): S171–S185

63. Moore RJ, Vernon-Roberts B, Fraser RD, et al. The origin and fate of herniated lumbar intervertebral disc tissue. Spine 1996;21(18): 2149–2155

64. Jackson H, Winkelman R, Bichel W. Nerve endings in the human lumbar spinal column and related structures. J Bone Joint Surg Am 1966;48:1272–1280

65. Koeller W, Muehlhaus S, Meier W, et al. Biomechanical properties of human intervertebral discs subjected to axial dynamic compression: influence of age and degeneration. J Biomech 1986;19: 807–816

66. Keller TS, Spengler DM, Hansson TH. Mechanical behavior of the human lumbar spine, I: Creep analysis during static compressive loading. J Orthop Res 1987;5(4):467–478

67. Kazarian LE. Creep characteristics of the human spinal column. Orthop Clin North Am 1975;6(1):3–18

68. Li S, Patwardhan AG, Amirouche F, Havey R, Meade KP. Limitations of the standard linear solid model of intervertebral discs subject to prolonged loading and low frequency vibration in axial compression. J Biomech 1995;28(7):779–790

5 The Mechanisms of Pain from Intervertebral Discs

Todd F. Alamin and Vijay Agarwal

Any therapeutic endeavor relies on an understanding of the mechanism by which the pain is produced. Is the pain originating in the intervertebral disc (IVD) an inflammatory process, or a purely mechanical one? From which part of the disc does the pain originate? The answers are critical to the patient for whom treatment is contemplated: the information put forth in this chapter will hopefully aid in this analysis.

Pain that originates at the level of the disc can be divided into two categories: radicular pain (typically manifested as leg pain caused by a process originating at the level of the root) and discogenic pain (typically manifested as axial back pain caused by mechanical loading of a pathologically degenerated disc). These broad categories of pain may have features in common, but their distinct clinical behavior warrants categorization when considering their pathophysiology.

The mechanism of pain production can be thought of first as the stimulation and firing of a nociceptive afferent, and second, as the conveyance of this signal through the signal processing pathway to the level of consciousness. This chapter begins with a description of the signal processing pathway, and then moves to the research area of focus: characteristics of relevant nociceptive afferents and the factors that lead to their firing. Radicular pain and discogenic pain will be addressed sequentially—deeper knowledge of one will facilitate a better understanding of the other.

■ Innervation

A comprehensive understanding of lumbar spine innervation from an anatomical point of view is critical when analyzing potential mechanisms of pain caused by the IVD. There are two pathways by which afferent information can be transmitted from the disc to the dorsal root ganglion: segmentally, via the sinuvertebral nerve,[1–3] and nonsegmentally, through the paravertebral sympathetic trunk.[2,3]

The spinal cord sends off a ventral and a dorsal root, which combine to form the spinal nerve. The ventral root is the efferent motor root; all motor fibers, both somatic and autonomic, leave the spinal cord via the ventral roots. The dorsal root is the afferent sensory root; at its distal end, before the formation of the spinal nerve, is the dorsal root ganglion (DRG), containing the soma of the afferent nerve fibers. DRG neurons are of the pseudo-unipolar type, conveying sensory information from the receptor to the soma, and from the soma to the junction in the dorsal horn of the spinal cord, via two independent axons. The dorsal and ventral roots combine to form the spinal nerve, which divides into the dorsal and ventral primary rami, each containing both motor and sensory fibers. The dorsal primary ramus then splits into the medial and lateral branches for the supply of the muscles and skin of the posterior trunk; the larger ventral primary ramus supplies the anterolateral trunk and limbs. Ventral primary rami from different levels combine in the cervical, lumbar, and sacral regions to form peripheral plexuses.

The sympathetic trunk is a group of nerve fibers that originates as the internal carotid nerve and runs from the carotid canal in the skull to the coccyx, anterolateral to the vertebral column, receiving contributions along the way from nerve roots exiting the spine through the thoracic and upper two lumbar segments. Cell bodies of preganglionic neurons in the sympathetic system reside in the intermediolateral cell column in the lateral horn of the spinal cord, from the T1–L2 levels. Preganglionic fibers travel via the ventral root at each spinal level, through the T1–L2 spinal nerves and ventral rami to join the sympathetic trunk via the communicating ramus (described below). Paravertebral ganglia that exist as fusiform expansions at the junction of the communicating ramus (and the sympathetic trunk along its course) are locations of interconnection among these autonomic fibers and contain the cell bodies of the postganglionic nerves. The sympathetic trunk travels superiorly with the internal carotid artery through the carotid canal into the skull. Inferiorly, the bilateral chains converge in front of the coccyx to form the ganglion impar. The two branches of the sympathetic trunk contributing to the spinal nerve are the gray ramus communicans (containing unmyelinated postganglionic sympathetic fibers) and white ramus communicans from the thoracic, first, and second lumbar nerves (containing myelinated preganglionic sympathetic fibers).

Each sinuvertebral nerve is formed by the union of a branch of the ventral ramus of the spinal nerve at that level and a branch of the sympathetic trunk via the segmental gray ramus communicans. The posterior and posterolateral anulus and posterior longitudinal ligament are innervated by the sinuvertebral nerve, direct sensory branches from the ventral primary ramus, and, to a lesser degree, rami communicantes from the sympathetic trunk.[4,5] The lateral and anterior aspects of the anulus, as well as the anterior longitudinal ligament, are innervated via rami communicantes from the sympathetic trunk, along with direct branches from the sympathetic trunk.[3,4,6,7] The innervation of the endplate is 2-fold: intraosseous nerves that are direct branches of the primary ventral rami follow vasculature channels into the endplate,[8] and the basivertebral nerve—a branch of the sinuvertebral nerve—enters the endplate centrally and posteriorly[9] via the posterior neurovascular foramen. In a nondegenerated sheep disc, Fagan et al[10] found a limited nerve supply confined to the outermost structures; there was no significant difference in overall density of endplate and anulus innervation, with the richest area of innervations in the superficial anulus. No innervation was found in the inner anulus or nucleus. In human patients with degenerative disc disease, Brown et al[11] presented similar findings, with no innervation detected in disc inner anulus or nucleus pulposus (NP).

Animal models have been the basis for extensive characterization of lumbar disc innervation.[12–17] The fluorogold injection technique, in which tracer is taken up at the level of the nerve ending and then transported up the afferent axon, has been used to establish the transmission pathway from the level of the disc.[18] Investigators have found that particles injected into the disc can then be detected in primary sensory neurons in the dorsal root ganglia and primary sensory fibers in the posterior horn of the spinal cord not only at the injected level but at multiple levels—clearly documenting the polysegmental nature of the afferent nerve supply of the disc. This polysegmental origin of innervation is not only the case for the somatic but also for the autonomic innervation of the disc via the sympathetic trunk. Vertebral endplate innervation, predominantly somatic via the sinuvertebral nerve and branches of the primary ventral ramus, is also polysegmental in origin. In both the somatic and autonomic pathways, stimulation of afferents results in contralateral dorsal root ganglia involvement.

The first comprehensive description of the source and pattern of lumbar IVD innervation in humans is based on the meticulous dissection of four adult cadaveric spines.[4] The sinuvertebral nerve was found to arise from both the ventral primary ramus (somatic origin) and a ramus communicans (sympathetic origin). The nerve was found to enter the vertebral canal through the intervertebral foramen by crossing the vertebral body just caudal to the pedicle. Lesser branches of the nerve passed medially and caudally from the intervertebral foramen and branched over the IVD at the level of the origin of the primary (or parent) nerve. The sinuvertebral nerve gives rise to both ascending and descending branches, but Bogduk and others found that the ascending branch was consistently much larger.[4] This major branch of the sinuvertebral nerve courses parallel to the posterior longitudinal ligament, giving off transverse branches that pass deep to the ligament to supply the anulus (**Fig. 5.1**).

Each ventral primary ramus receives at least one rami communicantes, but more often two or more rami extend from the sympathetic trunk around the vertebral body and through the psoas muscle. Bogduk described "paradiscal" rami as fibers that cross the IVD on its surface, instead of passing through the muscle belly of the psoas adjacent to the disc. These paradiscal rami are likely the

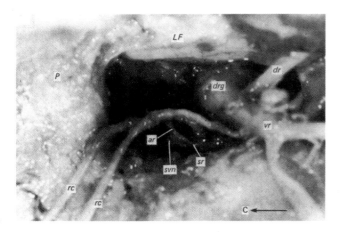

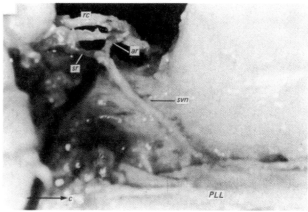

A   **B**

Fig. 5.1   The sinuvertebral nerves. The arrow (C) indicates the cranial end of the specimen. **(A)** Lateral view of a right L1 intervertebral foramen, showing the origin of the sinuvertebral nerve. **(B)** Medial view of the same foramen as in **A**, showing the recurrent course of the nerve through the foramen. The nerve has been lifted by a 0- to 75-mm probe.

(Continued on page 42)

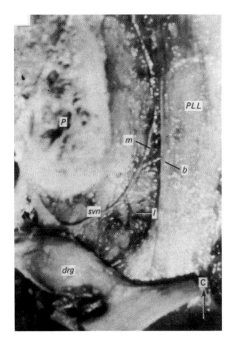

C

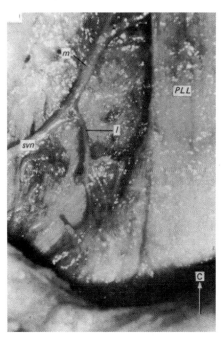

D

Fig. 5.1 *(Continued)* The sinuvertebral nerves. The arrow (C) indicates the cranial end of the specimen. **(C)** The course of a left L2 sinuvertebral nerve within the vertebral canal. **(D)** A close-up view of the lesser descending branch of the nerve in **C**. P, pedicle; LF, ligamentum flavum; PLL, posterior longitudinal ligament; IVD, intervertebral disc; drg, dorsal root ganglion; dr, dorsal ramus; vr, ventral ramus; rc: ramus communicans; svn, sinuvertebral nerve; ar, autonomic root of svn; sr, somatic root of svn; m, major ascending branch of svn; l, lesser descending branch of svn; b, branches to posterior longitudinal ligament. (From Bogduk N, Tynan W, Wilson AS. The nerve supply to the human lumbar intervertebral discs. J Anat 1981;132[Pt 1]: 39–56. Reprinted with permission.)

predominant source of autonomic input to the ventral primary ramus.

The autonomic component of disc innervation of lower lumbar levels is not affected by root blocks performed below the L2 level; these sympathetic fibers predominantly enter the spinal canal as part of the L2 root. Clinical reports of significant relief of low back pain via L2 selective nerve root blocks[1,14,19–25] suggest that these autonomic fibers may play a role in some patients with low back pain, but this role has not been clearly established. It seems likely that this autonomic innervation is important in patients with neuropathic pain states, and less so in patients with low back pain that is more clearly mechanical in nature.

■ Proximal Signaling Pathway

The sources of somatic afferent information from the disc are sinuvertebral nerve, basivertebral nerve, and direct branches of the primary ventral rami, which either supply the posterior anulus or course with the intraosseous vessels to the endplate. This information is collected polysegmentally via ipsilateral and contralateral DRGs and is then transmitted to the dorsal horn of the spinal cord. In the spinal cord, pain signals synapse on the superficial layer of the dorsal horn and travel via the spinothalamic tract to the thalamus and somatosensory and pain centers in the cortex. Information from the autonomic afferent innervation of the lower lumbar discs is predominantly collected at the level of the L2 dorsal root ganglia is transmitted to the

dorsal horn, and subsequently courses proximally into the central nervous system (**Fig. 5.2**).

■ Radicular Pain

In 1934, Mixter and Barr's description of sciatica caused by disc herniation hypothesized that this complaint was caused solely by the mechanical deformation of the root affected by the disc herniation.[26] Imaging studies and the finding of relief of sciatica with fragment removal have rendered the mechanical deformation of the root an obvious point of focus, but animal studies and clinical investigations have painted a more complex picture of the clinical syndrome.

Several animal models of sciatica have been developed that involve the simple application of NP material to the nerve root without mechanical deformation of the root; results show that this is sufficient to elicit pathophysiologic events which are likely closely related to the clinical complaint of sciatica. These findings have led investigators to attempt to determine the chemical basis of this pathologic response; a better understanding of this signaling may boost the effectiveness of targeted pharmaceutical therapy.

Another line of empirical evidence also leads to the conclusion that mechanical deformation of the root is not alone in its role in sciatica: purely physical deformation of nerves elsewhere in the body caused by spinal cord tumors, nerve root sheath tumors, and compressive neuropathies typically present predominantly with numbness and weakness without significant pain.[27] Why, then, would a herniated nucleus

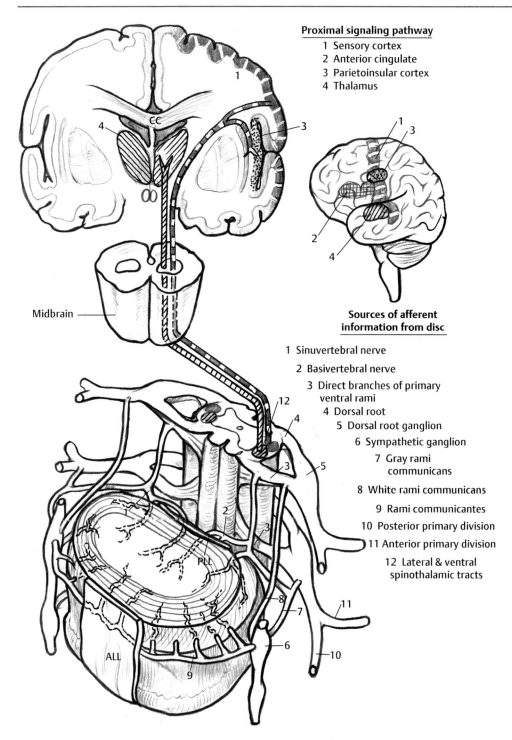

Proximal signaling pathway
1 Sensory cortex
2 Anterior cingulate
3 Parietoinsular cortex
4 Thalamus

Sources of afferent information from disc

1 Sinuvertebral nerve
2 Basivertebral nerve
3 Direct branches of primary ventral rami
4 Dorsal root
5 Dorsal root ganglion
6 Sympathetic ganglion
7 Gray rami communicans
8 White rami communicans
9 Rami communicantes
10 Posterior primary division
11 Anterior primary division
12 Lateral & ventral spinothalamic tracts

Fig. 5.2 Sources of somatic afferent innervation of the vertebral disc and the subsequent pain signaling pathway.

pulposus (HNP), if predominantly a lesion inducing mechanical deformation of the nerve root, almost always present first with pain as the chief complaint?

Different levels of information are available to investigators interested in the pathophysiology of sciatica. Animal studies, in which an experimental lesion is induced and followed by histologic assessments of proximal afferent structures, provide some information about structural changes that could be representative of inflammation or injury. Neurophysiologic studies of lesioned animals demonstrate, with more physiologic emphasis than anatomic studies, the effect of the lesion on structures in the signaling pathway. Animal behavioral studies are perhaps more compelling as these sorts of studies assess the effect of the lesion on the animal's overall behavior pattern and more closely model the clinical complaint of pain. Human experimental studies under local anesthesia can provide information regarding the pain sensitivity of particular anatomic structures, and histologic analysis of surgical specimens allows for an understanding of receptor presence and density in the tissue of origin. Finally, therapeutic trials allow for the assessment of the effect of a treatment strategy and represent the culmination of a long line of research into basic mechanisms.

Effect of Nucleus Pulposus

A series of articles by Olmarker et al[28-30] examined the effect of NP applied directly onto porcine spinal nerves without mechanical compression. On assessment of nerve conduction velocities of the NP-treated roots compared with the control roots, the NP-treated roots were noted to exhibit a pronounced decrease in nerve conduction velocities at 1, 3, and 7 days after treatment. These roots were then examined via light microscopy, and morphologic changes consistent with nerve fiber injury were noted in some of the NP-treated roots. A majority of the nerve fibers, however, exhibited no structural changes at the light microscopic level; thus, the changes noted in some fibers could not completely explain the changes in function seen in all.

Electron microscopy showed significant ultrastructural changes in the NP group, even in the myelinated fibers that did not show signs of axonal damage on light microscopy. Significant findings included an expanded Schwann cell cytoplasm and intracellular edema in the treated groups, which were thought to be related to the dramatic neurophysiologic changes in these groups. These findings were confirmed in a dog model by Kayama et al.[31] At 7 days from exposure to NP, nerve conduction velocities were 13 ± 14 m/second in the experimental group, and 73 ± 5 m/second in the control group. Similar to findings in the Olmarker et al study,[29] structural changes of the axons consistent with nerve fiber injury were noted, but the investigators felt that these were not dramatic enough to account for the observed neurophysiologic changes. Capillary stasis was also noted in the experimental group. NP has also been found to stimulate an autoimmune-like response: subcutaneous NP has been found in animal models to attract activated T and B cells.[32]

Olmarker et al[27] reported a new method of studying pain in the rat that focused on changes in behavior rather than changes in neurophysiologic thresholds. In this study, 40 rats were divided into four groups: exposure of L4 DRG, incision of L4/5 disc (causing leakage of NP onto the root), exposure and displacement of L4 DRG with an implanted needle, and combination of incision and displacement. These animals were assessed at 1, 3, 7, 14, and 21 days after operation, and significant behavioral differences were only noted in the series with both incision and displacement. These rats demonstrated behavior consistent with increased focal pain (lifting of the hind paw on the operated side and increased rotation of the head toward the operated side). No detectable differences were noted at 14 days; however, by 21 days after surgery, increased immobility and decreased locomotion were noted in this group. The investigators were not certain if this represented an additive effect of the two factors or if both were necessary for the condition to develop. An assessment of walking ability in rats—subjected to either laminectomy or laminectomy and exposure to NP via incision of the lumbar disc—revealed decreased walking ability in the disc incision group.[33]

In a unique report, Kuslich et al[34] described their findings in 193 consecutive patients treated for lumbar disc herniation with a microdiscectomy under local anesthetic. During the procedure, mechanical force was applied to various tissues in and around the exposed disc, and the patient's response to stimulus was recorded. The noteworthy findings showed that, whereas retraction of the affected nerve root caused pain in 99% of patients, retraction of an uncompressed or normal nerve produced significant pain in only 9% of cases. In concordance with the findings in the Olmarker et al[28] animal study, the Kuslich et al[34] findings suggest that in the clinical situation, an inflamed or stimulated root is necessary for mechanical stress to cause significant pain.

Effect of Inflammatory Cytokines

To determine the component of the NP responsible for the neurophysiologic changes noted in the root subsequent to its application, Olmarker et al[29] subjected porcine cauda equina to either fresh NP, NP kept at 37 degrees for 24 hours, NP kept at −20°C for 24 hours, or NP digested by hyaluronidase for 24 hours. Only the group that was subjected to lysis of the NP cells by freezing of the NP showed no reduction in conduction velocity. The researchers interpreted this to mean that the effect induced by NP was related to cell population, not the matrix, which should have been digested in the hyaluronidase group. In a follow-up study, this group demonstrated that live and dead NP cells induced similar neurophysiologic changes; the authors concluded that the effects were related to membrane-bound substances or structures.[35]

In a dog model of NP-induced nerve root injury investigating a potential vascular correlate of nerve conduction velocity changes, Otani et al[36] demonstrated a reduction in blood flow in the nerve root that began 1 day after disc incision and was maximal after 1 week, resolving by 1 month. Nerve conduction velocity was also reduced in the experimental group, but this did not begin until 3 days after incision and was not fully resolved until 2 months later. The authors hypothesized that the reduction in blood flow represents part of the mechanism of the NP-induced neurophysiologic changes.

To further investigate the mechanism of action of the NP-induced neurophysiologic effect on the nerve root, Olmarker and Larsson used a monoclonal antibody to determine whether tumor necrosis factor-α (TNF-α), an inflammatory cytokine, was present in porcine NP cells.[30] The authors found that TNF-α was present in the soma of NP cells. Application of NP to the root elicited the predicted decrease in nerve conduction velocity, but treatment with doxycycline (known to block TNF-α, as well as other cytokines such as interleukin-1 [IL-1], interferon-τ, and nitric oxide synthetase) completely blocked this effect, and local application of anti-TNF-α antibody induced a partial block of the effect.

Direct evidence that TNF-α is a significant element in this pathway has been reported by multiple investigators.[37–39] Direct application of TNF-α to rat nerve roots produces the characteristic neurophysiologic changes caused by NP application.[38] The exposure of rat L5 nerve roots to TNF-α has also been reported to result in a significant increase in the frequency of spontaneous discharges and enhanced responses of wide dynamic range neurons to noxious stimulation, as well as inflammatory changes in the ganglion.[39]

NP application to the nerve root has also been associated with an increase in brain-derived nerve growth factor (BDGF), a neuromodulator of nociceptive information in the dorsal horn, which is thought to play an important role in inflammatory pain states through its effect on NMDA receptor activity. BDGF has been found to be upregulated in both the DRG and the spinal cord after application of NP to the root; a follow-up study demonstrated that this upregulation could be blocked by the administration of infliximab (a monoclonal antibody to TNF-α).[40] Additional studies have demonstrated that the NP-induced effects may be blocked by methylprednisolone and cyclosporine A, and somewhat less efficiently by indomethacin and lidocaine.[30]

Murata and Olmarker et al[41] investigated the effect of intraperitoneal injection of TNF-α inhibitor (infliximab) either 1 day before or 3 hours after an induced disc herniation on histologic features of the root in a rat model. No staining for TNF-α was noted in rat NP cells 1 to 3 days after the injection, and weak staining was noted 7 days after injection. Positive staining was noted in all rats that were not injected. A characteristic semilunar enlargement of the DRG (an "inflammatory crescent") at the site of application of the NP was noted. This crescent was noted in all of the treatment groups and was particularly pronounced at 1 and 3 days after surgery. The groups treated with the inhibitor demonstrated a smaller number of deformed nuclei at the 1-, 3-, 7-, and 14-day time points; at 21 days after surgery, the crescent was thicker in the nontreatment group.

There has also been interest in the potential therapeutic effect of serotonin (5-HT) receptor antagonists due to the discovery of 5-HT receptors in the dorsal root ganglia, and the role of 5-HT in the hyperalgesia of acute inflammation demonstrated in animal models.[42,43] The effect of a 5-HT 2A receptor antagonist, sarpogrelate, was examined in a rat NP root exposure model. When administered daily between days 7 and 14 after exposure, measured mechanical allodynia was significantly reduced on days 11 and 15.

Clinical Studies of Sciatica and Selective Antiinflammatories

Two open-label studies assessing the results of treatment of patients with sciatica caused by lumbar disc herniation reported impressive results, with dramatic early relief of sciatica.[44] In the first study, 10 patients with HNP underwent infusion of 3 mg/kg infliximab over 2 hours; leg pain was found to decrease by 50% at 1 hour, 60% of patients were pain-free at 2 weeks, and 90% were pain-free at 3 months.[45] The control group was a historical group with sciatica caused by HNP that had been treated with periradicular injection of normal saline. A second study reported open-label use of three subcutaneous injections of a TNF-α inhibitor, etanercept (25 mg every 3 days), in 10 patients with sciatica caused by HNP.[46] Again, a historical cohort was used as a control; this group had been treated with standard care and intravenous (IV) methylprednisolone. All 10 patients in the treatment group improved by day 10 as measured by the Visual Analogue Score for Leg Pain (VASL), the Oswestry Disability Index (ODI), and the Roland–Morris Disability Questionnaire (RMDQ); and 9 out of 10 continued to show improvement at 5 weeks. These improvements were significantly better than those observed in the methylprednisolone group.

The findings in these open-label studies prompted a prospective, randomized clinical trial reported by Korhonen et al.[47] In this study, 40 subjects with sciatica caused by HNP were randomized to treatment with either placebo or a single injection of infliximab (monoclonal antibody against TNF-α; 5 mg/kg). No difference in leg pain, back pain, health-related quality of life scales, or rate of surgery was noted in the two groups at either 3 months or 1 year after treatment. A subset of 21 of these 40 patients was analyzed by magnetic resonance imaging (MRI) both before and at 2, 4, 12, and 26 weeks after the administration of either infliximab or placebo. In both groups, HNP volume diminished at 6 months, but no difference in volume change was detected between the groups. The authors noted a slight decrease in the amount of disc herniation resorption at 2 weeks from the time of infusion in the infliximab group, but no difference was observed at the other time points; therefore, it was concluded that infliximab did not inhibit overall hernia resorption.

Use of a different TNF-α antagonist, REN-1654, that belongs to a chemical class of compounds known as benzamide and has been shown to act as a functional TNF-α antagonist in vitro and in vivo, was reported by Carragee et al.[48] Administration of this oral compound at 100 mg per day for 3 weeks in a placebo-controlled, prospective randomized study of 64 patients did not demonstrate a significant benefit in the primary endpoint of the study (decrease in daily leg pain at 3 weeks). However, a slightly greater reduction in maximal leg pain was observed in the treatment group in the first 2 weeks.

The animal data suggesting a beneficial effect of a 5-HT2A receptor antagonist led to an NSAID-controlled, randomized trial in 40 patients with sciatica due to disc herniation.[49] The authors of this study found that within the limits set by the power of their study, the efficacy of the 5HTA receptor antagonist was similar to that of NSAID therapy.

Simple mechanical deformation of the nerve root is likely not sufficient to explain the clinical syndrome of sciatica related to disc herniation. Sensitization of the root, which may be related to exposure to inflammatory cytokines, seems to be necessary to induce in the root the property of signaling pain in response to the mechanical deformation caused by a disc herniation. It is likely that inflammatory cytokines such as TNF-α have a role in this process, as selective inhibitors can block the typical neurophysiologic effects elicited by NP in different animal models. It remains to be seen, however, whether this strategy of desensitization of the root via treatment with inflammatory inhibitors is useful in the treatment of radicular pain caused by disc herniation. Thus far, the few trials of this approach have not been successful in demonstrating a clinically significant effect.

■ Discogenic Pain

The mechanism of the second type of pain associated with the IVD, discogenic pain, is not well understood. The clinical and radiographic criteria by which the diagnosis of discogenic pain is established are disputed, and outcomes of operative treatment are not as successful as those for radicular pain. The uncertainty of diagnosis makes any investigation into the pathophysiologic mechanisms more challenging: without a firm understanding of what features are sufficient to cause the clinical problem, the appropriate pathophysiology to be investigated cannot be universally accepted. The goal here is to discuss mechanisms of pain generation at the level of the disc and not address other potential causes of low back pain; it will be assumed that axial back pain that arises from the disc is a significant clinical problem.

Two processes may be critical to explaining discogenic pain: (1) sensitization of the nociceptive afferents, which renders them susceptible to firing in response to applied loads; and (2) degenerative changes of the disc subjected to these loading conditions. Sensitization of the nociceptive afferents, which innervate the posterior anulus and vertebral endplate, may occur in the same manner as the nerve root is sensitized by exposure to the proinflammatory substances found in the NP. The effect may be different, however, as these nociceptive afferents are clearly different structures than the nerve root or dorsal root ganglion that is stimulated *and* compressed by an HNP. Similar to the animal pain behavioral models of HNP that require an inflammatory stimulus and mechanical deformation of the root,[50,51] axial pain arising from the disc may require both an inflammatory stimulus and mechanical loading of a degenerated disc.

Degenerated discs on imaging studies in asymptomatic subjects become increasingly more common as the subject population ages; these findings of disc degeneration are not distinguishable from those found in subjects with significant pain.[52] Common morphologic changes noted on imaging studies, then, are not able to differentiate painful from nonpainful disc degeneration. Many attempts have been made to identify a feature unique to painful degenerate discs compared with nonpainful degenerate discs, but there has been as yet no finding proven to have these characteristics.

An understanding of the mechanical component of the syndrome of discogenic pain relies on an analysis of the biomechanics and anatomy of the degenerative disc. In an effort to describe the kinematic and mechanical correlates of disc degeneration, Kirkaldy-Willis described three biomechanical stages of disc degeneration: temporary dysfunction, unstable phase, and stabilization phase.[53] The earlier phases of disc degeneration, in which the height of the disc is relatively preserved, but the nucleus has become dehydrated and the anulus has begun to degenerate, have been modeled experimentally. Significant findings of these cadaveric loading experiments are notable for increased segmental motion as a result of standard applied bending moments. In this early phase of disc instability, the flexion/extension resistance of the degenerate disc is reduced relative to its adjacent normal counterparts. Under such circumstances, an applied load and flexion moment to the spinal column (holding weight out in front of the body) will result in earlier and greater flexion at the degenerate disc relative to its counterparts with stiffer kinematics (**Fig. 5.3**). This situation is no longer the case in the stabilization phase, in which segmental stiffness is increased.

Discogenic pain is a fundamentally painful process: for it to exist, there must be a mechanism of transmission of a nociceptive signal from the disc to proximal portions of the nervous system. In vivo evidence for significant innervation of both the posterior anulus and the vertebral endplate was reported by Kuslich et al.[4] In this report, cited previously with regard to radicular pain, the anulus and vertebral endplate were stimulated during microdiscectomy under

Applied Flexion Moment

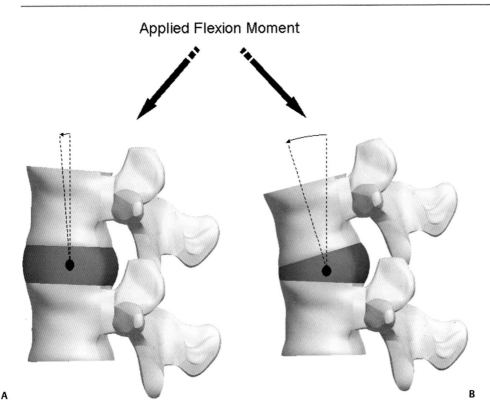

A   **B**

Fig. 5.3 In the early phase of disc instability, the flexion–extension resistance of the degenerate disc **(B)** is reduced relative to its adjacent normal counterpart **(A)**.

local anesthetic. It was found that stimulation of the anulus was noted to be painful in 73% of cases, and stimulation of the endplate was painful in 61% of cases. It has further been observed that the administration of small doses of short-acting local anesthetic, likely to stay confined to the intradiscal space, can quickly and dramatically improve pain thought to be discogenic in origin.[54] This observation implies the presence of nociceptors accessible to the locally applied anesthetic, which are in the endplate and anulus and visualized with contrast on discography.

The nucleus and inner anulus of a nondegenerated disc are not significantly innervated.[10] The outer anulus is innervated in normal discs superficially to a depth of up to 3.5 mm. The posterior anulus is always innervated, as is the anterolateral anulus; these are the two richest areas of innervation of the anulus. Nerve ingrowth along vascularized granulation tissue has been noted in both animal models and human discs through tears in the posterior anulus into more central regions of the disc. The endplate is the second critical structure of the disc that is extensively innervated. Its afferent nerve endings are found predominantly in the central regions of the endplate that adjoin the NP; several studies have demonstrated that degenerated discs have a more densely innervated endplate than normal controls.[10,11,55,56]

It is generally agreed that discogenic pain is exacerbated by loading conditions that increase the axial loads borne by the painful degenerated disc. Clinically, patients with presumed discogenic pain typically complain of pain in positions that involve flexion and loading of the lumbar spine. The load distribution of the spinal segment varies based on position. In extension, the loads are distributed to the disc and facet joints. In flexion, the loads are borne almost entirely through the disc.[57,58] Both the overall loads on the spine (determining the segmental loads) and the position of the spinal segment (determining the distribution of the segmental load between the disc and posterior elements) determine the magnitude of the load borne by the IVD. The likely origin of the predominance of flexion-related symptoms is the flexion moment exerted on the spine in flexion, which increases the overall loads on the spine, coupled with the segmental flexion of the affected segment seen in these positions.

The positions typically associated with symptoms of discogenic pain have been investigated, using disc pressures as a proxy for loads borne by the disc. The first of such studies was reported by Nachemson.[59] Findings of the pressure measurements in this study via an intradiscal manometer in 100 patients over 20 years show that reclined posture—compared with upright standing position—reduced intradiscal pressure by 50 to 80%; unsupported sitting (a common provocative position for patients with discogenic pain) increased intradiscal pressure by 40% compared with the standing position; and forward flexion holding 20 kg in front of the body increased pressure by 300% and added rotation, while decreasing the weight to 10 kg increased the pressure by 400%.

Sato et al[60] reported the results of intradiscal pressure monitoring in various positions in 8 healthy volunteers and 28 patients with ongoing low back pain or sciatica at L4/5. Findings in healthy subjects showed pressures of 91 kPa in the prone position, 151 kPa in the lateral, 539 kPa in the upright standing, 623 kPa in the upright sitting, and 1324 kPa in the flexed standing positions. Intradiscal pressure was found to be directly related to the degree of flexion of the motion segment. Recordings from degenerated discs were significantly lower, and the pressure varied inversely with the grade of degeneration. The lower values noted in degenerated discs coincide with cadaveric data that demonstrate disc pressure is not a useful proxy for disc loads in degenerated discs; this is likely related to the relative dehydration and nonfluid-like behavior of a degenerated disc.

It has been hypothesized that innervated, torn annular fibers, which are subject to shearing conditions during loading, may be the clinically important source of pain arising from annular portions of the disc. Loading in flexion, particularly in a hypermobile spinal segment in the early part of the degenerative cascade, leads to a posterior shift in the NP.[61] This posterior shift, coupled with radially directed forces caused by axial loads, exerts hoop stresses that are highest in the posterior anulus in this position of segmental flexion.[62] These hoop stresses are not resisted in the normal way by torn portions of the anulus—likely causing shearing or spreading of these annular tears, which, if innervated, could generate pain.

Similarly, type 1 Modic endplate changes have been suggested as demonstrating an identifiable endplate characteristic denoting an arthritic endplate (similar to chondral changes noted in an arthritic knee), unable to bear loads without generating significant pain.[63] Pain would be expected to vary directly with the load borne by the disc, manifested by increasing pain in positions of segmental lumbar flexion and overall applied load. However, these imaging findings have been noted in subjects with and without pain, calling their role in discogenic pain into question.

If structural features alone are not sufficient to make a disc painful on loading, then perhaps this can be explained by a combination of pathoanatomic characteristics, coupled with an element that increases the "sensitivity" of the nociceptors of the degenerated disc. Alterations in collagen content, fewer glycosaminoglycans, and a lower pH have been suggested as critical factors in painful disc degeneration.[64] Many investigators, however, have focused on alterations in the firing thresholds of disc nociceptive afferents as a way of accounting for the difference between painful and asymptomatic disc degeneration.

Afferent innervation can be grossly categorized into two types: those implicated in inflammatory pain, and those implicated in neuropathic pain. Those involved in inflammatory pain are thought to primarily function as nociceptors, susceptible to respond to decreases in receptor thresholds (e.g., increases in degree of inflammation) by firing more readily to stimuli (e.g., mechanical stresses). Innervation involved in neuropathic pain can be thought of as having a primary role other than pain perception; these nerves will only induce pain in an injury state. Differentiation of these two types of innervation can be performed by assessing receptor subtypes and morphological characteristics. Afferent neurons related to inflammatory pain are typically small, peptide-containing neurons that possess receptors for substance P and calcitonin gene-related peptide (CGRP). Conversely, neurons involved in neuropathic pain states can be small and nonpeptide-containing and typically bind to isolectin B4 (IB4).

Using such methods of analysis, innervation of the posterior anulus is predominantly inflammatory, and that of the anterior anulus is neuropathic.[11,16,65,66] Innervation of the endplate, transmitted by the basivertebral nerve, is also predominantly of the inflammatory subtype.[63] This line of investigation leads to the conclusion that posterior annular and endplate innervation is likely more important than anterior innervation in inflammatory (i.e., mechanical) pain states involving the disc. It is afferents of the inflammatory subtype (accounting for both radicular pain and mechanical discogenic pain) that are susceptible to inflammatory mediator-induced modification of neurophysiologic behavior.[65,67] Because of this fundamental similarity between radicular pain and mechanical discogenic low back pain, the pharmacologic strategies that seem promising in experimental models of radicular pain might be effective in discogenic pain (**Fig. 5.4**).

Clinical Studies of Discogenic Pain and Selective Anti-Inflammatories

Two open-label case series involving the use of TNF-α inhibitors for low back pain have been reported. Tobinick noted significant improvement in a cohort of 20 patients with chronic low back pain treated with 1 to 5 perispinal injections of a second TNF-α inhibitor, etanercept.[68] Also, an observational series of patients with inflammatory conditions treated with infliximab showed an 87% decrease in the Visual Analog Scale (VAS) scores for back pain.[69]

Two prospective, randomized, placebo-controlled studies of the use of selective antiinflammatories for chronic low back pain thought to be discogenic in origin had negative results. In a placebo-controlled, randomized trial of the matrix metalloproteinase inhibitor doxycycline (200 mg every day) in 50 patients with chronic low back pain, no beneficial effect was noted in the treatment group.[70] A second study entailed a placebo-controlled dose response trial of intradiscal etanercept in 36 patients with discogenic or radiculopathy; no significant benefit was noted in pain or disability in any of the patient groups.

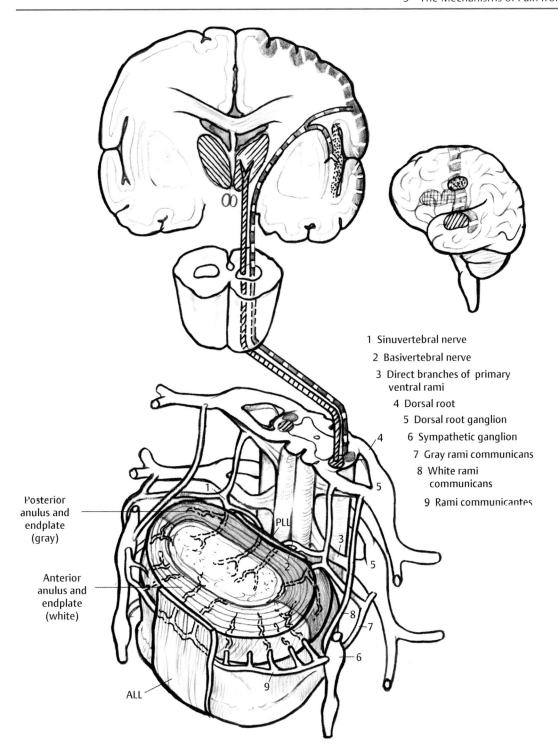

1 Sinuvertebral nerve

2 Basivertebral nerve

3 Direct branches of primary
ventral rami

4 Dorsal root

5 Dorsal root ganglion

6 Sympathetic ganglion

7 Gray rami communicans

8 White rami
communicans

9 Rami communicantes

Posterior
anulus and
endplate
(gray)

Anterior
anulus and
endplate
(white)

PLL

ALL

Fig. 5.4 Inflammatory versus neuropathic innervation of the vertebral endplate. ALL, anterior longitudinal ligament ; PLL, posterior longitudinal ligament.

■ Conclusion

Careful examination of the mechanisms of pain production at the level of the IVD leads to several conclusions. Mechanisms exist to allow for the generation of inflammatory pain but also for neuropathic pain. These types of pain are signaled by two distinct pain processing pathways and likely represent distinct clinical entities. It is likely that radicular pain and mechanical discogenic low back pain are both predominantly mediated by the inflammatory pain pathway, and that two features are important: sensitization of nociceptive afferents and mechanical stimulation of these sensitized afferents. We are currently able to assess the latter feature via static and dynamic imaging studies, but a method does not currently exist to objectively and clinically determine the degree of afferent sensitization. This degree of afferent sensitization

may be more critical in explaining the variability in the clinical course of patients with discogenic pain, compared with the more predictable presentation, natural history, and response to treatment of patients with radicular pain. It is our hope that the information presented here will aid in the assessment and treatment of patients with these clinical conditions.

References

1. Nakamura SI, Takahashi K, Takahashi Y, Yamagata M, Moriya H. The afferent pathways of discogenic low-back pain: evaluation of L2 spinal nerve infiltration. J Bone Joint Surg Br 1996;78(4):606–612
2. Wiberg G. Back pain in relation to the nerve supply of the intervertebral disc. Acta Orthop Scand 1949;19(2):211–221 illust.
3. Bogduk N. The innervation of the lumbar spine. Spine 1983;8(3):286–293
4. Bogduk N, Tynan W, Wilson AS. The nerve supply to the human lumbar intervertebral discs. J Anat 1981;132(Pt 1):39–56
5. Chen JD, Hou SX, Peng BG, Shi YM, Wu WW, Li L. Anatomical study of human lumbar spine innervation. Zhonghua Yi Xue Za Zhi 2007;87(9):602–605
6. Roofe PG. Innervation of annulus fibrosus and posterior longitudinal ligament. Arch Neurol Psychiatry 1940;44:100–103
7. Pedersen HE, Blunck CF, Gardner E. The anatomy of lumbosacral posterior rami and meningeal branches of spinal nerve (sinu-vertebral nerves), with an experimental study of their functions. J Bone Joint Surg Am 1956;38-A(2):377–391
8. Lotz JC, Ulrich JA. Innervation, inflammation, and hypermobility may characterize pathologic disc degeneration: review of animal model data. J Bone Joint Surg Am 2006;88(Suppl 2):76–82
9. Antonacci MD, Mody DR, Heggeness MH. Innervation of the human vertebral body: a histologic study. J Spinal Disord 1998;11(6):526–531
10. Fagan A, Moore R, Vernon Roberts B, Blumbergs P, Fraser R. ISSLS Prize winner. The innervation of the intervertebral disc: a quantitative analysis. Spine 2003;28(23):2570–2576
11. Brown MF, Hukkanen MV, McCarthy ID, et al. Sensory and sympathetic innervation of the vertebral endplate in patients with degenerative disc disease. J Bone Joint Surg Br 1997;79(1):147–153
12. Ohtori S, Inoue G, Koshi T, et al. Characteristics of sensory dorsal root ganglia neurons innervating the lumbar vertebral body in rats. J Pain 2007;8(6):483–488
13. Ohtori S, Takahashi K, Chiba T, Yamagata M, Sameda H, Moriya H. Sensory innervation of the dorsal portion of the lumbar intervertebral discs in rats. Spine 2001;26(8):946–950
14. Ohtori S, Takahashi Y, Takahashi K, et al. Sensory innervation of the dorsal portion of the lumbar intervertebral disc in rats. Spine 1999;24(22):2295–2299
15. Takahashi Y, Chiba T, Kurokawa M, Aoki Y, Takahashi K, Yamagata M. Stereoscopic structure of sensory nerve fibers in the lumbar spine and related tissues. Spine 2003;28(9):871–880
16. Aoki Y, Ohtori S, Takahashi K, et al. Innervation of the lumbar intervertebral disc by nerve growth factor-dependent neurons related to inflammatory pain. Spine 2004;29(10):1077–1081
17. Ozawa T, Aoki Y, Ohtori S, et al. The dorsal portion of the lumbar intervertebral disc is innervated primarily by small peptide-containing dorsal root ganglion neurons in rats. Neurosci Lett 2003;344(1):65–67
18. Zhang Y, Kerns JM, Anderson DG, et al. Sensory neurons and fibers from multiple spinal cord levels innervate the rabbit lumbar disc. Am J Phys Med Rehabil 2006;85(11):865–871
19. Takahashi Y, Nakajima Y, Sakamoto T, Moriya H, Takahashi K. Capsaicin applied to rat lumbar intervertebral disc causes extravasation in the groin skin: a possible mechanism of referred pain of the intervertebral disc. Neurosci Lett 1993;161(1):1–3
20. Higuchi K, Sato T. Anatomical study of lumbar spine innervation. Folia Morphol (Warsz) 2002;61(2):71–79
21. Morinaga T, Takahashi K, Yamagata M, et al. Sensory innervation to the anterior portion of lumbar intervertebral disc. Spine 1996;21(16):1848–1851
22. Takahashi Y, Morinaga T, Nakamura S, Suseki K, Takahashi K, Nakajima Y. Neural connection between the ventral portion of the lumbar intervertebral disc and the groin skin. J Neurosurg 1996;85(2):323–328
23. Suseki K, Takahashi Y, Takahashi K, et al. Innervation of the lumbar facet joints. Origins and functions. Spine 1997;22(5):477–485
24. Suseki K, Takahashi Y, Takahashi K, et al. CGRP-immunoreactive nerve fibers projecting to lumbar facet joints through the paravertebral sympathetic trunk in rats. Neurosci Lett 1996;221(1):41–44
25. Suseki K, Takahashi Y, Takahashi K, Chiba T, Yamagata M, Moriya H. Sensory nerve fibres from lumbar intervertebral discs pass through rami communicantes: a possible pathway for discogenic low back pain. J Bone Joint Surg Br 1998;80(4):737–742
26. Mixter W, Barr J. Rupture of intervertebral disc with involvement of the spinal canal. N Engl J Med 1934;211:210–214
27. Olmarker K, Storkson R, Berge OG. Pathogenesis of sciatic pain: a study of spontaneous behavior in rats exposed to experimental disc herniation. Spine 2002;27(12):1312–1317
28. Olmarker K, Blomquist J, Stromberg J, Nannmark U, Thomsen P, Rydevik B. Inflammatogenic properties of nucleus pulposus. Spine 1995;20(6):665–669
29. Olmarker K, Brisby H, Yabuki S, Nordborg C, Rydevik B. The effects of normal, frozen, and hyaluronidase-digested nucleus pulposus on nerve root structure and function. Spine 1997;22(5):471–475
30. Olmarker K, Larsson K. Tumor necrosis factor alpha and nucleus-pulposus-induced nerve root injury. Spine 1998;23(23):2538–2544
31. Kayama S, Konno S, Olmarker K, Yabuki S, Kikuchi S. Incision of the anulus fibrosus induces nerve root morphologic, vascular, and

functional changes: an experimental study. Spine 1996;21(22): 2539–2543

32. Geiss A, Larsson K, Rydevik B, Takahashi I, Olmarker K. Autoimmune properties of nucleus pulposus: an experimental study in pigs. Spine 2007;32(2):168–173

33. Rousseau MA, Ulrich JA, Bass EC, Rodriguez AG, Liu JJ, Lotz JC. Stab incision for inducing intervertebral disc degeneration in the rat. Spine 2007;32(1):17–24

34. Kuslich SD, Ulstrom CL, Michael CJ. The tissue origin of low back pain and sciatica: a report of pain response to tissue stimulation during operations on the lumbar spine using local anesthesia. Orthop Clin North Am 1991;22(2):181–187

35. Kayama S, Olmarker K, Larsson K, Sjögren-Jansson E, Lindahl A, Rydevik B. Cultured, autologous nucleus pulposus cells induce functional changes in spinal nerve roots. Spine 1998;23(20):2155–2158

36. Otani K, Arai I, Mao GP, Konno S, Olmarker K, Kikuchi S. Nucleus pulposus-induced nerve root injury: relationship between blood flow and motor nerve conduction velocity. Neurosurgery 1999; 45(3):614–619

37. Cohen SP, Wenzell D, Hurley RW, et al. A double-blind, placebo-controlled, dose-response pilot study evaluating intradiscal etanercept in patients with chronic discogenic low back pain or lumbosacral radiculopathy. Anesthesiology 2007;107(1):99–105

38. Igarashi T, Kikuchi S, Shubayev V, Myers RR. 2000 Volvo Award Winner in Basic Science Studies. Exogenous tumor necrosis factor-alpha mimics nucleus pulposus-induced neuropathology: molecular, histologic, and behavioral comparisons in rats. Spine 2000;25(23):2975–2980

39. Onda A, Hamba M, Yabuki S, Kikuchi S. Exogenous tumor necrosis factor-alpha induces abnormal discharges in rat dorsal horn neurons. Spine 2002;27(15):1618–1624

40. Onda A, Murata Y, Rydevik B, Larsson K, Kikuchi S, Olmarker K. Infliximab attenuates immunoreactivity of brain-derived neurotrophic factor in a rat model of herniated nucleus pulposus. Spine 2004;29(17):1857–1861

41. Murata Y, Onda A, Rydevik B, Takahashi K, Olmarker K. Selective inhibition of tumor necrosis factor-alpha prevents nucleus pulposus-induced histologic changes in the dorsal root ganglion. Spine 2004;29(22):2477–2484

42. Doi-Saika M, Tokunaga A, Senba E. Intradermal 5-HT induces Fos expression in rat dorsal horn neurons not via 5-HT3 but via 5-HT2A receptors. Neurosci Res 1997;29(2):143–149

43. Tokunaga A, Saika M, Senba E. 5-HT2A receptor subtype is involved in the thermal hyperalgesic mechanism of serotonin in the periphery. Pain 1998;76(3):349–355

44. Mulleman D, Mammou S, Griffoul I, Watier H, Goupille P. Pathophysiology of disk-related low back pain and sciatica. II. Evidence supporting treatment with TNF-alpha antagonists. Joint Bone Spine 2006;73(3):270–277

45. Karppinen J, Korhonen T, Malmivaara A, et al. Tumor necrosis factor-alpha monoclonal antibody, infliximab, used to manage severe sciatica. Spine 2003;28(8):750–753

46. Genevay S, Stingelin S, Gabay C. Efficacy of etanercept in the treatment of acute, severe sciatica: a pilot study. Ann Rheum Dis 2004; 63(9):1120–1123

47. Korhonen T, Karppinen J, Paimela L, et al. The treatment of disc-herniation-induced sciatica with infliximab: one-year follow-up results of FIRST II, a randomized controlled trial. Spine 2006; 31(24):2759–2766

48. Carragee E, Klapper J, Schaufele M, et al. Oral REN-1654 in sciatica: a phase 2, randomized, double-blind, placebo-controlled, multi-center study in subjects with pain due to lumbosacral radiculopathy. Spine J 2006;6(5):2S

49. Kanayama M, Hashimoto T, Shigenobu K, Oha F, Yamane S. New treatment of lumbar disc herniation involving 5-hydroxytryptamine 2A receptor inhibitor: a randomized controlled trial. J Neurosurg Spine 2005;2(4):441–446

50. Hou SX, Tang JG, Chen HS, Chen J. Chronic inflammation and compression of the dorsal root contribute to sciatica induced by the intervertebral disc herniation in rats. Pain 2003;105(1-2): 255–264

51. Omarker K, Myers RR. Pathogenesis of sciatic pain: role of herniated nucleus pulposus and deformation of spinal nerve root and dorsal root ganglion. Pain 1998;78(2):99–105

52. Boden SD. The use of radiographic imaging studies in the evaluation of patients who have degenerative disorders of the lumbar spine. J Bone Joint Surg Am 1996;78(1):114–124

53. Kirkaldy-Willis WH, Farfan HF. Instability of the lumbar spine. Clin Orthop Relat Res 1982;(165):110–123

54. Alamin T, Agarwal V, Carragee E. FAD vs provocative discography: comparative results and postoperative clinical outcome. Paper presented at North American Spine Society 22nd Annual Conference; October 23–27, 2007; Austin, TX

55. Freemont AJ, Jeziorska M, Hoyland JA, Rooney P, Kumar S. Mast cells in the pathogenesis of chronic back pain: a hypothesis. J Pathol 2002;197(3):281–285

56. Freemont AJ, Peacock TE, Goupille P, Hoyland JA, O'Brien J, Jayson MI. Nerve ingrowth into diseased intervertebral disc in chronic back pain. Lancet 1997;350(9072):178–181

57. Shirazi-Adl A. Biomechanics of the lumbar spine in sagittal/lateral moments. Spine 1994;19(21):2407–2414

58. Shirazi-Adl A, Drouin G. Nonlinear gross response analysis of a lumbar motion segment in combined sagittal loadings. J Biomech Eng 1988;110(3):216–222

59. Nachemson AL. Disc pressure measurements. Spine 1981;6(1):93–97

60. Sato K, Kikuchi S, Yonezawa T. In vivo intradiscal pressure measurement in healthy individuals and in patients with ongoing back problems. Spine 1999;24(23):2468–2474

61. Fennell AJ, Jones AP, Hukins DW. Migration of the nucleus pulposus within the intervertebral disc during flexion and extension of the spine. Spine 1996;21(23):2753–2757

62. Liu L, Pei F, Song Y, Zou L, Zhang C, Zhou Z. The influence of the intervertebral disc on stress distribution of the thoracolumbar vertebrae under destructive load. Chin J Traumatol 2002;5(5): 279–283

63. Ohtori S, Inoue G, Ito T, et al. Tumor necrosis factor-immunoreactive cells and PGP 9.5-immunoreactive nerve fibers in vertebral endplates of patients with discogenic low back pain and Modic type 1 or type 2 changes on MRI. Spine 2006;31(9): 1026–1031

64. Mooney V. What is going to happen to back pain? Discussion paper. J R Soc Med 1993;86(5):273–276

65. Ozawa T, Ohtori S, Inoue G, Aoki Y, Moriya H, Takahashi K. The degenerated lumbar intervertebral disc is innervated primarily by peptide-containing sensory nerve fibers in humans. Spine 2006; 31(21):2418–2422

66. Peng B, Wu W, Hou S, Li P, Zhang C, Yang Y. The pathogenesis of discogenic low back pain. J Bone Joint Surg Br 2005;87(1):62–67

degeneration involves a complex interplay of biologic and biomechanical events that are predisposed by genetic factors and modulated by environmental influences.

Degeneration of the spine is an inevitable consequence of aging. Miller et al reported an increase in disc degeneration from 16% at age 20 to ~98% at age 70 years based on macroscopic disc degeneration grades of 600 autopsy specimens. Interestingly, the authors noted that lumbar disc degeneration was already present in 11- to 19-year-old males and 10 years later in females.[2] Although spinal degeneration is inevitable with aging and invariably seen on MRI studies, it is typically asymptomatic.[3]

Kirkaldy-Willis et al postulated that injury or repetitive strain to the facet joint is a cardinal event in the spinal degenerative sequence.[1] More recently, the IVD has received considerable attention as the source of initial spinal motion segment dysfunction. Butler et al suggested that disc degeneration likely predates facet arthrosis based on a CT and MRI study.[4] The authors noted that in 68 patients (330 discs/390 facet joints) there were 144 degenerated discs and 41 levels with facet osteoarthritis. Disc degeneration without facet osteoarthritis was found at 108 levels, whereas all but one of 41 levels with facet degeneration also had disc degeneration.[4]

The widespread acceptance that spinal pain is thought to originate from the IVD is evidenced by the host of diagnostics (including discography) and therapeutic interventions directed toward the disc. Most treatments for painful discs, however, have met with inconsistent clinical outcomes,[5] probably reflecting a relatively unsophisticated approach to understanding spinal pain. Recent data supporting the idea of facet (zygapophyseal) joint mediated pain have come from studies of patients sustaining cervical whiplash injuries.[6,7] Lord et al evaluated cervical zygapophyseal joint pain after whiplash in a diagnostic double-blind study using placebo-controlled local anesthetic blocks. Sixty-eight patients with a predominant complaint of neck pain and headaches after a whiplash injury were evaluated. The authors noted that among patients with dominant headache, comparative blocks revealed that the prevalence of C2–C3 zygapophyseal joint pain was 50%. Overall, the prevalence of cervical zygapophyseal joint pain was 60%.[6,7] These studies support the complex interplay of the IVD and facet joints in health and disease of the spine.

Our understanding of spinal degeneration has advanced as we have appreciated that the degenerative cascade involves interplay of both biologic and biomechanical factors. Biochemical events are important in the pathogenesis of the degenerative process as well as in the pain-signaling pathways responsible for the clinical features of the condition. As we better appreciate the biologic aspects of spinal degeneration, less invasive, nonablative treatments designed to reverse these biologic processes and restore the disc and facet functioning may become a reality.

■ Intervertebral Disc Degeneration

IVD degeneration is a major cause of musculoskeletal disability in humans.[8–10] Degeneration has been linked to low back pain; however, the exact relationship between the two remains uncertain.[11,12] The macroscopic features characterizing disc degeneration include the formation of tears within the anulus fibrosus (AF), and progressive fraying and dehydration of the nucleus pulposus (NP) with eventual loss of the anular–nuclear distinction.[8,9,13] These pathologic alterations result in substantial changes in the functioning of the disc. Unquestionably, disc degeneration is a multifactorial process influenced by genetics, lifestyle conditions (including obesity, occupation, and smoking), biomechanical loading, and biochemical event.[14,15]

Intervertebral Disc Biomechanics

The disc is capable of converting axial spinal loads into tensile hoop stresses in the outer AF, while allowing motion of the vertebral segment. This behavior of the IVD is dependent on the distinct biomechanical properties of the NP and AF. The proteoglycan (PG)-rich NP acts as an internal semifluid mass, whereas the collagen-rich AF acts as a laminar fibrous container.[16] The hydrostatic properties of the disc arise from its high water content, which allows it to support such large loads.[17,18]

The NP in a young adult acts as a viscid fluid under applied pressure but also exhibits considerable elastic rebound, assuming its original physical state upon release.[19] Whereas a major function of the NP is to resist and redistribute compressive forces within the spine, the major function of the AF is to withstand tension. The unique combination of biochemical and biomechanical properties of the AF and NP allows the IVD to absorb and disperse the normal loading forces experienced by the spine.[19,20] When one of these two units, either the AF or NP, is compromised, degenerative changes ensue because of the alteration in mechanical force distribution across the functional spinal unit.

Horst and Brinckmann found that the stress distribution across the IVD and vertebral endplate depends on the degree of disc degeneration.[21] Under pure compressive and eccentric-compressive loading, the healthy lumbar IVD demonstrated a uniform stress distribution across the entire endplate area. Severely degenerated discs demonstrated the same uniform shape of stress distribution under compressive loading but a nonuniform stress distribution when loaded eccentrically. The asymmetry of the stress distribution in degenerated discs was found to increase with both angle of inclination and degree of degeneration. The asymmetric stress distribution was presumed to occur because of the relatively solid nature of the degenerated disc and its inability to conform to the eccentric loads. These results have been further supported by more recent studies as well.[22,23]

With advancing degeneration, it appears that the proportion of load transmission shifts to the posterior elements. Yang and King indirectly measured facet forces by using an intervertebral load cell to measure the load transferred through the disc.[11] The model predicted a significant increase in facet load for segments with degenerated discs. The increase was more prominent as the eccentricity of the applied compressive load increased posteriorly. This biomechanical sequence of disc degeneration leading to posterior element load bearing may, in fact, be what is observed clinically in that disc degeneration typically precedes facet arthrosis.[4]

Clinically, a common observation is that disc degeneration creates instability of the lumbar spine and, therefore, increases range of motion.[24] The interplay between the IVD geometric and material properties as well as facet joint competence is important in defining the stability of the involved motion segment.[25] Biomechanical studies suggest that changes in stability with disc degeneration are quite complex. The kinematic behavior of a simulated degenerative model under compressive and shear loading was studied by Frei et al.[26] The authors found greater axial translations under compression in the degenerated model (nucleotomy) compared with the normal disc. In anterior shear, the anterior translation was smaller in the degenerated specimens versus the normal specimens. Anterior shear was accompanied by a significant increase in coupled flexion rotation in the degenerative model, which could explain the counterintuitive decrease in translation. This was attributed to an increase in facet load in degenerated specimens during anterior shear loading. In addition, Fujiwara et al[27] found that in vitro cadaveric specimens had segmental motion changes, which were much greater in axial rotation compared with lateral bending, flexion, and extension. Ochia et al[28] also found an increase in torsional and flexion and extension movements in vivo. These kinematic studies ultimately can be related clinically to the concept that excessive motion beyond normal soft tissue or bony constraints causes compression or stretching of the neural elements, or deformation of the soft tissue.[29] These instabilities can cause abnormal motion and contact forces, as well as accelerate facet degeneration and osteoarthritis. Eventually as pointed out by Kirkaldy-Willis, with advancing degeneration the motion segment ultimately becomes less mobile, although the remaining motion may certainly be painful.[24] As the disc becomes less mobile, this may, in turn, decrease the intrinsic disc strength and may decrease nutrition to the disc.[30]

Besides spinal instability creating degenerative disc disease, another competing biomechanical cause for disc degeneration is the "wear and tear" hypothesis. In this mechanism, a series of minor mechanical traumas to the disc accumulate, eventually creating disc weakening. This weakening results in further injury, and a vicious cycle

ensues ultimately leading to disc degeneration.[31,32] If this model was the main reason for disc degeneration, a logical assumption would be that those who experienced heavy physical disc loading, particularly laborers, would have an elevated risk of disc degeneration. Most studies have shown an association between heavy physical loading and disc degeneration.[33–42] A study by Friberg and Hirsch, however, did not find an association between occupational and spine degeneration radiographically.[43] Other studies as well have not demonstrated a clear association.[33,44–48]

Whatever the biomechanical etiology for disc degeneration, researchers have attempted to define a relationship between biomechanical IVD alterations and symptomatology. More recently, disc dysfunction associated with axial back pain giving rise to so-called internal disc derangement has received considerable attention. MRI is a valuable diagnostic tool in assessing for internal disc derangement.[49] MRI allows determination of the proton density of the disc indicative of the state of hydration and can also identify the presence of annular tears. Aprill and Bogduk described the MRI high-intensity zone (HIZ), which they believe to be representative of an annular tear extending to the periphery of the disc.[50] The HIZ can be seen on spin echo T2-weighted (T2W) MRI scans as a high-intensity signal located in the substance of the posterior AF (**Figs. 6.2, 6.3**). The HIZ has been suggested as, but by no means confirmed to be, associated with discogenic axial back pain.[51,52]

Modic et al described adjacent bony endplate changes that occur with degeneration of the IVD.[53,54] Type 1 changes (decreased signal intensity on T1-weighted [T1W] spin-echo MRI scans and increased signal intensity on T2W MRI scans) were identified in 20 patients, type 2 changes (increased signal intensity on T1W MRI scans and isointense or slightly increased signal intensity on T2W MRI scans) in 77 patients, and type 3 changes (decreased signal on T1W and T2W MRI scans) in 16 patients. Histopathologic sections in cases of type 1 change demonstrated disruption and fissuring of the endplates and vascularized fibrous tissue, type 2 changes demonstrated yellow marrow replacement, and type 3 changes demonstrated loss of marrow and advanced bony sclerosis. These signal intensity changes appear to reflect a spectrum of vertebral body marrow changes associated with degenerative disc disease.[53]

Mechanical Treatments

As disc degeneration progresses, the resulting abnormal motion or instability is believed to be a cause of spinal pain, likely related to stretching of soft tissues and stimulation of free nerve endings.[24,25,55] Although a precise understanding of what constitutes spinal "instability" remains elusive, numerous treatments aimed at reducing painful spinal motion have been described. Physical therapy using stabilizing exercises has been proposed as an attempt to restabilize the

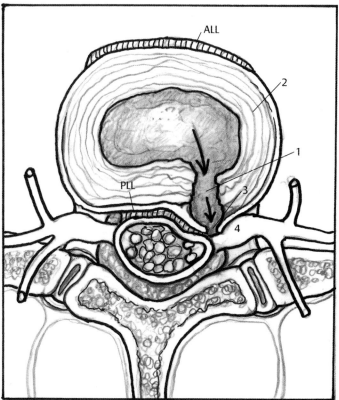

1 Nucleus pulposus:
phospholipase A2
PGs, No
Metalloproteinases
Inflammatory agents

2 Anulus

3 Fissure

4 Dorsal root
ganglion

Fig. 6.2 Biology of disc disruption. ALL, anterior longitudinal ligament; PLL, posterior longitudinal ligament.

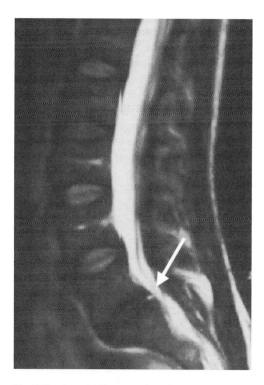

Fig. 6.3 A sagittal magnetic resonance imaging scan demonstrating a degenerated, collapsed L5–S1 disc space as evidenced by the loss of disc height and decreased T2-weighted signal. The white arrow points to an area along the posterior anulus exhibiting an increased T2-weighted signal representative of a high intensity zone.

"unstable" spine.[56,57] This approach may be more effective when painful segmental motion is the consequence of injury and dysfunction of the paraspinal muscle system that renders the motion segment biomechanically vulnerable in the neutral zone. The clinical diagnosis is based on the report of pain and the observation of movement dysfunction within the neutral zone and the associated finding of excessive intervertebral motion at the symptomatic level.

Other reported techniques for restabilizing the spine include intradiscal therapies such as intradiscal electrothermal therapy (IDET), which purportedly attempt to stiffen the motion segment by altering collagen fibers within the IVD.[58,59] Histologic studies of IVD material after IDET have reported histologic changes of collagen fibril denaturation in the posterior AF.[60] Another restabilization approach involves the use of posteriorly implanted "dynamic devices" that limit, but do not eliminate motion. These devices have been extensively implanted in patients in Europe for select cases of mechanical back pain with "instability." Total disc replacement, which provides axial stability while allowing for motion, is being increasingly used for the treatment of painful disc degeneration.

■ Facet Joint Biomechanics

Facet joints are true synovial articulations and undergo degenerative changes similar to those of osteoarthritis seen in other synovial joints.[11,61] The facet joints are one of the primary stabilizing structures of the spinal motion segment.[62,63] As the degenerative cascade progresses and anterior column support is lost, the facet joints bear more weight and the fulcrum moves dorsally to balance the motion segment.[64] With progressive spinal degeneration, the load-bearing patterns of the facet joints are altered.[27]

Fujiwara et al performed a biomechanical and imaging study of human cadaveric spinal motion segments to determine the effect of disc degeneration and facet joint osteoarthritis on the segmental flexibility of the lumbar spine.[27] The authors noted that axial rotation was most affected by disc degeneration. Facet cartilage degeneration, especially thinning of the cartilage, causes capsular ligament laxity, which may allow abnormal motion or hypermobility of the facet joint. The authors noted a significant linear correlation between facet cartilage thinning and disc degeneration in the male cadavers. Cartilage degeneration appeared to further increase the segmental movements already present in the hypermobile, degenerated disc.

Facetectomy studies have been performed by Sullivan et al in the lumbar spine of immature white rabbits to create a facet-mediated degenerative model.[65] The researchers resected the inferior articular process on one side at a selected vertebral level and on the opposite side at the adjacent level. The disc height was decreased at the surgical level in 50% of the discs at 6 months and 74% at 12 months. At 9 to 12 months, the discs showed thinning of the posterior AF, circumferential slits in the peripheral AF, and an increased area as well as decreased organization of the NP. The facet joints opposite the facetectomy began to show degeneration at 6 months. The authors concluded that the facet joint protects the IVD from rotational stresses.

Unquestionably, the facet joint complex has an important role in stabilizing the segmental spinal unit.[27,32,62,66,67] As disc disease progresses, increased stress is applied posteriorly accelerating facet osteoarthrosis. The resultant facet joint osteoarthrosis is likely to change the segmental spinal motion, altering the mechanical forces experienced by the IVD.

■ Biologic Factors

Cells residing in both the AF and NP actively regulate the homeostasis of IVD tissue. These cells maintain a balance between anabolism and catabolism by modulating a variety of substances including cytokines, enzymes, enzyme inhibitors, and growth factors in a paracrine and/or autocrine fashion.[13,68–70] Anabolic regulators include polypeptide growth factors, such as insulin-like growth factor (IGF), transforming growth factor-β (TGF-β), and bone morphogenetic proteins (BMPs). Other small molecules such as the synthetic peptide of link proteins have also been reported to

be regulators of matrix synthesis.[13,70,71] The catabolic process is also mediated by various enzymes, such as matrix metalloproteinases, aggrecanases, and cytokines.[72,73] The degeneration of an IVD results from an imbalance between the anabolic and catabolic processes, or the loss of steady-state metabolism that is maintained in the normal disc.

This delicate homeostatic balance affects the biomechanics of the IVD as well. A healthy IVD is populated by at least two morphologically distinct cell types.[74–79] Most cells are small and round, similar to chondrocytes. The second cell type is thought to be a remnant of the primitive notochord and has a vacuolated appearance and prominent intracellular glycogen deposits. Surrounding these cells is a matrix rich in large aggregating PGs. This matrix imbibes water allowing the NP to resist compressive forces. With disc degeneration, chondrocytic cells are replaced by fibrocytes synthesizing type I collagen.[9] The baseline synthesis of type II collagen also declines, altering collagen fiber cross-linking.[72,73,80] Additionally, a progressive loss of the PG matrix occurs, resulting in IVD dehydration and desiccation within the NP. These changes create a weaker biomechanical construct to resist compression and shear forces.[81] Last, an overall decrease in disc cell density with age and degeneration is seen. In studies of human IVDs, Gruber et al reported that apoptosis, or programmed cell death, largely accounts for this depopulation over time, and that interventions which delay or halt apoptotic cell death may constitute a means of treating degenerative disc disease.[74]

In addition to mediating disc degeneration, biochemical events appear to play a significant role in producing disabling spinal pain.[13,81,82] Biochemical events involved in discogenic pain production appear to include the production and release of inflammatory mediators and cytokines from the disc, vascular ingrowth into annular fissures, and the stimulation of free nerve endings in the outermost region of the disc.[83–85]

Studies have suggested nutrition as an important factor in the pathogenesis of disc disease.[9] To maintain the steady-state metabolism of cells, the IVD requires proper nutrition, which is accomplished by diffusion of nutrients through the endplates and into the IVD. Trauma, cigarette smoking, and other factors that affect the integrity of the endplates and endplate vasculature may affect diffusion and disturb the nutrition of the disc cells.[86] Vascular channels in the endplate of the IVD are particularly vital for maintaining the nutrition of the avascular NP. In degenerative discs, the diffusion capacity decreases creating a lower oxygen tension, decreased pH, and accumulation of catabolic byproducts. Typically, vascular channels at the endplate proliferate to maintain adequate nutrition of the disc. It has been claimed that the induction of new blood vessels in the endplate is facilitated by the activation of enzymes such as matrix metalloproteinases[87]; leading to the belief that with IVD injury the activation of these enzymes is the cause of increasing inflammation within the disc. This inflammation is the harbinger of further degeneration, culminating in a vicious cycle of accelerated degeneration. There are also reports that these channels ultimately disappear with disc degeneration and eventually become obliterated with calcification.[88,89] Further research using microangiography and immunohistochemical analysis is needed to determine if the loss in vascularity at the endplate can be reversed.

Genetic factors play a significant role in the degenerative spinal cascade. A twin study by Sambrook et al examined the hypothesis that disc degeneration has a major genetic component. Spine MRI scans were obtained for 86 pairs of monozygotic (MZ) twins and 154 dizygotic (DZ) twins. A substantial genetic influence on disc degeneration was found.[90] Further genetic predispositions to disc degeneration have been suggested by other studies on vitamin D receptor gene polymorphism.[91,92] The authors noted that in

205 young adults, allelic variation (*Tt* allele) in the vitamin D receptor gene was associated with multilevel and severe disc degeneration. Unquestionably, the genetic effect on the disc degeneration cascade requires further analysis.

Premise for Biologic Treatment

Current treatment options for degenerative disc disease address its clinical symptom, pain, as opposed to the pathophysiologic root of the disorder. Furthermore, traditional strategies such as fusion of the involved motion segment are not reliable and may even create instability at adjacent levels or even adjacent level degeneration.[93] In recent years, technologies such as disc replacement, aimed at restoring some degree of motion at the involved segment while eliminating pain, have begun to be studied.[94] However, these motion preserving techniques are appropriate for more advanced stages of spinal degeneration. With a better understanding of the sequence of biologic and biomechanical events associated

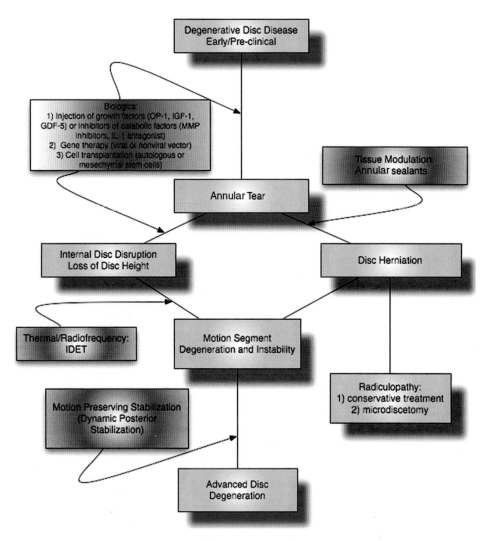

Fig. 6.4 Schematic depictions of therapeutic options for spinal degeneration, including biologic and traditional treatments.

with spinal degeneration comes the opportunity for earlier interventions (**Fig. 6.4**). With early disc and/or facet degeneration, biologic strategies aimed at reversing or retarding the degenerative process are appealing.

Biologic therapies can be considered to be structural modifying therapies (those that reverse or retard disc or facet degeneration) and/or symptom modifying therapies (those that provide relief from pain). Various biologic strategies to repair or regenerate the disc have been suggested.[5,60,95] Because the disc has only a limited intrinsic capacity for regeneration, the therapeutic approaches are generally geared toward the enhancement of matrix production by injecting proteins or using gene therapy. Some researchers have begun to increase the intrinsic capacity for regeneration by transplanting cells to the disc to repair the damaged disc matrix.[96–98]

One strategy for preventing, arresting, or reversing IVD degeneration is to increase the accumulation of the extracellular matrix by enhancing its synthesis and/or inhibiting its degradation through the introduction of biologic proteins directly into the IVD. Various candidates exist that fulfill these requirements; however, a complete understanding of all the factors involved is far from being complete. Factors that enhance synthesis include TGF-β1, BMP-2, and BMP-7. In vitro studies have already demonstrated that exogenous application of these growth factors can increase extracellular matrix synthesis by IVD cells.[99–102] In addition to increasing the synthesis of PGs, application of BMP-7 has been shown to increase disc height in normal rabbits and delay loss of disc height in a lapine model of IVD degeneration.[100,103] Blocking the effect of catabolic factors also holds promise. Matrix metalloproteinase 13 (MMP-13), otherwise known as collagenase-3, is recognized to be the most potent degrading enzyme of type II collagen, a principal component of IVD.[104,105] Degradation of the disc collagen, in turn, alters disc homeostasis and affects the IVD's ability to resist compressive and tensile stresses. For example, activation of MMPs can result in as much as 80% loss of tissue glycosaminoglycan content and destruction of the collagen matrix.[106] These changes result in matrix swelling and

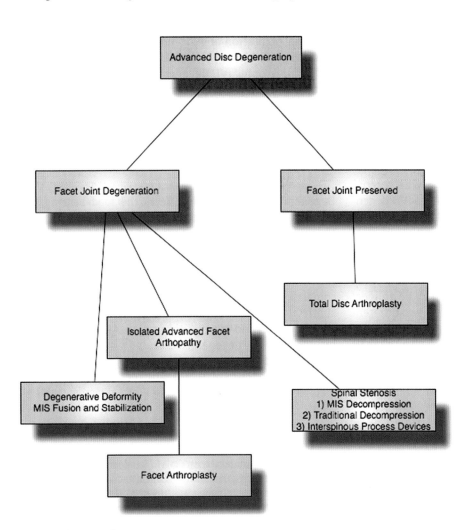

Fig. 6.4 (Continued)

48. Burns J, Loecker T, Fischer J, Bauer D. Prevalence and significance of spinal disc abnormalities in an asymptomatic acceleration subject panel. Aviat Space Environ Med 1996;67:849–853

49. Narvani A, Tsiridis E, Ishaque M, Wilson L. "Pig tail" technique in intradiscal electrothermal therapy. J Spinal Disord Tech 2003; 16:280–284

50. Aprill C, Bogduk N. High-intensity zone: a diagnostic sign of painful lumbar disc on magnetic resonance imaging. Br J Radiol 1992;65:361–369

51. Lam K, Carlin D, Mulholland R. Lumbar disc high-intensity zone: the value and significance of provocative discography in the determination of the discogenic pain source. Eur Spine J 2000; 9:36–41

52. Schellhas K. HIZ lesions. Spine 1997;22:1538

53. Modic M, Steinberg P, Ross J, Masaryk T, Carter J. Degenerative disk disease: assessment of changes in vertebral body marrow with MR imaging. Radiology 1988;166:193–199

54. Mitra D, Cassar-Pullicino V, McCall I. Longitudinal study of high intensity zones on MR of lumbar intervertebral discs. Clin Radiol 2004;59:1002–1008

55. Niosi C, Oxland T. Degenerative mechanics of the lumbar spine. Spine J 2004;4:202S–208S

56. O'Sullivan P. Lumbar segmental "instability": clinical presentation and specific stabilizing exercise management. Man Ther 2000;5: 2–12

57. McGill S. Low back stability: from formal description to issues for performance and rehabilitation. Exerc Sport Sci Rev 2001;29:26–31

58. Lee J, Lutz G, Campbell D, Rodeo S, Wright T. Stability of the lumbar spine after intradiscal electrothermal therapy. Arch Phys Med Rehabil 2001;82:120–122

59. Davis T, Delamarter R, Sra P, Goldstein T. The IDET procedure for chronic discogenic low back pain. Spine 2004;29:752–756

60. Shah R, Lutz G, Lee J, Doty S, Rodeo S. Intradiskal electrothermal therapy: a preliminary histologic study. Arch Phys Med Rehabil 2001;82:1230–1237

61. Yang K, An H, Ochia R, Lorenz E, Inoue N. In vivo measurement changes in lumbar facet joint width during torsion. Paper presented at 51st Annual Meeting of the Orthopaedic Research Society; February 20–23, 2005; Washington, DC

62. Adams M, Hutton W. Cadaver lumbar intervertebral joints. Spine 1980;5(5):483–484

63. Adams M, Hutton W. The mechanical function of the lumbar apophyseal joints. Spine 1983;8:327–330

64. Panjabi M, Goel V, Oxland T, et al. Human lumbar vertebrae: quantitative three-dimensional anatomy. Spine 1992;17:299–306

65. Sullivan J, Farfan H, Kahn D. Pathologic changes with intervertebral joint rotational instability in the rabbit. Can J Surg 1971; 14:71–79

66. Panjabi M, Oxland T, Yamamoto I, Crisco J. Mechanical behavior of the human lumbar and lumbosacral spine as shown by three-dimensional load-displacement curves. J Bone Joint Surg Am 1994; 76:413–424

67. Adams M, Hutton W, Stott J. The resistance to flexion of the lumbar intervertebral joint. Spine 1980;5:245–253

68. Roberts S, Caterson B, Menage J, Evans E, Jaffray D, Eisenstein S. Matrix metalloproteinases and aggrecanase: their role in disorders of the human intervertebral disc. Spine 2000;25:3005–3013

69. Oegema T. The role of disc cell heterogeneity in determining disc biochemistry: a speculation. Biochem Soc Trans 2002;30:839–844

70. Oegema T. Biochemistry of the intervertebral disc. Clin Sports Med 1993;12:419–439

71. Cadderdon R, Shimer A, Gilbertson L, Kang J. Advances in gene therapy for intervertebral disc degeneration. Spine J 2004;4: 341S–347S

72. Mwale F, Demers C, Petit A, et al. A synthetic peptide of link protein stimulates the biosynthesis of collagens II, IX, and proteoglycans by cells of the intervertebral disc. J Cell Biochem 2003; 88:1202–1213

73. Mwale F, Roughley P, Antoniou J. Distinction between the extracellular matrix of the nucleus pulposus and hyaline cartilage: a requisite for tissue engineering of intervertebral disc. Eur Cell Mater 2004;8:58–64

74. Gruber H, Norton H, Hanley E. Anti-apoptotic effects of IGF-1 and PDGF on human intervertebral disc cells in vitro. Spine 2000;25: 2153–2157

75. Gruber H, Leslie K, Ingram J, Norton H, Hanley E. Cell-based tissue engineering for the intervertebral disc: in vitro studies of human disc cell gene expression and matrix production within selected cell carriers. Spine J 2004;4:44–55

76. Gruber H, Leslie K, Ingram J, Hoelscher G, Norton H, Hanley E. Colony formation and matrix production by human anulus cells: modulation in three-dimensional culture. Spine 2004;29: E267–E274

77. Gruber H, Ingram J, Leslie K, Norton H, Hanley E. Cell shape and gene expression in human intervertebral disc cells: in vitro tissue engineering studies. Biotech Histochem 2003;78:109–117

78. Gruber H, Hanley E. Biologic strategies for the therapy of intervertebral disc degeneration. Expert Opin Biol Ther 2003;3:1209–1214

79. Gruber H, Hanley E. Observations on morphologic changes in the aging and degenerating human disc: secondary collagen alterations. BMC Musculoskelet Disord 2002;3:9

80. Pokharna H, Phillips F. Collagen crosslinks in human lumbar intervertebral disc aging. Spine 1998;23:1645–1648

81. Fujita K, Nakagawa T, Hirabayashi K, Nagai Y. Neutral proteinases in human intervertebral disc: role in degeneration and probable origin. Spine 1993;18:1766–1773

82. Takahashi M, Hoshino H, Ishihara C, Kushida K, Inoue T. The effect of prostaglandin E1 on human bone metabolism: evaluation by biochemical markers for bone turnover. Endocr Res 2000;26: 119–128

83. Kääpä E, Zhang L, Muona P, Holm S, Vanharanta H, Peltonen J. Expression of type I, III, and VI collagen mRNAs in experimentally injured porcine intervertebral disc. Connect Tissue Res 1994; 30:203–214

84. Kääpä E, Holm S, Han X, Takala T, Kovanen V, Vanharanta H. Collagens in the injured porcine intervertebral disc. J Orthop Res 1994;12:93–102

85. Kääpä E, Gronblad M, Holm S, Liesi P, Murtomaki S, Vanharanta H. Neural elements in the normal and experimentally injured porcine intervertebral disk. Eur Spine J 1994;3:137–142

86. Cinotti G, Della Rocca C, Romeo S, Vittur F, Toffanin R, Trasimeni G. Degenerative changes of porcine intervertebral disc induced by vertebral endplate injuries. Spine 2005;30:174–180

87. Crean J, Roberts S, Jaffray D, Eisenstein S, Duance V. Matrix metalloproteinases in the human intervertebral discs: role in disc degeneration and scoliosis. Spine 1997;22:2877–2884

88. Katz M, Hargens A, Garfin S. Intervertebral disc nutrition: diffusion versus convection. Clin Orthop Relat Res 1986;210:243–245

89. Holm S, Nachemson A. Nutrition of the intervertebral disc: acute effects of cigarette smoking. An experimental animal study. Ups J Med Sci 1988;93:91–99

90. Sambrook P, MacGregor A, Spector T. Genetic influences on cevical and lumbar disc degeneration: a magnetic resonance imaging study in twins. Arthritis Rheum 1999;42:366–372

91. Videman T, Leppavuori J, Kaprio J, et al. Intragenic polymorphisms of the vitamin D receptor gene associated with intervertebral disc degeneration. Spine 1998;23:2477–2485

92. Kawaguchi Y, Kanamori M, Ishihara H, Ohmori K, Matsui H, Kimura T. The association of lmbar disc disease with vitamin-D receptor gene polymorphism. J Bone Joint Surg Am 2002;84: 2022–2028

93. Ghiselli G, Wang J, Bhatia N, Hsu W, Dawson E. Adjacent segment degeneration in the lumbar spine. J Bone Joint Surg Am 2004;86: 1497–1503

94. Carl A, Ledet E, Yuan H, Sharan A. New developments in nucleus pulposus replacement technology. Spine J 2004; 4(6, Suppl) 325S–329S

95. Phillips F, Reuben J, Wetzel FT. Intervertebral disc degeneration adjacent to a lumbar fusion: an experimental rabbit model. J Bone Joint Surg Br 2002;84:289–294

96. Walsh A, Bradford D, Lotz J. In vivo growth factor treatment of degenerated intervertebral discs. Spine 2004;29:156–163

97. Nishida K, Doita M, Takada T, et al. Biological approach for treatment of degenerative disc diseases. Clin Calcium 2005;15:399–406

98. Moon S, Gilbertson L, Nishida K, et al. Human intervertebral disc cells are genetically modifiable by adenovirus-mediated gene transfer: implications for the clinical management of intervertebral disc disorders. Spine 2000;25:2573–2579

99. Takegami K, An H, Kumano F, et al. Osteogenic protein-1 is most effective in stimulating nucleus pulposus and annulus fibrosus cells to repair their matrix after chondroitinase ABC-induced chemonucleolysis. Spine J 2005;5:231–238

100. An H, Takegami K, Kamada H, et al. Intradiscal administration of osteogenic protein-1 increases intervertebral disc height and proteoglycan content in the nucleus pulposus in normal adolescent rabbits. Spine 2005;30:25–30

101. Li J, Kim K, Park J, Elmer W, Hutton W, Yoon S. BMP-2 and CDMP-2: stimulation of chondrocyte production of proteoglycans. J Orthop Sci 2003;8:829–835

102. Thompson J, Oegema T, Bradford D. Stimulation of mature canine intervertebral disc by growth factors. Spine 1991;16:253–260

103. An H, Masuda K. Relevance of in vitro and in vivo models for intervertebral disc degeneration. J Bone Joint Surg Am 2006;88:88–94

104. Reboul P, Pelletier J, Tardif G, Cloutier J, Martel-Pelletier J. The new collagenase, collagenase-3, is expressed and synthesized by human chondrocytes but not by synoviocytes, a role in osteoarthritis. J Clin Invest 1996;97:2011–2019

105. Mitchell P, Magna H, Reeves L, et al. Cloning expression, and type II collagenolytic activity of matrix metalloproteinase-13 from human osteoarthritic cartilage. J Clin Invest 1996;97:761–768

106. Bonassar L, Stinn J, Paguio C, et al. Activation and inhibition of endogenous matrix metalloproteinases in articular cartilage: effects on composition and biophysical properties. Arch Biochem Biophys 1996;333:359–367

107. Handa T, Ishihara H, Ohshima H, Osada R, Tsuji H, Obata K. Effects of hydrostatic pressure on matrix synthesis and matrix metalloproteinase production in the human lumbar intervertebral disc. Spine 1997;22:1085–1091

108. Risbud M, Shapiro I, Vaccaro A, Albert T. Stem cell regeneration of the nucleus pulposus. Spine J 2004;4:348S–353S

109. Franceschi R, Wang D, Krebsbach P, Rutherford R. Gene therapy for bone formation: in vitro and in vivo osteogenic activity of an adenovirus expressing BMP7. J Cell Biochem 2000;78:476–486

110. Ratko T, Cummings J, Blebea J, Matuszewski K. Clinical gene therapy for nonmalignant disease. Am J Med 2003;115:560–569

111. Nishida K, Kang J, Gilbertson L, et al. Modulation of the biological activity of the rabbit intervertebral disc by gene therapy: an in vivo study of adenovirus-mediated transfer of the human transforming growth factor beta 1 encoding gene. Spine 1999;24:2419–2425

112. Moon S, Nishida K, Gilbertson J, et al. Responsiveness of human intervertebral disc cells to adenovirus mediated transfer of TGF-B1 cDNA in 2D and 3D culture systems: comparison to exogenous TGF-B1. Paper presented at International Society for the Study of the Lumbar Spine Meeting; 2002; Adelaide, Australia

113. Larson J, Levicoff E, Gilbertson L, Kang J. Biologic modification of animal models of intervertebral disc degeneration. J Bone Joint Surg Am 2006;88:83–87

114. Paul R, Haydon R, Cheng H, et al. Potential use of Sox9 gene therapy for intervertebral degenerative disc disease. Spine 2003;28: 755–763

115. Moon S, Nishida K, Gilbertson L, Hall R, Robbins P, Kang J. Biologic response of human intervertebral disc cell to gene therapy cocktail. Paper presented at Orthopedic Research Society Meeting; 2001; San Francisco, CA

116. Prockop D. Marrow stromal cells as stem cells for nonhematopoietic tissues. Science 1997;276:71–74

117. Shimer A, Chadderdon R, Gilbertson L, Kang J. Gene therapy approaches for intervertebral disc degeneration. Spine 2004;29: 2770–2778

118. Liu L, Wang G, Lee K, et al. Expression of soluble TNF-RII from transduced human mesenchymal stem cells: in vitro and in vivo efficacy. Blood 1999;94:32

II Disc Herniation

7 Pathophysiology and Etiology of Intervertebral Disc Herniation

Cary R. Templin, Yu-Po Lee, and Steven R. Garfin

Herniation of the intervertebral disc (IVD) is the most common cause of radicular leg pain in working-age adults.[1] More than 250,000 elective lumbar spine operations are performed each year in the United States, and lumbar discectomy is the most common procedure.[2] The absolute incidence of disc herniation, however, is probably underestimated given the high rate of asymptomatic disc herniations observed in magnetic resonance imaging (MRI) studies.[3,4] Despite the common prevalence of disc herniation, much still remains unknown. It is unclear exactly what causes some herniations to present with pain and neurologic symptoms, whereas others are asymptomatic. In addition, what changes occur in a normal IVD that ultimately lead to a disc herniation?

The purpose of this chapter is to review the structure and function of the IVD and its surrounding structures as they relate to the pathophysiology of disc herniation. The etiology of disc herniation, and the biomechanical aspects of disc herniation, both degenerative and traumatic, will also be reviewed.

■ Pathophysiology

The state of the IVD is dynamic over its lifetime. Changes in the vascularity, nutrition, and cellular and molecular structure vary from early youth through adulthood. Physiologically, these changes seem to be patterned changes with age as the disc matures; however, "early degeneration" occurs quite frequently. This degenerative process leads to an increased inability of the disc to withstand physiologic loading. This can precipitate annular tearing and subsequent disc herniation. Disc degeneration, which commonly begins in early adulthood, may directly predispose the disc to herniation.[5]

Prior to the onset of the degenerative process, the nucleus pulposus (NP) is a homogeneous structure that serves a vital role in maintaining the mechanical function and structure of the disc. The healthy disc, with abundant hydration, largely hydrophilic proteoglycans, and a competent anulus, is ideal for absorbing complex loads early in life and in young adulthood. Beginning in the second decade, however, as the nucleus begins to lose its strongly hydrophilic proteoglycans, the disc becomes more solid and less adept at absorbing these loads and dispersing them to the surrounding structures.[5–8] As a result of the degenerative process, the nucleus becomes heterogeneous and absorbs axial loads in a nonuniform manner, with an altered transfer of load to the anulus and vertebral endplate. Loading moves from the more central endplate to the peripheral regions including the anulus (**Fig. 7.1**).[9] This uneven distribution of forces across the endplate increases as the degenerative process progresses. Subsequently, increased compressive and shear forces are transmitted to the anulus, stressing its fibers.[10,11] With continued strain on the annular fibers the result is fissuring and rupture of the annular complex. Stress concentration in the posterior anulus may predispose this region to disc prolapse.[10] Fissuring and concentration of stress to the posterolateral region permit the migration of nuclear fragments to the periphery of the disc and herald the herniation of disc material. This migration of nuclear material may occur in a gradual, or stepwise, fashion.[12]

Although the nucleus becomes less homogeneously structured through changes in its collagen framework and proteoglycan structure, it may become fragmented. The fragmented nucleus, when placed under load, typically follows the path of least resistance through radial annular fissures and is prone to protrusion or extrusion through the anulus (**Fig. 7.2**).[13] Mechanically induced herniation commonly occurs in patients around the age of 30 to 40 years.[14] Such patients have degenerated discs that have maintained some degree of hydration. This explains why herniation is much more likely in this age group than in those who are older. Conversely, the disc in the older population has typically become hardened, solidified, and stiff, and is less prone to herniation.

The inciting etiology of the herniation process is not fully understood but is thought to be multifactorial. Genetic inheritance, nutritional and metabolite supply, and mechanical forces are factors in the process.

Genetic Influences

Recent studies have implicated genetic influences as a major factor in early-onset disc degeneration.[15] Although physical loading in the form of lifting, torsional loading (e.g., lifting

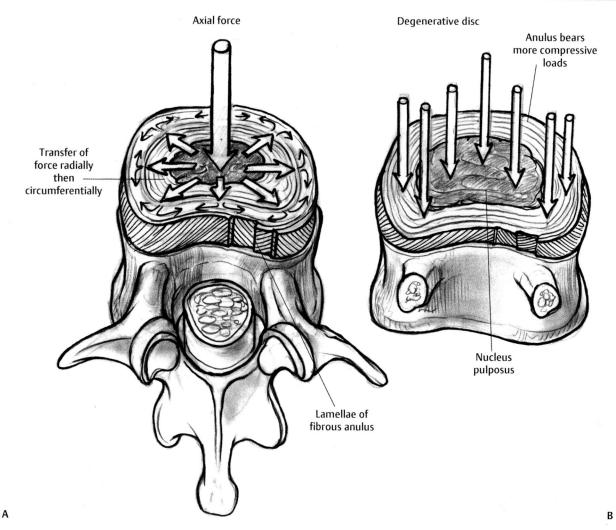

Axial force

Transfer of
force radially
then
circumferentially

Lamellae of
fibrous anulus

Degenerative disc

Anulus bears
more compressive
loads

Nucleus
pulposus

A   B

Fig. 7.1 **(A)** Depicts the transfer of force from an axial load in the central nucleus pulposus radially to the anulus fibrosus, where the force is directed circumferentially. Note the lamellar structure of the anulus with an alternating directional pattern of fibers, which resists multidirectional tensile forces. **(B)** With degeneration, the disc loses height, the nucleus has decreased potential for absorption and transfer of load, and the anulus bears more compressive loads.

and twisting or golfing), and driving have been identified as risk factors for disc degeneration and subsequent herniation,[16–18] some authors feel that these factors play only a minor role in the process in addition to genetic predisposition.[19–21] Twin and family studies have shown a strong genetic predisposition to disc disease.[20,22–26] Genotypical differences in collagen type IX have been shown to display advanced degenerative changes that may affect the crosslinking of type II collagen.[27,28] Kawaguchi et al[29] showed that multilevel disc degeneration occurred more frequently in a subset of patients with less genetic potential to form large aggrecan molecules. They did not, however, find an increased incidence of disc herniation in this population. This may be due to the loss of hydration and resultant increased stiffness of the disc.[15] In addition, vitamin D receptor and matrix metalloproteinase-3 alleles have been shown to predispose certain populations to disc disease. Virtanen and colleagues have mapped a possible location of the gene responsible to chromosome 21q, a finding that may offer further insight into the genetic influences of disc degeneration.[30]

Disc Biomechanics

The cellular morphology of the disc is distinct, based upon the region of the disc. Cells of the anulus are largely fibroblast-like cells, which are aligned parallel to the collagen within the lamella. In the nucleus, the cells, which resemble chondrocytes, become less abundant, more rounded, and less structured, forming clusters. In the inner annular layers, the cells display characteristics of both the nuclear and annular cells and appear fibrocartilaginous in nature.[14,31] Cells of the disc are responsive to mechanical loading and

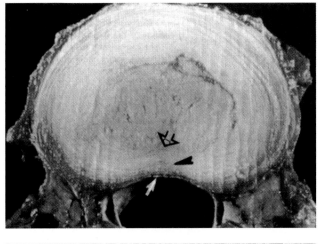
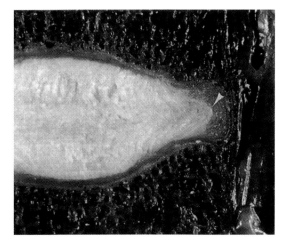
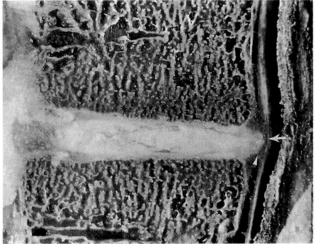

Fig. 7.2 **(A)** A transverse section of a well-preserved disc showing the posterior extent of the nucleus pulposus, which lies in a more posterior position. The annular fibers are less abundant posteriorly and the thin posterior longitudinal ligament is also present. **(B)** A fairly well preserved disc specimen displaying a disc prolapse into the anulus. The material has passed through the inner layers but is still confined by the outer layers of the anulus. **(C)** A degenerated disc specimen with extrusion of nuclear material. Note the fragmented nucleus has passed beyond the outer fibers of the anulus. (From Resnick D. Degenerative disease of the spine. In: Resnick D, ed. Diagnosis of Bone and Joint Disorders, 4th ed. Philadelphia: Saunders, 2002:1434–1435. Reprinted with permission.)

respond to both the type of load (i.e., compression or strain) as well as the direction and magnitude of the load.[32] Based on their typical loading patterns, disc cells are responsible for the processes that maintain the extracellular matrix through continued degradation and regeneration. In the healthy disc, these processes are balanced and serve to maintain the disc.[31] In the degenerate disc, however, the cells are unable to maintain and repair the degraded disc.

As the degenerative process takes place, there is alteration of the load pattern as areas of the anulus experience greater compressive loads, whereas a decompressed and heterogeneous nucleus is loaded irregularly. The response is an alteration of cellular signaling and thus in protein production. Herniated discs have been shown to contain increased matrix metalloproteinases (MMPs), nitric oxide, prostaglandin E2 (PGE-2), and interleukin-6 (IL-6).[33] The cells of the nucleus and the anulus respond differently to variable loads depending upon the intensity, duration, frequency, and direction of loading.[34–39] These cellular responses can affect the structure and composition of the extracellular matrix by stimulating the production of specific collagen types, as well as proteases

and proteoglycans that alter the disc's structural properties. Though paradoxical, the disc's attempts to fortify its structure cause it to become stiffer and thus alter its loading mechanics. Alteration of loads can lead to annular disruption and eventual disc collapse.

As the degenerated discs become structurally altered, they do not function optimally; hence, the NP becomes more susceptible to herniation. Degenerative discs have been shown to have a 25% decreased resistance to torsion, likely because of loss of tension in the collapsed nucleus and annular tissues.[40] Mimura et al[41] demonstrated that disc degeneration leads to increased laxity in motion in flexion–extension, axial rotation, and lateral bending. The anulus is also altered in degenerated discs, specifically posterolaterally, where the elastic modulus is found to be decreased in relation to the severity of the degeneration.[42] It is reasonable to think that increased strain on the anulus is likely a large factor in producing the annular defects necessary for herniation.

In a human cadaveric study Iencean found that herniation occurs at a significantly lower intradiscal pressure in discs with preexisting degeneration.[43] They also found that discs with more advanced degeneration sustained even lower pressures prior to herniation than those discs with early degenerative changes. Positioning in flexion further reduced the pressure required for herniation by additionally stressing the already degenerated fibers. Herniations in this study were found to occur most frequently in a paramedian direction.[43]

Tsuji et al[44] found that the paramedian or posterolateral aspect of the anulus had a less structured collagen arrangement, possibly predisposing it to annular tear and particulate herniation. Ohshima et al[45] suggested that the morphology of lumbar disc herniation was dependent on the size and development of the posterior longitudinal ligament (PLL). In the lower lumbar spine the PLL is less developed, and posterolateral disc displacement with PLL rupture was common.

Kuga and Kawabuchi[46] studied the effects of repetitive flexion and axial rotation in the IVD of the rat, which is histologically similar in structure to the human disc. They found histologically that the anulus of herniated discs showed disorganization of the lamellar structure with rupture, and that herniation occurred despite absence of focal compression to the nucleus.[46] Previously, in a similar study involving human discs in vitro, Gordon et al[47] developed a reliable model of disc herniation by repetitive loading in flexion, axial rotation, and compression. Discs failed by annular protrusion of the nucleus through annular tears, supporting the hypothesis that disc prolapse is peripheral in origin, with the anulus fibrosus serving as the primary site of pathologic change.[47]

Flexion–extension and lateral bending of the spine generates alteration of steady-state pressure in the IVD (**Fig. 7.3**). Flexion causes migration of the nucleus to the posterior aspect of the disc, whereas lateral bending causes the nucleus to be displaced contralateral to the side of bending as the tissues move from the area of high pressure to low.[48-50] Concurrently, the anulus, which is weaker dorsally than ventrally, is stretched, further lowering its ability to resist herniation.[48] Axial loading of the spine in conjunction with flexion–extension and rotational moments combine to induce disc herniation.[51] Torsional movements cause shifting of the spine's center of rotation to the posterolateral portion of the disc, and torsional loads have been proposed to induce lateral herniation.[52,53]

Certainly, although in vitro studies suggest the anulus as the primary site responsible for herniation, it is the combination of nuclear degeneration coupled with these complex forces upon the anulus that account for herniation. As the nucleus degenerates and more stress is transferred to the anulus and its lamellar structure, the disc has a greater propensity for peripheral breakdown and rupture. Degenerated annular fibers have a 30% decrease in yield and ultimate stress when compared with normal discs.[54] Reuber

et al[55] showed that degenerated discs subjected to combined compression and lateral bending were more prone to annular bulging than normal-appearing discs, showing their decreased structural integrity.

Brinckmann suggested that degeneration and fragmentation of the NP with its separation from the endplate is a prerequisite for herniation.[56] In his study, after radial sectioning of the anulus with the spine placed into complex loading positions, without fragmentation of the nucleus or separation from the endplate, herniation did not occur. Radial annular fissuring alone was not sufficient to cause herniation.[56] Simunic et al, however, showed that healthy discs that were compressed while fully flexed and fully hydrated were highly susceptible to intraannular prolapse through an existing annular division.[57] They found that flexion is a primary risk factor in disruption of the healthy disc nucleus. This is consistent with other literature in that flexion is a risk factor for herniation, primarily in discs that maintain their hydration, as in the young adult population.[49,58,59] Simunic et al further contend that degeneration which occurs in herniated disc specimens may occur after the prolapse event, rather than before, suggesting that the nucleus may be healthy and well hydrated prior to herniation.[57]

Using finite element analysis, Schmidt et al[60] found that combined moments in flexion-extension, lateral bending, and axial torsion led to higher stresses than pure moments alone, especially posterolaterally. Shear strain was maximal with lateral bend and flexion, whereas fiber strain was maximized with lateral bending with axial rotation.[60] It has been previously shown in cadaveric testing that peak stresses develop at the posterior anulus lateral to the midline of the disc.[61] It is a combination of moments to which the in vivo spine is most commonly subjected that likely predisposes to disc failure, especially posterolaterally.

In addition to complex directional loading causing herniation, Wilder et al[62] studied the disc's response to static and vibration loading in the seated position. A 1-hour seated exposure to vibration was able to produce significant changes in the mechanical properties of the lumbar disc. Static loading in this position was able to incite sudden motion segment instability in flexion or lateral bending and could apply tensile impact loading on the posterolateral aspect of the disc. They also found that loading after sustained vibration was sufficient to cause tracking tears proceeding from the nucleus to the peripheral posterolateral anulus.[62] This study emphasizes the role that both vibration and static loads may play in the etiology of disc herniation and helps to explain the increased incidence of disc herniation in truck drivers and others exposed to vibrational loads.

Ninomiya and Muro[63] studied the pathoanatomy of lumbar disc herniation using computed tomographic (CT)

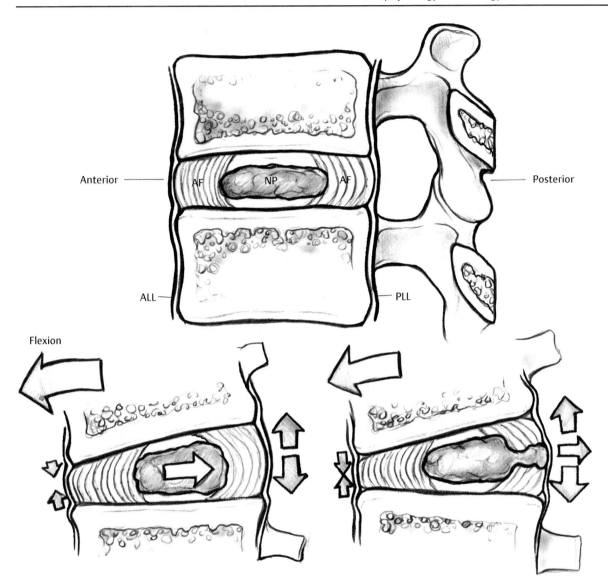

Fig. 7.3   This drawing of the intervertebral disc highlights the effect of flexion on the nucleus and anulus. When flexed, the posterior aspect of the anulus is loaded in tension, while anteriorly there is compression. Concurrently, the nucleus is forced posteriorly. With progressive gradual disruption of the anulus from complex loading posteriorly and posterolaterally, nuclear tissue herniates through annular fissures. AF, anulus fibrosus; NP, nucleus pulposus; ALL, anterior longitudinal ligament; PLL, posterior longitudinal ligament.

discography. They found that as the disc degenerates, radial fissures develop, and the path of herniation proceeds directly parallel to the sagittal plane at the central or paracentral portion of the disc (**Fig. 7.4**). Herniations following this path protruded to the dura and nerve roots. Herniations in the foraminal and extraforaminal region proceed obliquely to the sagittal plane at the posterolateral portion of the disc. Discography has shown that most herniations occurred in the inferior aspect of the disc.[63] The development of radial fissures was proposed to occur with the confluence of posterior annular circumferential fissures and perinuclear annular fissures. Discograms can confirm the pathway of migration of nuclear material to the spinal canal (**Fig. 7.5**).

■ Etiology of Symptoms

After the disc is prolapsed, it may affect the nerve roots in many ways. First of all, the fragment may cause direct compression of the nerve root. This may lead to alteration of the physiologic function of the nerve and may manifest as pain, weakness, or sensory disturbance in the nerve's distribution. The amount of canal compromise has been found to correlate

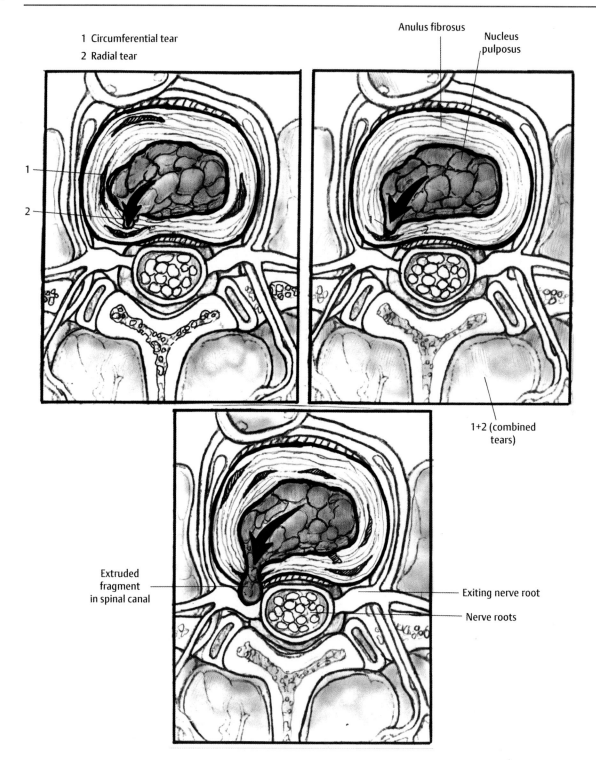

1 Circumferential tear
2 Radial tear

Anulus fibrosus
Nucleus pulposus

1+2 (combined tears)

Extruded fragment in spinal canal
Exiting nerve root
Nerve roots

Fig. 7.4 Progression of the herniation process. Circumferential and radial annular disruptions combine to allow propagation of nuclear material (shaded) to the disc periphery (disc protrusion). Continued mechanical stress and structural disruption of the disc result in migration of the nuclear material beyond the anulus (extruded fragment) and can eventually completely separate from the disc to lie free within the spinal canal as a sequestrated fragment.

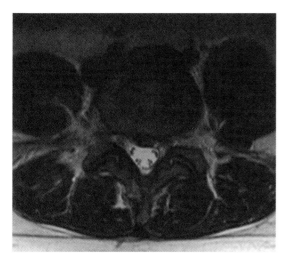 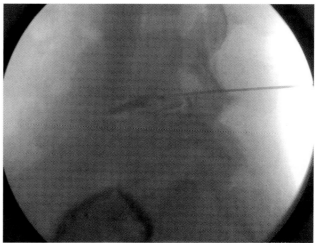

Fig. 7.5 **(A)** This lateral fluoroscopic image after the injection of contrast material into the disc shows the degeneration in the disc of a 23-year-old female patient. Annular disruption is evident with contrast extravasation from the nucleus to the periphery. The pathway of migration through the inferior aspect of the disc is apparent. The outline of the herniated fragment is evident within the spinal canal. **(B)** This axial T2-weighted magnetic resonance imaging scan in the same patient shows a centrally extruded disc fragment. The migration pathway of the herniated fragment is evident by the right paracentral annular disruption.

with the clinical success with surgical intervention, but the location of the herniation and its relation to the nerve root is an important factor in the symptomatology.[64,65]

The inflammatory cascade is believed to play a role in the production of symptoms after disc herniation. Aside from direct compression of the nerve root, herniated disc fragments have been shown to incite an inflammatory reaction in animal studies and in human specimens obtained at surgery.[66–68] The inflammatory cascade is believed to play a role in the production of symptoms after disc herniation.[69] Inflammatory cytokines such as IL-1 and tumor necrosis factor-α (TNF-α) have been implicated in inciting the pain response.[8,70]

Because of the inflammatory aspect of the herniated disc, directed antiinflammatory therapy has been attempted. Transforaminal injection of steroid has shown success in decreasing the symptoms of disc herniation.[71,72] Efforts to use infliximab (Centocor, Malvern, PA), a TNF-α blocker, however, have not shown strongly positive results despite success in decreasing inflammation in vitro.[73,74]

■ Conclusion

Although lumbar disc herniation can occur in the young healthy disc when overwhelming stress is place upon it, this rarely occurs. Typically, lumbar disc herniation occurs in individuals with preexisting disc degeneration, which may or may not be symptomatic. Given the pathophysiology of disc degeneration with alteration in metabolite transport and structure, the pathway toward disc herniation can be understood, but the inciting factors are currently unknown. The potential for the lumbar disc to heal once structural changes have occurred is minimal. This process is further complicated by the loss of nutritional support and paradoxical loading of the disc. Such paradoxical loads serve to affect the disc's cellular responses and further promote the degenerative process leading to further annular fissuring and fragmentation of the nuclear tissues.

Adams et al point out that the loss of structural integrity of the disc is truly the definition of degeneration.[14] An MRI study of asymptomatic patients showed that the presence of a more extensive disc herniation is a risk factor for advancing degeneration, thus highlighting the lack of structural support that presents with disc degeneration and subsequent herniation.[75] This finding suggests that once the disc is damaged structurally, the degenerative process is likely inevitable.

The biomechanics of the lumbar spine place the greatest stresses on the posterolateral aspect of the disc through flexion–extension, lateral bending, and torsional loads. With alterations in the structural integrity of this area of the anulus, the disc can no longer meet its physiologic demands. Compressive forces normally transmitted into tensile forces within the anulus can no longer be resisted and annular failure ensues. As the nucleus is repetitively loaded, fragmented tissue follows the path of least resistance, culminating in herniation of the disc.

References

1. Frymoyer JW. Back pain and sciatica. N Engl J Med 1988;318(5): 291–300

2. Weinstein JN, Tosteson TD, Lurie JD, et al. Surgical vs nonoperative treatment for lumbar disk herniation: the Spine Patient Outcomes Research Trial (SPORT): a randomized trial. JAMA 2006;296(20): 2441–2450

3. Boden SD, Davis DO, Dina TS, Patronas NJ, Wiesel SW. Abnormal magnetic-resonance scans of the lumbar spine in asymptomatic subjects: a prospective investigation. J Bone Joint Surg Am 1990;72(3):403–408

4. Jensen MC, Brant-Zawadzki MN, Obuchowski N, et al. Magnetic resonance imaging of the lumbar spine in people without back pain. N Engl J Med 1994;331(2):69–73

5. Hadjipavlou AG, Simmons JW, Pope MH, Necessary JT, Goel VK. Pathomechanics and clinical relevance of disc degeneration and annular tear: a point-of-view review. Am J Orthop 1999;28(10):561–571

6. Buckwalter JA. Aging and degeneration of the human intervertebral disc. Spine 1995;20(11):1307–1314

7. Miller JA, Schmatz C, Schultz AB. Lumbar disc degeneration: correlation with age, sex, and spine level in 600 autopsy specimens. Spine 1988;13(2):173–178

8. Anderson DG, Tannoury C. Molecular pathogenic factors in symptomatic disc degeneration. Spine J 2005;5(6, Suppl):260S–266S

9. Kurowski P, Kubo A. The relationship of degeneration of the intervertebral disc to mechanical loading conditions on lumbar vertebrae. Spine 1986;11(7):726–731

10. Adams MA, McNally DS, Dolan P. "Stress" distributions inside intervertebral discs: the effects of age and degeneration. J Bone Joint Surg Br 1996;78(6):965–972

11. Adams MA, McMillan DW, Green TP, Dolan P. Sustained loading generates stress concentrations in lumbar intervertebral discs. Spine 1996;21(4):434–438

12. Adams MA, Hutton WC. Gradual disc prolapse. Spine 1985;10(6): 524–531

13. Moore RJ, Vernon-Roberts B, Fraser RD, Osti OL, Schembri M. The origin and fate of herniated lumbar intervertebral disc tissue. Spine 1996;21(18):2149–2155

14. Adams MA, Roughley PJ. What is intervertebral disc degeneration, and what causes it? Spine 2006;31(18):2151–2161

15. Ala-Kokko L. Genetic risk factors for lumbar disc disease. Ann Med 2002;34(1):42–47

16. Heliovaara M, Impivaara O, Sievers K, et al. Lumbar disc syndrome in Finland. J Epidemiol Community Health 1987;41:251–258

17. Heliovaara M. Risk factors for low back pain and sciatica. Ann Med 1989;21:257–264

18. Kelsey JL, Githens PB, O'Conner T, et al. Acute prolapsed lumbar intervertebral disc: an epidemiologic study with special reference to driving automobiles and cigarette smoking. Spine 1984;9: 608–613

19. Kuh DJ, Coggan D, Mann S, Cooper C, Yusuf E. Height, occupation and back pain in a national prospective study. Br J Rheumatol 1993;32:911–916

20. Battieá MC, Videman T, Gibbons LE, Fisher LD, Manninen H, Gill K. 1995 Volvo Award in Clinical Sciences. Determinants of lumbar disc degeneration: a study relating lifetime exposures and magnetic resonance imaging findings in identical twins. Spine 1995; 20:2601–2612

21. Virtanen IM, Karppinen J, Taimela S, et al. Occupational and genetic risk factors associated with intervertebral disc disease. Spine 2007;32(10):1129–1134

22. Sambrook PN, MacGregor AJ, Spector TD. Genetic influences on cervical and lumbar disc degeneration: a magnetic resonance imaging study in twins. Arthritis Rheum 1999;42:366–372

23. Heikkilaü JK, Koskenvuo M, Heliovaara M, et al. Genetic and environmental factors in sciatica: evidence from a nationwide panel of 9365 adult twin pairs. Ann Med 1989;21:393–398

24. Varlotta GP, Brown MD, Kelsey JL, Golden AL. Familial predisposition for herniation of a lumbar disc in patients who were less than twenty-one years old. J Bone Joint Surg Am 1991;73:124–128

25. Matsui H, Terahata N, Tsuji H, Hirano N, Naruse Y. Familial predisposition and clustering for juvenile lumbar disc herniation. Spine 1992;17:1323–1328

26. Scapinelli R. Lumbar disc herniation in eight siblings with a positive family history for disc disease. Acta Orthop Belg 1993;59:371–376

27. Annunen S, Paassilta P, Lohiniva J, et al. An allele of COL9A2 associated with intervertebral disc disease. Science 1999;285:409–412

28. Paassilta P, Lohiniva J, Goring HHH, et al. Identification of a novel common genetic risk factor for lumbar disc disease. JAMA 2001; 285:1843–1849

29. Kawaguchi Y, Osada R, Kanamori M, et al. Association between an aggrecan gene polymorphism and lumbar disc degeneration. Spine 1999;24(23):2456–2460

30. Virtanen IM, Noponen N, Barral S, et al. Putative susceptibility locus on chromosome 21q for lumbar disc disease (LDD) in the Finnish population. J Bone Miner Res 2007;22(5):701–707

31. Bibby SR, Jones DA, Lee RB, Yu J, Urban JPG. The pathophysiology of the intervertebral disc. Joint Bone Spine 2001;68(6):537–542

32. Setton LA, Chen J. Mechanobiology of the intervertebral disc and relevance to disc degeneration. J Bone Joint Surg Am 2006; 88(Suppl 2):52–57

33. Kang JD, Stefanovic-Racic M, McIntyre LA, Georgescu HI, Evans CH. Toward a biochemical understanding of human intervertebral disc degeneration and herniation: contributions of nitric oxide, interleukins, prostaglandin E2, and matrix metalloproteinases. Spine 1997;22(10):1065–1073

34. Hutton WC, Toribatake Y, Elmer WA, Ganey TM, Tomita K, Whitesides TE. The effect of compressive force applied to the intervertebral disc in vivo: a study of proteoglycans and collagen. Spine 1998;23(23):2524–2537

35. Terahata N, Ishihara H, Ohshima H, Hirano N, Tsuji H. Effects of axial traction stress on solute transport and proteoglycan synthesis in the porcine intervertebral disc in vitro. Eur Spine J 1994;3(6):325–330

36. Ishihara H, McNally DS, Urban JP, Hall AC. Effects of hydrostatic pressure on matrix synthesis in different regions of the intervertebral disk. J Appl Physiol 1996;80(3):839–846

37. Rannou F, Maite C, Michel R, Poiraudeau S. Disk degeneration and disk herniation: the contribution of mechanical stress. Joint Bone Spine 2001;68:543–546

38. Matsumoto T, Kawakami M, Kuribayashi K, Takenaka T, Tamaki T. Cyclic mechanical stretch stress increases the growth rate and collagen synthesis of nucleus pulposus cells in vitro. Spine 1999; 24(4):315–319

39. Handa T, Ishihara H, Ohshima H, Osada R, Tsuji H, Obata K. Effects of hydrostatic pressure on matrix synthesis and matrix

metalloproteinase production in the human lumbar intervertebral disc. Spine 1997;22(10):1085–1091

40. Farfan HF, Cossette JW, Robertson GH, Wells RV, Kraus H. The effects of torsion on the lumbar intervertebral joints: the role of torsion in the production of disc degeneration. J Bone Joint Surg Am 1970;52(3):468–497

41. Mimura M, Panjabi MM, Oxland TR, Crisco JJ, Yamamoto I, Vasavada A. Disc degeneration affects the multidirectional flexibility of the lumbar spine. Spine 1994;19(12):1371–1380

42. Umehara S, Tadano S, Abumi K, Katagiri K, Kaneda K, Ukai T. Effects of degeneration on the elastic modulus distribution in the lumbar intervertebral disc. Spine 1996;21(7):811–819

43. Iencean SM. Lumbar intervertebral disc herniation following experimental intradiscal pressure increase. Acta Neurochir (Wien) 2000;142(6):669–676

44. Tsuji H, Hirano N, Ohshima H, Ishihara H, Terahata N, Motoe T. Structural variation of the anterior and posterior anulus fibrosus in the development of human lumbar intervertebral disc: a risk factor for intervertebral disc rupture. Spine 1993;18(2):204–210

45. Ohshima H, Hirano N, Osada R, Matsui H, Tsuji H. Morphologic variation of lumbar posterior longitudinal ligament and the modality of disc herniation. Spine 1993;18(16):2408–2411

46. Kuga N, Kawabuchi M. Histology of intervertebral disc protrusion: an experimental study using an aged rat model. Spine 2001; 26(17):E379–E384

47. Gordon SJ, Yang KH, Mayer PJ, Mace AH Jr, Kish VL, Radin EL. Mechanism of disc rupture: a preliminary report. Spine 1991; 16(4):450–456

48. Benzel EC. Degenerative and inflammatory diseases of the spine. In: Benzel EC, ed. Biomechanics of Spine Stabilization. Rolling Meadows, IL: American Association of Neurological Surgeons; 2001

49. Adams MA, Hutton WC. 1981 Volvo Award in Basic Science. Prolapsed intervertebral disc: a hyperflexion injury. Spine 1982;7(3): 184–191

50. Krag MH, Seroussi RE, Wilder DG, Pope MH. Internal displacement distribution from in vitro loading of human thoracic and lumbar spinal motion segments: experimental results and theoretical predictions. Spine 1987;12(10):1001–1007

51. Goel VK, Voo LM, Weinstein JN, Liu YK, Okuma T, Njus GO. Response of the ligamentous lumbar spine to cyclic bending loads. Spine 1988;13(3):294–300

52. Cossette JW, Farfan HF, Robertson GH, Wells RV. The instantaneous center of rotation of the third lumbar intervertebral joint. J Biomech 1971;4(2):149–153

53. Bogduk N. Pathology of lumbar disc pain. J Manag Med 1990;5: 72–79

54. Fujita Y, Duncan NA, Lotz JC. Radial tensile properties of the lumbar annulus fibrosus are site and degeneration dependent. J Orthop Res 1997;15(6):814–819

55. Reuber M, Schultz A, Denis F, Spencer D. Bulging of lumbar intervertebral disks. J Biomech Eng 1982;104(3):187–192

56. Brinckmann P. Injury of the annulus fibrosus and disc protrusions: an in vitro investigation on human lumbar discs. Spine 1986;11(2): 149–153

57. Simunic DI, Broom ND, Robertson PA. Biomechanical factors influencing nuclear disruption of the intervertebral disc. Spine 2001;26(11):1223–1230

58. Andersson GB, Schultz AB. Effects of fluid injection on mechanical properties of intervertebral discs. J Biomech 1979;12(6):453–458

59. Nachemson A. The load on lumbar disks in different positions of the body. Clin Orthop Relat Res 1966;45:107–122

60. Schmidt H, Kettler A, Heuer F, Simon U, Claes L, Wilke HJ. Intradiscal pressure, shear strain, and fiber strain in the intervertebral disc under combined loading. Spine 2007;32(7):748–755

61. Edwards WT, Ordway NR, Zheng Y, McCullen G, Han Z, Yuan HA. Peak stresses observed in the posterior lateral annulus. Spine 2001;26(16):1753–1759

62. Wilder DG, Pope MH, Frymoyer JW. The biomechanics of lumbar disc herniation and the effect of overload and instability. J Spinal Disord 1988;1(1):16–32

63. Ninomiya M, Muro T. Pathoanatomy of lumbar disc herniation as demonstrated by computed tomography/discography. Spine 1992;17(11):1316–1322

64. Carlisle E, Luna M, Tsou PM, Wang JC. Percent spinal canal compromise on MRI utilized for predicting the need for surgical treatment in single-level lumbar intervertebral disc herniation. Spine J 2005;5(6):608–614

65. Carragee EJ, Kim DH. A prospective analysis of magnetic resonance imaging findings in patients with sciatica and lumbar disc herniation: correlation of outcomes with disc fragment and canal morphology. Spine 1997;22(14):1650–1660

66. Hasegawa T, An HS, Inufusa A, Mikawa Y, Watanabe R. The effect of age on inflammatory responses and nerve root injuries after lumbar disc herniation: an experimental study in a canine model. Spine 2000;25(8):937–940

67. Gronblad M, Virri J, Tolonen J, et al. A controlled immunohistochemical study of inflammatory cells in disc herniation tissue. Spine 1994;19(24):2744–2751

68. Habtemariam A, Gronblad M, Virri J, Seitsalo S, Karaharju E. A comparative immunohistochemical study of inflammatory cells in acute-stage and chronic-stage disc herniations. Spine 1998;23(20): 2159–2165

69. Nygaard OP, Mellgren SI, Osterud B. The inflammatory properties of contained and noncontained lumbar disc herniation. Spine 1997;22(21):2484–2488

70. Yoshida M, Nakamura T, Sei A, Kikuchi T, Takagi K, Matsukawa A. Intervertebral disc cells produce tumor necrosis factor alpha, interleukin-1beta, and monocyte chemoattractant protein-1 immediately after herniation: an experimental study using a new hernia model. Spine 2005;30(1):55–61

71. Riew KD, Yin Y, Gilula L, et al. The effect of nerve-root injections on the need for operative treatment of lumbar radicular pain: a prospective, randomized, controlled, double-blind study. J Bone Joint Surg Am 2000;82-A(11):1589–1593

72. Wang JC, Lin E, Brodke DS, Youssef JA. Epidural injections for the treatment of symptomatic lumbar herniated discs. J Spinal Disord Tech 2002;15(4):269–272

73. Korhonen T, Karppinen J, Paimela L, et al. The treatment of disc-herniation-induced sciatica with infliximab: one-year follow-up results of FIRST II, a randomized controlled trial. Spine 2006;31(24):2759–2766

74. Autio RA, Karppinen J, Niinimaki J, et al. The effect of infliximab, a monoclonal antibody against TNF-alpha, on disc herniation resorption: a randomized controlled study. Spine 2006;31(23): 2641–2645

75. Elfering A, Semmer N, Birkhofer D, Zanetti M, Hodler J, Boos N. Risk factors for lumbar disc degeneration: a 5-year prospective MRI study in asymptomatic individuals. Spine 2002;27(2):125–134

8 Clinical Features of Herniated Nucleus Pulposus

Stewart M. Kerr, Deepan N. Patel, and Alexander R. Vaccaro

Intervertebral discs (IVDs) provide for a segmental arrangement to the spinal column which allows for movement and flexibility in what would otherwise be an immobile rigid column of bone. The IVD, like most connective tissue, consists of a sparse cell population. It is comprised of the outer and inner anulus fibrosus (AF) and a central gelatinous, semicompressible core—the nucleus pulposus (NP). These structures are composed largely of proteoglycans and the fibrillar collagens (type I and II), the ratio of which favors a preponderance of type II collagen with increasing proteoglycan concentration toward the disc center.[1–5]

With aging, the AF collagen fibers become more disorganized and also can harden; fissures can form within these fibers and occasionally extend full thickness. This may allow for protrusion of the inner, gelatinous nucleus pulposus. A herniated nucleus pulposus (HNP) usually occurs in a posterior or posterolateral direction as a result of relative interface weakness between the outer AF, its vertebral body insertion, and the posterior longitudinal ligament. Herniated tissue frequently results in compression of neural or neurovascular structures potentially causing pain and neurologic dysfunction.[6]

In this chapter, we will review the risk factors and clinical features of herniated lumbar nucleus pulposus, which may include axial pain and a wide array of sensory–motor dysfunction. We additionally will discuss cauda equina syndrome (CES) and specific imaging modalities helpful in the evaluation of HNP.

■ Types of Nucleus Pulposus Herniation

The predominance of posterior-lateral herniations (aside from the previously mentioned weak points in the anulus adjacent to the midline posterior longitudinal ligament [PLL]), may also result from circumferential variations in annular material properties; the anterior portions have both a larger tensile modulus of elasticity and ultimate

stress.[7] It is also likely that posterior herniations are more symptomatic than are anterior herniations and are therefore brought to clinical attention more frequently.

In addition to posterior or posterolateral herniations, the nucleus pulposus may herniate into a far lateral position or through the endplates and into adjacent vertebral bodies (Schmorl's node) (**Fig. 8.1**). Contained herniations occur when the NP remains trapped within the outer fibers of the AF and has not breached the posterior longitudinal ligament (PLL).[8] When the HNP extends through the AF, it is considered to be extruded and can be further classified as either a free fragment or sequestered.[8] Rarely, the HNP may migrate intradurally (**Fig. 8.2**). Symptoms typically present when the extruded NP compresses neural tissue resulting in both a mechanical and cytokine-induced inflammatory effect frequently causing pain and dysfunction.[9]

■ Herniation Risk Factors

True soft disc herniations most commonly occur in the third to fourth decades of life while the nucleus still has high water turgor.[10] Skeletal biomechanics, occupation, and some lifestyle factors likely play a role in the development of an HNP. Symptomatic disc herniations are seen more commonly in men with exposure to prolonged vehicle or industrial vibrations and in those that engage in repetitive pulling or lifting work. Sagittal spine imbalance, pregnancy, obesity, and sedentary lifestyle have also been shown to contribute to the risk of disc herniation.[11]

The NP is capable of swelling to roughly 200% of its initial volume.[12] Prolonged recumbency retards water egress from the NP and is associated with higher hydrostatic pressure and for some patients greater disc volumes. This explains why many disc herniations occur shortly after disc loading during the transition from a recumbent to upright posture.[13]

■ Clinical Features of a Herniated Nucleus Pulposus

The clinical presentation of an HNP varies from no symptoms to rapid paralysis; the severity of symptoms often

The views expressed in this chapter are those of the authors and do not necessarily reflect the official policy or position of the Department of the Navy, Department of Defense, or the United States Government.

correlate with the acuity and degree of compression to the neural and vascular elements.

In the lumbar spine, herniations are most common at L4–L5 and L5–S1. Common presenting features include radicular pain and numbness, dysesthesias, motor weakness, and even muscle atrophy from prolonged compression or disuse. The lumbar spine is the most common location for symptomatic disc herniations accounting for 80% of all disc herniations. Common symptoms of symptomatic lumbar disc herniations are varied and include lower back and buttock pain, with or without radicular leg pain and sensory dysesthesias. These symptoms may be partially relieved with rest, activity modification, or change in position. Trunk flexion, prolonged standing or sitting, and straining maneuvers (i.e., Valsalva, cough), commonly increase the symptoms of disc herniation.[14]

Manifestations of herniated discs range from progressive motor weakness to conditions adversely affecting bladder, bowel, and sexual function such as conus medullaris and cauda equina syndromes.[15]

Axial pain may result from a disc herniation at any level within the spine. The cause and effect relationship, however, is unclear. In some patients, prodromal pain is experienced before a disc herniates. On the other end of the spectrum, an estimated one-third of people do not develop pain or other symptoms in the presence of HNP. Pain subsides in over 90% of symptomatic patients within 12 weeks of presentation.[16] The pain is presumed to result from both mechanical pressure and chemical inflammation of the nerve root by the HNP. Pain generation from disruption of the AF

is thought to be mediated via branches of the sinuvertebral nerves as the posterior anulus and PLL are the most highly innervated structures in the functional spinal unit.[6] Willburger and colleagues[17] investigated the histologic composition of herniated fragments and found higher pain intensity values correlated with increased NP and cartilage percentages. However, the individual contributions to pain from direct pressure, chemical inflammation, the composition of herniated tissue and disrupted anulus are likely variable and remain unclear.[8] Fortunately, most patients do not require operative management of lumbar HNPs.[18]

Radicular leg pain radiating below the knee is a helpful clinical pearl favoring the diagnosis of lumbar disc herniation. Classic lumbar NPH findings are shown in **Table 8.1**. Herniations typically result in impingement of the adjacent, traversing nerve root. In the setting of associated inflammation, the patient may develop discomfort in a dermatomal or radicular distribution.[19] Far lateral herniations, unlike a posterolateral herniation, characteristically compress the exiting rather than the traversing nerve root (i.e., a far lateral L4–L5 HNP will compress the L4 *not* the L5 nerve root).[9,20]

An HNP at L4–L5 or L5–S1 is suggested by a positive straight-leg raise or tension test. This is performed by elevating the symptomatic straight leg in a supine patient or extending the flexed knee in a seated patient. A positive test occurs when the patient experiences below-the-knee pain in a dermatomal or myotomal distribution correlating with the anatomic location of the herniated disc. During the performance of this test in a seated patient, the patient may feel the need to slump or lean back and assume a tripod

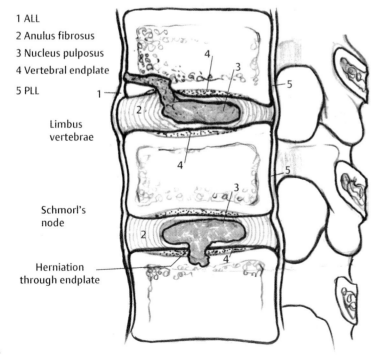

1 ALL
2 Anulus fibrosus
3 Nucleus pulposus
4 Vertebral endplate
5 PLL

Limbus vertebrae

Schmorl's node

Herniation through endplate

Fig. 8.1 **(A)** Two lumbar motion segments (sagittal view) showing a herniated nucleus pulposus (HNP) anterior to the vertebral body/anterior longitudinal ligament (limbus vertebrae), and herniation through the vertebral endplate and into the vertebral body (Schmorl's node).

(Continued on page 78)

A

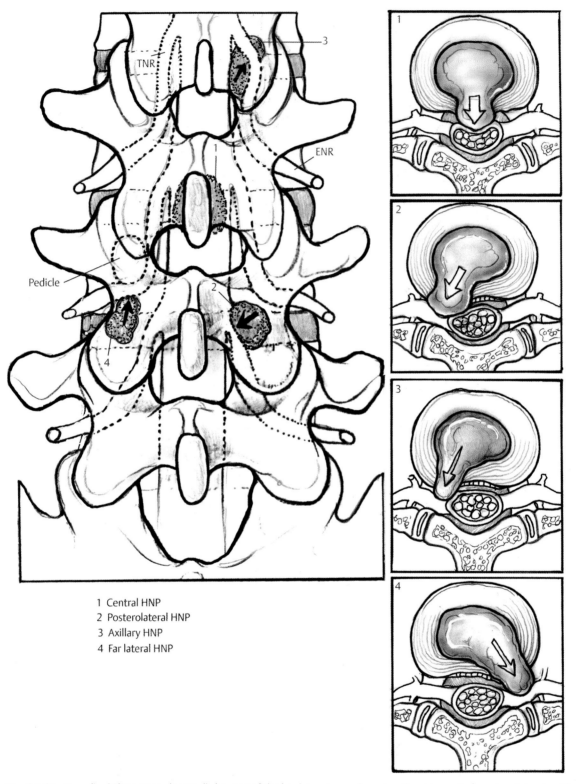

1 Central HNP
2 Posterolateral HNP
3 Axillary HNP
4 Far lateral HNP

Fig. 8.1 *(Continued)*   **(B)** Posterior (coronal) drawing of the lumbar spine and sacrum showing central, posterolateral, axillary, and far lateral HNP locations. ALL, anterior longitudinal ligament; PLL, posterior longitudinal ligament. TNR, traversing nerve root; ENR, exiting nerve root.

stance by balancing on their outstretched hands to relieve the pain. A positive contralateral straight-leg test occurs when straight-leg raising on the uninvolved side reproduces neural tension radicular pain in the opposite leg. Some clinicians anecdotally assume that a contralateral straight-leg test is often pathognomonic for the presence of a clinically significant disc herniation. However, the accuracy of the straight-leg and contralateral straight-leg tests in diagnosing a clinically significant HNP are limited by low specificity. Meta-analysis studies report sensitivity/specificity values of 0.85/0.52 and 0.30/0.84 for the straight-leg test and cross straight-leg tests, respectively.[21] The tension maneuver for an upper lumbar disc herniation involves the

femoral nerve stretch test.[22] This is performed by extending the hip on the symptomatic side with the knee in the flexed position performed with the patient standing or in the prone position.

A L1–L2 or L2–L3 disc herniation typically results in compression of the L2 or L3 nerve roots, respectively. Patients may complain of varying degrees of sensory disturbance along the anterior or anteromedial thigh. Lower extremity motor weakness is most commonly observed in the hip flexors, but can include subtle motor deficits in the quadriceps. Muscle atrophy is not usually observed. Patellar tendon reflexes may be normal or slightly decreased; Achilles deep tendon reflexes are normal.[23]

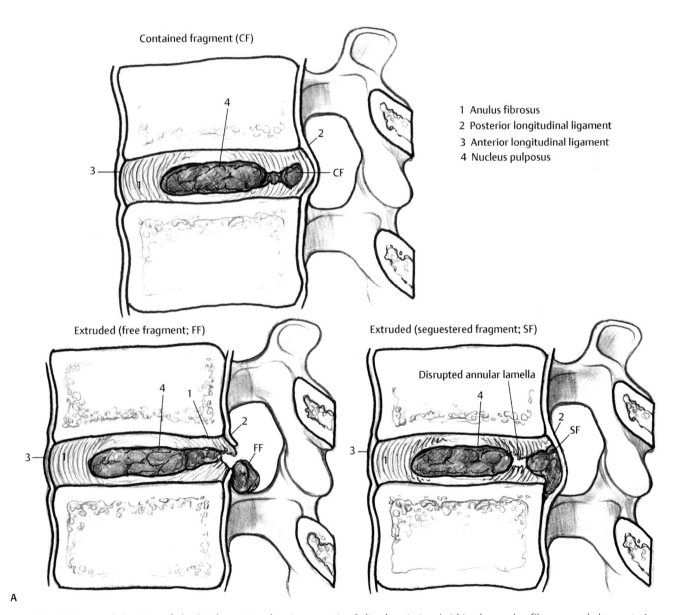

1 Anulus fibrosus
2 Posterior longitudinal ligament
3 Anterior longitudinal ligament
4 Nucleus pulposus

Fig. 8.2 **(A)** Sagittal drawing of the lumbar spine showing contained disc herniation (within the anulus fibrosus and the posterior longitudinal ligament) and extruded (both free and sequestered subtypes) disc herniation.

(Continued on page 80)

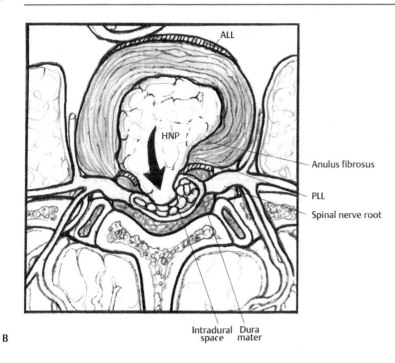

Fig. 8.2 *(Continued)* **(B)** Axial drawing of the lumbar spine showing herniated nucleus pulposus (HNP) beyond the anulus fibrosus, posterior longitudinal ligament (PLL), and dura mater, within the intradural space. ALL, anterior longitudinal ligament.

B

Compression of the L4 nerve root secondary to a posterolateral L3–L4 HNP or a far lateral L4–L5 HNP may result in quadriceps and tibialis anterior motor weakness.[9] Sensory deficits or dysesthesias may be perceived along the medial gastrocnemius or calf region.[24] Patellar deep tendon reflexes may be decreased or absent.

A posterolateral L4–L5 disc herniation results in compression of the fifth lumbar nerve root (**Fig. 8.3**). Sensory deficits (numbness or dysesthesias) may extend along the L5 dermatome involving the anterolateral leg and dorsolateral foot. Motor weakness, when present, involves the extensor hallucis longus and extensor digitorum longus. In most cases, reflexes will remain unchanged.

A posterolateral L5–S1 herniated disc results in compression of the S1 nerve root. Pain and numbness may be experienced along the lateral malleolus, lateral hindfoot, and plantar aspect of the foot and toes. Motor weakness is most prominent in the gastrocnemius–soleus complex and peroneal muscles. The ankle jerk reflex will be reduced or absent. In general, a lower lumbar posterolateral herniation most commonly affects one rather than both lower extremities.

■ Cauda Equina Syndrome

A large posterocentral, and at times, posterolateral lumbar disc herniation may result in significant compression of the cauda equina or conus medullaris. The incidence of CES is estimated to be 1 in 33,000 to 100,000.[25] This may cause findings such as bilateral lower extremity radicular pain and weakness, bowel and bladder dysfunction, and saddle or perineal anesthesia. Urologic and sexual dysfunction are common following untreated CES. Podnar et al[26] reported on 65 patients with chronic lesions and noted dysfunctional

Table 8.1 Lumbar Nerve Root Impingement with Associated Clinical Findings

Nerve Root	Sensory Findings	Motor Findings	Reflex Findings
L3	L3 dermatome pain/numbness (or quadriceps myotome pain)	Decreased quadriceps strength	Possible decreased patellar tendon deep tendon reflex
L4	L4 dermatome pain/numbness (or tibialis anterior myotome pain)	Decreased tibialis anterior strength	Possible decreased patellar tendon reflex
L5	L5 dermatome pain/numbness (or anterior leg myotome pain)	Decreased extensor hallucis longus strength	None
S1	S1 dermatome pain/numbness (or posterior leg myotome pain)	Decreased gastrocnemius-soleus and peroneal strength	Decreased Achilles tendon deep tendon reflex

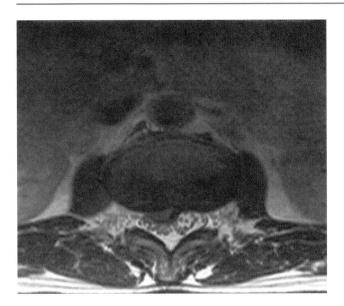

Fig. 8.3 A T2-weighted axial magnetic resonance imaging scan of an L4–L5 posterolateral herniated nucleus pulposus with neural element compression. This patient had L5 distribution radicular dysesthesias and right extensor hallucis longus weakness.

bladder emptying in 92% of females and 95% of males. Urinary dysfunction interfered with sexual function in 67% of the women and 72% of the men who were sexually active.

The timing for surgical decompression in CES is controversial; the literature includes heterogeneous patient populations with varied follow-ups. As a result, determining long-term outcomes following decompression with respect to various time intervals has been difficult. Further, there are potential medicolegal ramifications associated with delays in surgical decompression due to the likely urologic and sexual morbidity associated with CES.

McCarthy and colleagues[27] reported on 42 patients with CES who underwent surgical decompression. Five patients underwent decompression within 24 hours of urologic dysfunction onset and 21 patients were operated on within 48 hours. The remaining 16 patients underwent surgery more than 48 hours from sphincteric symptom onset. Urinary retention, urinary incontinence, and reduced perianal sensation was experienced by 60, 55, and 76% of the 42 patients on initial presentation. At a mean of 60 months follow-up (range 25 to 114 months), 12% of those with initial retention continued to have retention. These problems did not resolve in patients presenting with urinary incontinence and reduced perianal sensation in 43% and 66%, respectively. A significantly higher incidence of urinary incontinence was seen in females at follow-up. Also, bowel dysfunction at initial presentation was correlated with sexual dysfunction at follow-up. In this group of patients, outcomes were not different with respect to acuity of symptom onset or

the time to surgical decompression.[27] These findings differ from those reported by Shapiro. Twenty-four of the 44 patients in his cohort underwent delayed decompression, with 17 patients (71%) delayed an average of 3.7 days. Statistically significant persistent bladder dysfunction, motor deficit, pain, and sexual dysfunction occurred with surgical delays.[28]

Additional reports by Kennedy et al[29] have correlated delayed decompression with poor outcome. This was seen in 5 of 19 patients reported to have undergone decompression at a mean of 30 hours (range 20 to 72 hours). The 14 of 19 patients with satisfactory recovery all underwent early decompression (mean 14 hours, range 16 to 24 hours).

In 2000, Ahn and colleagues[30] reported the results of their meta-analysis, which studied the data from 322 patients. Surgical decompression did not show statistically significant improvement when performed within 24 hours compared with those patients operated on within 48 hours from the onset of CES. Patients decompressed within 48 hours were found to have improved sensory-motor, bladder, and bowel function when compared with those surgically managed more than 48 hours after onset of symptoms. Interestingly, in 2004, Kohles and colleagues repeated the meta-analysis performed by Ahn et al and found that there was an outcome difference in those decompressed within 48 hours that favored surgical decompression within 24 hours.[31]

■ Imaging Modalities for Herniated Nucleus Pulposus

The favored imaging modality to evaluate for the presence and extent of an intervertebral HNP is magnetic resonance imaging (MRI) as it is noninvasive and does not expose the patient to radiation. Jackson et al[32] published the results of 59 patients that prospectively underwent MRI, computed tomography (CT), and CT-myelography and showed a sensitivity of 76.5%, 73%, and 76%, respectively. False-negative rates were 35.7%, 40.2%, and 27.2%, respectively. In another investigation by Janssen and colleagues,[33] MRI accurately predicted the operative findings in 96% (98 of 102 disc levels). CT-myelography was significantly less at 57%. CT-myelography is most beneficial when MRI is contraindicated or may be distorted because of imaging artifact.

In all imaging modalities, caution should be applied when evaluating abnormal findings as many asymptomatic patients may have, depending on age, the pre-sence of spinal pathology.[34,35] Therefore MRI, CT, or CT-myelography findings should be carefully viewed within the context of a patient's presenting complaints and physical findings.[36]

■ Conclusion

Age-related degenerative changes to lumbar IVDs are common. HNPs also occur frequently and most often affect the lower lumbar intervertebral segments. Prompt surgeon evaluation of patients with saddle anesthesia, urologic dysfunction, and progressive lower extremity motor weakness is necessary. A thorough history, physical examination, and correlation with MRIstudies will allow for timely and efficient management of patients with a symptomatic IVD herniation.

References

1. Buckwalter JA. The fine structure of human intervertebral disc. In: White AA III, Gordon SL, eds. Proceedings of the American Academy of Orthopaedic Surgeons Symposium on Idiopathic Low Back Pain. Rosemont, IL: American Academy of Orthopaedic Surgeons; 1982:108–143
2. Eyre DR, Muir H. Quantitative analysis of types I and II collagens in human intervertebral discs at various ages. Biochim Biophys Acta 1977;492:29–42
3. Buckwalter JA, Mow VC, Boden SD, Eyre DR, Weidenbaum M. Intervertebral disk aging, degeneration and herniation. In: Buckwalter JA, et al, eds. Orthopaedic Basic Science. 2nd ed. Rosemont, IL: American Academy of Orthopaedic Surgeons; 2000:558–566
4. Buckwalter JA, Mow VC, Boden SD, Eyre DR, Weidenbaum M. Intervertebral disk structure, composition and mechanical function. In: Buckwalter JA, et al, eds. Orthopaedic Basic Science. 2nd ed. Rosemont, IL: American Academy of Orthopaedic Surgeons; 2000:548–556
5. Roberts S, Evans H, Trivedi J, Menage J. Histology and pathology of the human intervertebral disc. J Bone Joint Surg Am 2006;88(Suppl 2):10–14
6. Coppes MH, Marani E, Thomeer RT, Groen GJ. Innervation of "painful" lumbar discs. Spine 1997;22:2342–2350
7. Boden SD, Wiesel SW, Laws ER Jr, Rothman RM. The pathophysiology of the aging spine. In: The Aging Spine: Essentials of Pathophysiology, Diagnosis, and Treatment. Philadelphia: WB Saunders; 1991:21–38
8. Ito T, Takano Y, Yuasa N. Types of lumbar herniated disc and clinical course. Spine 2001;26(6):648–651
9. Erhard RE, Welch WC, Liu B, Vignovic M. Far-lateral disk herniation: a case report, review of the literature, and a description of nonsurgical management. J Manipulative Physiol Ther 2004;27(2):3
10. Ahn Y, Lee SH, Chung SE, Park HS, Shin SW. Percutaneous endoscopic cervical discectomy for discogenic cervical headache due to soft disc herniation. Neuroradiology 2005;47(12):924–930
11. Cummins J, Lurie JD, Tosteson TD, et al. Descriptive epidemiology and prior healthcare utilization of patients in the Spine Patient Outcomes Research Trial's (SPORT) three observational cohorts: disc herniation, spinal stenosis, and degenerative spondylolisthesis. Spine 2006;31(7):806–814
12. Ishihara H, Warensjo K, Roberts S, Urban JP. Proteoglycan synthesis in the intervertebral disk nucleus: the role of extracellular osmolality. Am J Physiol 1997;272(5 Pt 1):C1499–C1506
13. Urban JP, Maroudas A. Swelling of the intervertebral disc in vitro. Connect Tissue Res 1981;9:1–10
14. Rhee JM, Schaufele M, Abdu WA. Radiculopathy and the herniated lumbar disk: controversies regarding pathophysiology and management. Instr Course Lect 2007;56:287–299
15. Arce CA, Dohrman GJ. Herniated thoracic discs. Neurol Clin 1985;3:383–392
16. Morgan G Jr, Mikhail M, Murray M. Pain management. In: Clinical Anesthesiology. 4th ed. New York, NY: McGraw-Hill; 2002:309–343
17. Willburger RE, Ehiosun UK, Kuhnen C, Krämer J, Schmid G. Clinical symptoms in lumbar disc herniations and their correlation to the histological composition of the extruded disc material. Spine 2004;29(15):1655–1661
18. Benoist M. The natural history of lumbar disc herniation and radiculopathy. Joint Bone Spine 2002;69(2):155–160
19. Podichetty VK. The aging spine: the role of inflammatory mediators in intervertebral disc degeneration. Cell Mol Biol (Noisy-le-grand) 2007;53(5):4–18
20. Park JB, Chang H, Kim KW, Park SJ. Facet tropism: a comparison between far lateral and posterolateral lumbar disc herniations. Spine 2001;26(6):677–679
21. Devillé WL, van der Windt DA, Dzaferagić A, Bezemer PD, Bouter LM. The test of Lasègue: systematic review of the accuracy in diagnosing herniated discs. Spine 2000;25(9):1140–1147
22. Kobayashi S, Suzuki Y, Asai T, Yoshizawa H. Changes in nerve root motion and intraradicular blood flow during intraoperative femoral nerve stretch test: report of four cases. J Neurosurg 2003;99(3, Suppl):298–305
23. Tokuhashi Y, Matsuzaki H, Uematsu Y, Oda H. Symptoms of thoracolumbar junction disc herniation. Spine 2001;26(22):E512–E518
24. Williams KD, Park AL. Lower back pain and disorders of intervertebral discs. In: Canale ST, ed. Campbell's Operative Orthopedics. 10th ed. St. Louis, MO: Mosby; 2003:1982–2013
25. O'Connell JEA. Protrusions of the lumbar intervertebral discs: a clinical review based on five hundred cases treated by excision of the protrusion. J Bone Joint Surg Br 1951;33:8–30
26. Podnar S, Trsinar B, Vodusek DB. Bladder dysfunction in patients with cauda equina lesions. Neurourol Urodyn 2006;25(1):23–31
27. McCarthy MJ, Aylott CE, Grevitt MP, Hegarty J. Cauda equina syndrome: factors affecting long-term functional and sphincteric outcome. Spine 2007;32(2):207–216
28. Shapiro S. Medical realities of cauda equina syndrome secondary to lumbar disc herniation. Spine 2000;25(3):348–351
29. Kennedy JG, Soffe KE, McGrath A, Stephens MM, Walsh MG, McManus F. Predictors of outcome in cauda equina syndrome. Eur Spine J 1999;8(4):317–322
30. Ahn UM, Ahn NU, Buchowski JM, Garrett ES, Sieber AN, Kostuik JP. Cauda equina syndrome secondary to lumbar disc herniation: a meta-analysis of surgical outcomes. Spine 2000;25(12):1515–1522

31. Kohles SS, Kohles DA, Karp AP, Erlich VM, Polissar NL. Time-dependent surgical outcomes following caude equina syndrome diagnosis: comments on a meta-analysis. Spine 2004;29(11):1281–1287

32. Jackson RP, Cain JE Jr, Jacobs RR, Cooper BR, McManus GE. The neuroradiographic diagnosis of lumbar herniated nucleus pulposus. II. A comparison of computed tomography (CT), myelography, CT-myelography, and magnetic resonance imaging. Spine 1989;14(12):1362–1367

33. Janssen ME, Bertrand SL, Joe C, Levine MI. Lumbar herniated disk disease: comparison of MRI, myelography, and post-myelographic CT scan with surgical findings. Orthopedics 1994;17(2):121–127

34. Boden SD, Davis DO, Dina TS, Patronas NJ, Wiesel SW. Abnormal magnetic-resonance scans of the lumbar spine in asymptomatic subjects: a prospective investigation. J Bone Joint Surg Am 1990;72A:403–408

35. Borenstein DG, O'Mara JW Jr, Boden SD, et al. The value of magnetic resonance imaging of the lumbar spine to predict low-back pain in asymptomatic subjects: a seven-year follow-up study. J Bone Joint Surg Am 2001;83:1306–1311

36. Pevsner PH, Ondra S, Radcliff W, et al. Magnetic resonance imaging of the lumbar spine: a comparison with computed tomography and myelography. Acta Radiol Suppl 1986;369:706–707

9 Nonsurgical Treatment of Herniated Nucleus Pulposus

April Fetzer and Daphne R. Scott

Most cases of herniated nucleus pulposus (HNP) respond favorably to nonoperative treatment. This is because the natural history of the HNP is quite favorable regarding resolution of symptoms over time. Approximately 80% of patients have full improvement of symptoms within 6 weeks of onset, and 90% of patients show improvement within 12 weeks.[1] Most HNPs diminish in size over time, and 80% decrease by 50% or more.[1,2]

Accepted indications for proceeding with nonoperative treatment of the HNP include the absence of a progressive neurologic deficit and cauda equina syndrome.[1]

It is generally accepted that nonoperative management of the HNP may help avoid unnecessary surgery in many patients. Favorable outcomes for nonoperative treatment include the absence of pain on crossed straight leg raise, the absence of lower extremity pain with spinal extension, the absence of spinal stenosis on MRI, previous favorable response to steroids, the absence of a workman's compensation claim, a motivated and physically fit patient, and a normal psychological profile.[3]

The goals of nonoperative treatment are to educate patients, to relieve pain, to improve function, and to prevent chronicity of the problem.

Nonoperative treatments for the HNP include medications, bracing, physical therapy, and epidural steroid injections. Usually one, or any combination of the noted treatments, is applied to the patient with HNP. Each treatment option will be discussed and evaluated in this chapter.

■ Medications

Nonsteroidal Antiinflammatory Drugs

Nonsteroidal antiinflammatory drugs (NSAIDs) are a first-line treatment for the pain associated with the HNP. Both cyclo-oxygenase (COX) inhibitors, COX-I and COX-II, play a role in alleviating pain associated with inflammation. In the United States, however, current use of COX-II is limited to celecoxib secondary to cardiovascular side effects.[4] Although there are no studies on NSAIDs specifically in patients with HNP, NSAIDs have been found to be more effective than placebo for relieving pain. Evidence exists to support NSAID

efficacy when compared with placebo for chronic low back pain (LBP).[5]

Steroids

Steroids are typically prescribed either by oral, intramuscular, or injection routes[1] for pain associated with the HNP. They are indicated for short-term use for alleviation of pain associated with radiculopathy.[4] Although steroids are considered the standard of care, there are limited studies to support oral steroid use in this patient population. One published study on oral dexamethasone use reported no superiority to placebo for acute or long-standing pain, but did help patients with a positive straight leg raise alleviate pain.[1] Two studies on intramuscular injection revealed no benefit versus a modest benefit for pain relief.[4] Injection routes will be explored later in this chapter.

Nonopioid Analgesics

Acetaminophen has been found to be efficacious for mild to moderate pain.[4] It is safe, inexpensive, and sold over the counter. To avoid liver toxicity, the dosage limit is no more than 4 grams per day.

Tramadol is a centrally acting analgesic that has a weak effect on monoamine oxidase receptors.[4] Studies have shown that tramadol has improved pain control over placebo.[5] Neither acetaminophen nor tramadol has been specifically studied for pain control in patients with HNP.

Opioid Analgesics

Opioids are used to treat pain associated with acute or chronic radiculopathy, but there are no trials evaluating efficacy in patients with HNP.[1] Opioids are not recommended beyond a short period for first-line treatment secondary to addictive potential.[4] In general, opioids have been shown to be effective in relieving pain in patients with chronic LBP.[5]

Muscle Relaxants

Muscle relaxants may be used for patients with acute LBP, but like other medications, there are no studies on their effectiveness for HNP or radiculopathy.[1] It is thought that muscle relaxants may have additional benefits when used in combination with NSAIDs.[4] One high-quality study reported a significant difference between tetrazepam and placebo.[5]

Adjuvant Pain Medications

Although antidepressants are not recommended for routine use in patients with acute LBP, there is moderate evidence for the efficacy of tricyclic antidepressants in patients with chronic LBP.[4,5] Antiepileptics such as gabapentin or pregabalin may be helpful in treating neuropathic pain associated with radiculopathy, but these medications are not currently U.S. Food and Drug Administration (FDA) approved for this indication. Like other pain medications, there are no specific trials to support either antidepressants or antiepileptics for the specific treatment of the HNP.

■ Bracing

There is limited evidence to support the use of lumbar corsets in patients with LBP.[1] Bracing is not thought to improve lumbosacral biomechanics or enhance dynamic lifting capacity, and its use is controversial.[4]

■ Physical Therapy

Nonsurgical management of patients with LBP accounts for nearly half of all patients receiving treatment in outpatient physical therapy centers.[6,7] Traditionally, investigations of rehabilitation for low back disorders have demonstrated a dissension among rehabilitation approaches; a wide variety of treatment interventions are currently employed.[8,9] Currently, patients with LBP are seen as a homogeneous group and thus are treated similarly. No uniform identification of patient subgroups exists. For example, patients with LBP secondary to HNPs who may require individualized and specific treatments are not separated from patients with LBP secondary to other causes, such as degenerative disc disease.[10–15]

Difficulty in grouping patients based on pathoanatomic mechanisms, such as the HNP, is also difficult. A treatment-based classification system has been developed, which has demonstrated favorable results over a nonclassification-based approach.[16] The system classifies LBP patients into "specific exercise," "manipulation," "stabilization," or "traction treatment" groups.

Patients with HNPs fall into the "specific exercise" treatment group. Within this group, the basic clinical criteria for classification include patient preference for a specific position or movement and the ability to centralize distal extremity symptoms to the spine. Specifically, the physical therapist is able to obtain "centralization" by utilizing specific motions, either flexion or extension, of the lumbar spine.[17] Centralization itself refers to a phenomenon where patients' symptoms progress proximally from the distal extremity to the spine.[18,19] Rehabilitation of the patient subgroup who centralizes symptoms with extension movement of the lumbar spine is addressed in this section.

McKenzie originally observed the centralization phenomenon in 1959; he published his book on the mechanical standardized assessment and treatment of this patient group in 1981.[19] This system of assessment and treatment may also be referred to as mechanical diagnosis and therapy. Operational definitions have varied as to the time and place when centralization occurs within the mechanical assessment and intervention of the patient. As detailed above, however, it is generally accepted that centralization occurs when the symptoms move from a distal location in the extremity to a more central location in the extremity or in the spine with specific end-range movement.[20] Specifically, end-range extension movement of the lumbar spine (**Fig. 9.1**) has been found to relieve lower extremity symptoms in specific patient populations presenting with radicular symptoms.[21–27]

Recognition of centralization of symptoms in patients with HNPs provides physical therapists with the ability to classify patients for individualized treatment, as opposed to following traditional or general guidelines. Supporting evidence for the use of specific exercise in this patient population is emerging.[28,29]

The most common lumbar motion used with patients in the McKenzie-based "specific exercise" classification group is end-range lumbar extension (**Figs. 9.1 and 9.2**). Extension-based treatments have been studied with the greatest frequency in the literature. The study by Long[26] included 230 patients with LBP and/or sciatica. Subjects were randomly assigned to receive exercises either matching or not matching their directional preference for centralizing symptoms. Eighty-three percent of the patients reported

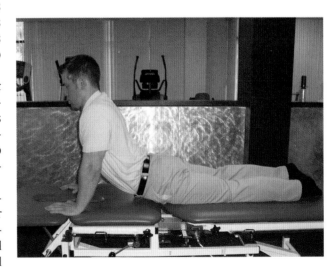

Fig. 9.1 Active prone press-up with end-range lumbar extension.

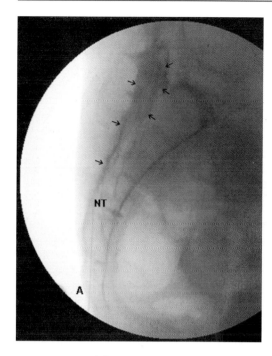

Fig. 9.5 Lateral fluoroscopic image detailing a caudal epidural steroid injection. Arrows indicate the contrast dye pattern within the caudal epidural space. A, sacral hiatus; NT, distal needle tip within the caudal epidural space.

Caudal Epidural Steroid Injections

Caudal ESIs yield steroid spread in the epidural space with entrance via the sacral hiatus (**Fig. 9.5**). There have been reports of increased incidence of vascular uptake of injectate, and increased subarachnoid injection with this approach. There are no studies available to delineate the efficacy of the caudal approach in regard to treatment of radiculopathy with HNP.

■ Percutaneous Disc Decompression

Percutaneous intradiscal therapies have been utilized since the 1970s to treat back and leg pain secondary to the HNP.[45] The percutaneous discectomy techniques treat contained HNPs via central decompression of the disc, typically removing ~7 to 10% of disc material, thus achieving relief of neural compression.[46,47] Percutaneous disc decompression has become popular with interventionalists, as it provides good short-term pain relief, but does not preclude the possibility of a future surgery, if necessary. The leading percutaneous disc decompression technologies are disc nucleoplasty, the DeKompressor, and percutaneous laser disc decompression (PLDD).

Nucleoplasty relies on radiofrequency energy to ablate and then coagulate nuclear material by creating small channels in the disc. Two small population-based clinical trials on nucleoplasty in patients who have small or medium herniations report significantly decreased pain and increased functional status following nucleoplasty at 6- and 12-month follow-up.[48,49]

DeKompressor technology relies on volume reduction to decrease intradiscal pressure. One study reports a decrease in pain of 70% in 72% of cases.[47] An additional prospective study using the decompressor in combination with a selective nerve root block yields a decrease in VAS scores from 7 to 1.5 at 6 months.[50]

Laser decompression (PLDD) utilizes vaporization of the nucleus pulposus via an optical fiber to achieve relief of neural compression from an HNP.[51] There is currently no consensus on the type of laser used, the energy applied, or the duration of application. There are several clinical trials published, but none with controls. Most studies report "immediate improvement" in 60 to 80% of patients, with return to work of 60% of patients at 4-week follow-up.[51] Given the low number of patient populations studied, weak methodology, the lack of long-term follow-up, and no controlled studies, laser decompression clearly needs multiple additional trials to evaluate clinical efficacy.

Patient Selection

Percutaneous microdiscectomy techniques yield promising outcomes for patient populations with contained HNPs (<6 mm) on magnetic resonance imaging (MRI).[49,51] Additional patient selection criteria include failure of conservative treatment for at least 6 weeks, neurologic findings limited to a single nerve root distribution, maintenance of disc height by over 50%, and leg greater than back pain.[51] Exclusion criteria include spondylolisthesis, spinal stenosis, previous surgery at the indicated disc level, secondary gain, and cauda equina syndrome.

■ Alternative Treatments

Tumor Necrosis Factor-Alpha

Tumor necrosis factor-alpha (TNF-α) is established to be an important inflammatory mediator in intervertebral disc herniation–induced sciatica in animal models. Infliximab (Remicade, Centocor, Malvern, PA) is a monoclonal antibody against TNF-α and has been utilized as an intravenous infusion for the treatment of acute sciatica from the HNP.[1] Although it sounds promising, the FIRST II (Finnish Infliximab Related STudy) trial does not support use of infliximab compared with placebo at 1-year follow-up.[52] Additional clinical trials are warranted for further investigation of this alternate treatment.

Ozone

In Italy, percutaneous oxygen-ozone (O_2-O_3) has been used as a treatment for HNP as a type of chemodiscolysis.[53] Ozone is an unstable form of oxygen that causes an oxide reduction called ozonolysis; this promotes progressive degeneration of the disc with fibrous replacement, and eventual disc shrinkage.[53] The ozone acts as an analgesic with antiinflammatory activity. There are few studies analyzing ozone therapies; those studies available have a low study population and short-term follow-up. These studies report 70 to 80% improvement in pain and, when used in combination with ESIs, report more effective pain relief than with steroid alone. Ozone therapy clearly needs more studies performed to fully understand its appropriate indication and outcomes.

■ Nonsurgical versus Surgical Treatment

There have been few studies examining surgical versus nonoperative treatment with long-term follow-up. The Weber trial[54] reported that surgery had statistically significant better outcomes at 1 year and 4 years, with outcomes diminishing at 10-year follow-up.[1] The Maine Lumbar Spine Study reported that both 1- and 10-year outcomes are better in surgically treated patients, with the greatest improvement at 2 years.[55-57] Despite overall symptomatic improvement in surgically treated patients, the Maine study reports that both work and disability outcomes are similar for operative and nonoperative management.

Recently, the Spine Patient Outcomes Research Trial (SPORT) reported that "patients with persistent sciatica from lumbar disc herniation improved in both operated and usual care groups." SPORT reports a small difference in favor of discectomy at 2-year follow-up when compared with standard nonoperative care.[58,59]

■ Conclusion

HNP with radiculopathy can be treated successfully with aggressive nonoperative care.[60] NSAIDs are found to help predominant LBP rather than radiculopathy. Intramuscular steroid injections and transforaminal ESIs are helpful for short-term relief and earlier improvement in function. Preference-based classification subgroups and centralization techniques within physical therapy regimens may provide significant improvement in patients' pain and function. ESIs are most beneficial via the transforaminal route, providing faster pain relief and restoration of function than natural history alone. Percutaneous discectomy techniques claim decreased pain and increased function at 12-month follow-up. Other alternate treatments such as ozone yield some positive outcomes, but clearly more advanced studies are needed.

References

1. Rhee JM, Schaufele M, Abdu WA. Radiculopathy and the herniated lumbar disc: controversies regarding pathophysiology and management. J Bone Joint Surg Am 2006;88(9):2070–2080
2. Saal JA, Saal JS, Herzog RJ. The natural history of lumbar intervertebral disc extrusions treated nonoperatively. Spine 1990;15(7):683–686
3. DePalma MJ, Bhargava A, Slipman CW. A critical appraisal of the evidence for selective nerve root injection in the treatment of lumbosacral radiculopathy. Arch Phys Med Rehabil 2005;86(7):1477–1483
4. Shen FH, Samartzis BS, Andersson GB. Nonsurgical management of acute and chronic low back pain. J Am Acad Orthop Surg 2006;14(8):477–487
5. Schnitzer TJ, Ferraro A, Hunsche E, Kong SX. A comprehenxive review of clinical trials on the efficacy and safety of drugs for the treatment of low back pain. J Pain Symptom Manage 2004;28(1):72–95
6. Di Fabio RP, Boissonnault W. Physical therapy and health-related outcomes for patients with common orthopedic diagnoses. J Orthop Sports Phys Ther 1998;27:219–230
7. Jette AM, Delitto A. Physical therapy treatment choices for musculoskeletal impairments. Phys Ther 1997;77:145–154
8. American Physical Therapy Association. Guide to Physical Therapist Practice. 2nd ed. Alexandria, VA: APTA; 2001
9. Hayden JA, van Tulder MW, Tomlinson G. Systematic review: strategies for using exercise therapy to improve outcomes in chronic low back pain. Ann Intern Med 2005;142:776–785
10. Abenheim L, Rossignol M, Valat JP, et al. The role of activity in the therapeutic management of back pain: report of the International Paris Task Force on Back Pain. Spine 2000;25(Suppl):1–33
11. Delitto A. Research in low back pain: time to stop seeking the elusive "magic bullet." Phys Ther 2005;85:206–208
12. Faas A. Exercises: which ones are worth trying, for which patients and when? Spine 1996;21:2874–2878
13. Koes B, Boutar L, Beckerman H, et al. Physiotherapy exercises and back pain: a blinded review. BMJ 1991;302:1572–1576
14. Spitzer W, LeBlanc F, Dupuis M. Scientific approach to the assessment and management of activity-related spinal disorders (the Quebec Task Force). Spine 1987;12(Suppl):16–21
15. Van Tulder MW, Koes B, Malmivaara A. Outcome of non-invasive treatment modalities on back pain: an evidence-based review. Eur Spine J 2006;15(Suppl 1):S64–S81
16. Fritz JM, Delitto A, Erhard RE. Comparison of classification-based physical therapy with therapy based on clinical practice guidelines for patients with acute low back pain: a randomized clinical trial. Spine 2003;28:1363–1371

17. Fritz JM, Cleland JA, Childs JD. Subgrouping patients with low back pain: evolution of a classification approach to physical therapy. J Orthop Sports Phys Ther 2007;37:290–302

18. Brennan GP, Fritz JM, Hunter SJ, Thackeray A, Delitto A, Erhard RE. Identifying subgroups of patients with acute/subacute "nonspecific" low back pain: results of a randomized clinical trial. Spine 2006;31(6):623–631

19. McKenzie RA. The Lumbar Spine: Mechanical Diagnosis and Therapy. Waikanae, New Zealand: Spinal Publications Ltd; 1989

20. Werneke M, Hart DL, Cook D. A descriptive study of the centralization phenomenon. A prospective analysis. Spine 1999;24(7):676–683

21. Delitto A, Cibulka M, Erhard R, et al. Evidence for an extension mobilization category in acute low back syndrome: a prescriptive validation pilot study. Phys Ther 1993;73:216–228

22. Fritz J, Delitto A, Vignovic M, et al. Interrater reliability of judgments of the centralization phenomenon and status change during movement testing in patients with low back pain. Arch Phys Med Rehabil 2000;81:57–61

23. Donelson R, Aprill C, Medcalf R, et al. A prospective study of centralization of lumbar and referred pain: a predictor of symptomatic discs and anular competence. Spine 1997;22:1115–1122

24. Donelson R, Silva G, Murphy K. The centralization phenomenon: its usefulness in evaluating and treating referred pain. Spine 1990;15:211–213

25. Karas R, McIntosh G, Hall H, et al. The relationship between nonorganic signs and centralization of symptoms in the prediction of return to work for patients with low back pain. Phys Ther 1997;77:354–360

26. Long A. The centralization phenomenon: its usefulness as a predictor of outcome in conservative treatment of chronic low back pain. Spine 1995;20:2513–2521

27. Sufka A, Hauger B, Trenary M, et al. Centralization of low back pain and perceived functional outcome. J Orthop Sports Phys Ther 1998;27:205–212

28. Browder DA, Childs JD, Cleland JA, Fritz JM. Effectiveness of an extension oriented treatment approach in a subgroup of patients with low back pain: a randomized clinical trial. [Abstract] J Orthop Sports Phys Ther 2007;37:A12–A13

29. Machado LA, de Souza MS, Ferreira PH, Ferreria ML. The McKenzie method for low back pain: a systematic review of the literature with a metanalysis approach. Spine 2006;31:E254–E262

30. Petersen T, Kryger P, Ekdal C, Olsen S, Jacobsen S. The effect of McKenzie therapy as compared with that of intensive strengthening training for the treatment of patients with sub-acute or chronic low back pain: a randomized controlled trial. Spine 2002;27:1702–1709

31. Aina A, May S, Clare H. The centralization phenomenon of spinal symptoms: a systematic review. Man Ther 2004;9:134–143

32. Mixter WJ, Barr JS. Rupture of the intervertebral disk with involvement of the spinal canal. N Engl J Med 1934;211:210–215

33. Chen B, Foye PM. Epidural steroid injections. emedicine 2005, August. Accessed April 2007

34. Vad VB, Bhat AL, Lutz GE, Cammisa F. Transforaminal epidural steroid injections in lumbosacral radiculopathy. Spine 2002;27(1):11–16

35. Armon C, Argoff CE, Samuels J, Backonja MM. Assessment: use of epidural steroid injections to treat radicular lumbosacral pain. Report of the Therapeutics and Technology Assessment Subcommittee of the American Academy of Neurology. Amer Acad Neuro 2007;68:723–729

36. Hooten MW, Mizerak A, Carns PE, Huntoon MA. Discitis after lumbar epidural corticosteroid injection: a case report and analysis of the case report literature. Pain Med 2006;7(1):46–51

37. Derby R, Bogduk N, Kine G. Precision Percutaneous Blocking procedures for localizing spinal pain. Part 2. The lumbar neuratial compartment. Pain Digest 1993;3:175–188

38. Derby R, Kine G, Saal JA, et al. Response to steroid and duration of radicular pain as predictors of surgical outcome. spine 1992;17:5176–5183

39. Lutz GE, Vad VB, Wisneski RJ. Fluoroscopic transforaminal lumbar epidural steroids: an outcome study. Arch Phys Med Rehabil 1998;79:1362–1366

40. Kraemr J, Ludwig J, Bickert U, et al. Lumbar epidural perineural injection: a new technique. Eur Spine J 1997;6:357–361

41. Kolgi I, Delecrin J, Berthelot JM, et al. Efficacy of nerve root versus interspinous injections of glucocorticoids in the treatment of disk-related sciatica: a pilot, prospective randomized, double blind study. J Bone Spine 2000;67:113–118

42. Riew KD, Yin Y, Gilula L, et al. The effect of nerve-root injections on the need for operative treatment of lumbar radicular pain. J Bone Joint Surg Am 2000;82:1589–1593

43. Thomas E, Cyteval C, Abiad L, Picot MC, Taourel P, Blotman F. Efficacy of transforaminal versus interspinous corticosteroid injection in discal radiculagia: a prospective, randomized, double-blind study. Clin Rheumatol 2003;22:299–304

44. Iwamoto J, Takeda T, Sato Y, Wakano K. Short term outcome of conservative treatment in athletes with symptomatic lumbar disc herniation. Am J Phys Med Rehabil 2006;85(8):667–674

45. Singh V, Derby R. Percutaneous lumbar disc decompression. Pain Physician 2006;9(2):139–146

46. Pomerantz SR, Hirsch JA. Intradiscal therapies for discogenic pain. Semin Musculoskelet Radiol 2006;10(2):125–135

47. Amoretti N, David P, Grimaud A, et al. Clinical follow-up of 50 patients treated by percutaneous lumbar discectomy. Clin Imaging 2006;30(4):242–244

48. Yakovlev A, Tamimi MA, Liang H, Eristavi M. Outcomes of percutaneous disc decompression utilizing nucleoplasty for the treatment of chronic discogenic pain. Pain Physician 2007;10(2):319–328

49. Mirzai H, Tekin I, Yaman O, Bursali A. The results of nucleoplasty in patients with lumbar herniated disc: a prospective clinical study of 52 consecutive patients. Spine J 2007;7(1):88–92

50. Slipman C, Menkin S, Garvan C, Bender F. Percutaneous lumbar disc decompression using the deKompressor: preliminary results. Poster presented at American Academy of Pain Medicine 22nd Annual Meeting, San Diego, February 22–25, 2008

51. Goupille P, Mulleman D, Mammou S, Griffoul I, Valat JP. Percutaneous laser disc decompression for the treatment of lumbar disc herniation: a review. Semin Arthritis Rheum 2007;37(1):20–30

52. Timo K, Jaro K, Leena P, et al. The treatment of disc herniation-induced sciatica with infliximab: one-year follow-up results of FIRST II, a randomized controlled trial. Spine 2006;31(24):2759–2766

53. Gallucci M, Lumbucci N, Zugaro L, et al. Sciatica: treatment with intradiscal and intraforaminal injections of steroid and oxygen-ozone versus steroid only. Radiology 2007;242(3):907–913

54. Weber H. Lumbar disc herniation: A controlled, prospective study with ten years of observation. Spine 1983;8:131–140

55. Atlas S, Deyo R, Keller R, et al. The Maine Lumbar Spine Study. Part II, 1-year outcomes of surgical and nonsurgical management of sciatica. Spine 1996;21(15):1777–1786

56. Atlas S, Deyo R, Keller RB, et al. The Maine Lumbar Spine Study. Part III.1-year outcomes of surgical and nonsurgical management of lumbar spinal stenosis. Spine 1996;21(15):1787–1794

57. Atlas SJ, Keller RB, Wu YA, Deyo RA, Singer DE. Long-term outcomes of surgical and nonsurgical management of sciatica secondary to a lumbar disc herniation: 10 year results from the Maine Lumbar Spine Study. Spine 2005;30(8):927–935

58. Weinstein JN, Lurie JD, Tosteson TD, et al. Surgical vs nonoperative treatment for lumbar disc herniation. The Spine Patient Outcomes Research Trial (SPORT). Spine 2006;20:2451–2459

59. Weinstein JN, Tosteson TD, Lurie JD, et al. Surgical vs nonoperative treatment for lumbar disc herniation. The Spine Patient Outcomes Research Trial (SPORT): a randomized trial. Spine 2006;20:2441–2450

60. Saal JA, Saal JS. Nonoperative treatment of herniated lumbar intervertebral disc with radiculopathy: an outcome study. Spine 1989;14(4):431–437

10 Percutaneous Decompression

Christopher A. Yeung, Christopher P. Kauffman, and Anthony T. Yeung

Throughout much of the late 20th century, surgical specialists have pursued less invasive techniques for the treatment of spinal problems. The patient benefits from these less invasive techniques have been well documented through the literature and have become the gold standard for numerous surgical procedures.

Advances in the ability to perform endoscopic discectomy have paralleled these other specialties; yet percutaneous spinal surgery has not met with the same peer recognition as the other fields. This is due, in part, to the high success rate and relative low morbidity of the current gold standard, posterior microscopic lumbar discectomy. This approach, however, still requires a 1-inch midline or paramedian incision, muscle and ligament stripping, muscle retraction, partial facet and lamina resection, and neural retraction. This can weaken the muscular lumbar stabilizers, create instability and facet arthrosis, cause traction neuropraxia, promote epidural scarring, and make revision surgery more difficult.

Today's endoscopic technology allows for visualized discectomy and decompression of the traversing and exiting nerve roots from a percutaneous posterolateral/transforaminal approach. This is safe and equally efficacious to microscopic discectomy in properly selected patients. The patients may also reap the benefits of the less-invasive approach.

Anterior and posterior interbody fusions are possible through percutaneous approaches. Pilot studies have begun using percutaneous delivery of autograft and allograft contained in an annular fence (Ouroboros Medical, San Diego, CA) and into a mesh bag (Optimesh, Spineology, St. Paul, MN) supplemented by facet or pedicle screw posterior stabilization. The progress made on percutaneous discectomy and decortication of the endplate will lead the way for future progress in percutaneous fusion. The percutaneous posterolateral endoscopic approach is also ideally suited for nucleus replacement and nucleus augmentation procedures. Future advances in the use of biomaterials and gene therapy may open the door to anular reinforcement and tissue repair or regeneration.

■ History

The basis for percutaneous lumbar disc procedures stemmed from the use of a Craig needle to perform a posterolateral biopsy for neoplastic conditions.[1,2]

■ Anatomy

Percutaneous lumbar surgery is performed through what has been named the triangular working zone, or Kambin's triangle (**Fig. 10.1**). This triangular zone is defined as a safe zone in the posterolateral anulus between the exiting and traversing nerve roots. The exiting nerve root forms the anterior border of the triangular zone as it exits under the cephalad pedicle. The superior endplate of the caudal vertebral body forms the inferior border, and the articular process and superior articulating facet of the caudal vertebra form the posterior border. The working zone is bordered medially by the traversing nerve root and dura. From cadaveric measurements it was determined that cannulas ranging from 4 to 10 mm could be safely used in the triangular working zone.[3–6] A thorough knowledge of the three-dimensional anatomy is necessary to understand and perform posterior percutaneous lumbar surgery.

■ Types of Percutaneous Lumbar Discectomy

Enzymatic Discectomy

Lyman W. Smith, MD, pioneered the use of chymopapain for the enzymatic degradation of the nucleus pulposus (NP) and coined the term *chemonucleolysis*. After obtaining permission from the FDA in 1963, Smith reported his first 10 patients' results in 1964. Two of the next 20 patients treated sustained paralysis.[7–9] Following its introduction chymopapain has been used on an inconsistent basis. In 1982, the FDA approved the use of a new formulation of the drug, Chymodiactin (Knoll Pharmaceutical Company, North Olive, NJ). Satisfactory results were reported in 82% of treated patients; however, media attention focused on 55 patients out of 100,000 who had catastrophic complications, 6 of them resulting in paraplegia secondary to acute transverse myelitis. Nordby et al[10] reviewed the adverse effects of chymopapain over a 10-year history. In this period, most of the complications occurred from 1982 to 1984, with a 50% decrease in complications from 1984 to 1988. The early experience with higher complications was attributed to poor technique, including injection of chymopapain directly into the subarachnoid space. After the

1 Exiting nerve root (hypotenuse)
2 Traversing nerve root (side)
3 Superior endplate caudal vertebra (base)

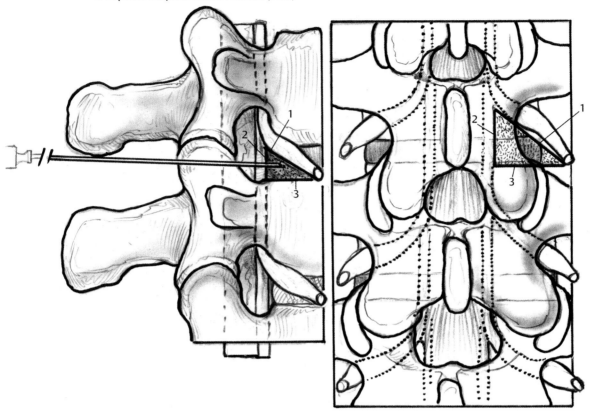

A

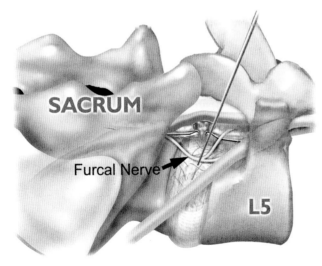

B

Fig. 10.1 (A) Triangular working zone at L5–S1 (Kambin's triangle; area of stippling). This is the access point for posterolateral disc access. **(B)** Instrument entry angle in Kambin's triangle. Accessory branches of the nerves can be found here and are named Furcal nerves.

development and use of preoperative sensitivity testing and preinjection discography, the complication rate has dropped significantly.[10]

Chymopapain is the only percutaneous modality to date to undergo prospective double-blind randomized trials.[11] The longest follow-up comes from an Australian study comparing chymopapain with saline injection. At 10 years, the patients remained blinded to which treatment they had received. The results showed that 80% of the patients who received chymopapain considered their surgery successful compared with only 34% of patients who received saline injection. Twenty percent of the chymopapain-treated patients went on to have open surgical intervention versus 47% of the patients receiving saline.[11] Other studies comparing chemonucleolysis with placebo injections reported success rates from 71 to 80%.[12–14]

There have been indirect comparisons of open discectomy and chemonucleolysis in the literature, but few direct comparisons. One small study prospectively compared the two. There were 46 patients in each group. Early results favored surgery, although at 1 year the two groups showed no statistically significant difference. One significant difference was that nine patients receiving chymopapain went on to have surgical intervention and only one in the surgical group underwent reexploration.[15] In a review of 45 clinical studies involving over 7000 patients, Nordby et al[10] reported an average success rate of 76% for chemonucleolysis versus an average of 88% for laminectomy and discectomy. In a meta-analysis of 43,662 patients treated with chemonucleolysis the overall complication rate was 3.7% with only 0.45% being severe complications. The study also looked at 2051 surgical patients with an overall complication rate of 26% and a severe complication rate of 4.2%.[16] Currently, chymopapain is not commercially available in the United States.

Automated Percutaneous Lumbar Discectomy

Onik et al[17] introduced automated percutaneous lumbar discectomy (APLD), in 1985, after developing an automated Nucleotome (Clarus Medical, LLC, Minneapolis, MN). The procedure involved introduction of an 8-inch Nucleotome with a blunt end into the center of the disc space. There were three available diameters: 2.0, 2.5, and 3.5 mm. The Nucleotome had a cutting blade and suction. It was driven by nitrogen gas and operated under fluoroscopic control. There was no direct visualization of the disc space or neural structures. It was operated in the disc space for ~10 minutes.[17,18]

The results of APLD have been mixed in the literature with few authors other than Onik et al being able to achieve their reported results. Initial results were 80% good to excellent, but only over a 6-month follow-up.[19] A multicenter study reported a 75% success rate when proper inclusion criteria were met.[20] The difficulty comes in interpretation of the imaging studies as they relate to contained disc herniations. Many of the failures were determined to be in noncontained herniations. In retrospectively reviewing their results at 5-year follow-up, Maroon found a success rate of 59%.[18]

Chatterjee et al[21] performed a randomized prospective trial comparing APLD and microdiscectomy for contained herniations. The herniations could be no larger than 30% of the canal size. The results of this study demonstrated a success rate of 29% for APLD versus 80% for microdiscectomy. The authors concluded that APLD was not as successful for

small, contained herniations as previously reported.[21] In a separate study out of the United Kingdom, Grevitt et al[23] reported on the long-term follow-up of initially successful APLD patients. The original study group had a 72% good to excellent result.[22] However, on longer follow-up (55 months), 33% of patients deteriorated into a fair or poor group making the overall success rate 45%.[23] Another study of long-term results showed that 38% of patients required subsequent open surgery within 5 years.[24]

Percutaneous Laser Discectomy

The use of a laser (light amplification by stimulated emission of radiation) is predicated on the ability of the laser to ablate tissue and achieve hemostasis. Lasers have been used extensively throughout multiple surgical specialties with success. There are several types of lasers used in medicine, including infrared, light, and ultraviolet lasers. Lasers that have been used successfully in the lumbar spine include the CO_2, potassium titanyl phosphate (KTP), Holmium: yttrium-aluminum-garnet (YAG), and neodymium:YAG. Only the KTP laser and the Holmium:YAG laser are FDA approved for use in the spine.

The underlying principle of laser lumbar surgery was that through tissue ablation intradiscal pressure could be substantially lowered. This was based on the work of Hirsh et al[25] and their postulated relationship between intradiscal pressure, disc herniation, and low back pain. They hypothesized that lowering this pressure in an injured disc could be efficacious in the relief of sciatica.[25] Based on this and early results of chymopapain and APLD, studies were performed to see how much disc could be ablated with the laser. Multiple studies described decreases in intradiscal pressures of 50% or greater.[26–28]

The results of laser discectomy fall within a similar range to that of chemonucleolysis and early results of APLD. Using the KTP laser, Davis[28a] reported a success rate of 80%. In a larger study, Choy and colleagues looked at 333 patients with herniated discs diagnosed by magnetic resonance imaging (MRI) or computed tomography (CT) and treated with percutaneous laser discectomy. At an average follow-up of 26 months, they reported a 78.4% overall success rate.[29]

Percutaneous laser discectomy, like its predecessors, was a fluoroscopically guided, nondirectly visualized procedure performed with a laser guide or partially visualized with smaller endoscopes. The inability to see the decompressed nerve or the targeted pathoanatomy consistently has limited its use. At this time, with newer operating or working channel spine endoscopes, the laser is used mainly as an adjunctive tool for hemostasis and targeted tissue ablation during endoscopic lumbar procedures.

Endoscopic Lumbar Discectomy

Endoscopic surgery developed out of fluoroscopically guided percutaneous procedures that initially used working cannula with modified instruments designed for disc removal. The first surgeon credited with percutaneous nucleotomy was Hijikata in 1975.[30] The evolution of endoscopic techniques followed a series of transitions. Initially, an arthroscope was used to inspect the disc and anulus intermittently through the cannula, while the mechanical nuclectomy was done under fluoroscopic guidance. The introduction of a biportal approach allowed for direct visualization of instruments introduced through a cannula inserted into the disc from the opposite posterolateral portal. The later development of an operating spine scope with a working channel allowed for surgical removal of disc material and visualization of foraminal anatomy under direct visualization via a uniportal approach.

Parviz Kambin performed the first true endoscopic lumbar procedures. The arthroscope was at first used intermittently through the working cannula. At certain stages of the procedure, such as perforating the disc in the triangular working zone, the arthroscope would be placed in the cannula. The nonworking channel scope was used for identification of the anulus and periannular structures and to ensure the nerve was not in the way prior to advancement of the cannula. Once the cannula was safely within the disc, the Nucleotome, an arthroscopic shaver, and pituitary rongeurs were passed through the cannula to perform mechanical disc removal. The majority of the procedure was only fluoroscopically visualized.[31] Kambin reported an 88% success rate in his first 100 patients.[32,33]

The early endoscopic procedures were limited by the absence of a working channel arthroscope. This led Kambin to the development of a biportal technique in which the scope was inserted on one side and the working cannula on the opposite side. Kambin's indications for a biportal approach included large subligamentous herniations, extraligamentous herniations, and arthroscopic interbody fusion.[5] In later studies, Kambin reports results from both uniportal and biportal procedures together. Overall results ranged from 85 to 92% satisfactory results at a minimum 2-year follow-up. There was no differentiation made between the results of uniportal versus biportal approaches.[34–36]

Kambin's first prototype of the working channel scope was not fully developed and was not successfully marketed. The problems with the initial scope included fragility, limited degree of angulation for the working instruments, and the inability to establish adequate inflow or outflow for adequate visualization.[37] Anthony Yeung developed the first working channel endoscope to become widely available. The scope was developed in 1997 and was approved for use by the FDA in March of 1998. The YESS (Yeung endoscopic spine surgery) system (Richard Wolf Surgical Instruments, Vernon Hills, IL) modified the scope by adding multichannel integrated irrigation, specialized beveled cannulas, a two-hole obturator, and newly designed discectomy tools,

which allowed for constant real-time visualization with a uniportal technique (**Fig. 10.2**).[38]

Another major change, which allowed for advancement in the field of endoscopic spinal surgery, was the emphasis on placement of the cannula closer to the epidural space and the base of the targeted disc herniation. This enabled surgeons to target extruded herniations in addition to contained herniations. Previous percutaneous modalities all focused on entry through Kambin's triangle and working within the center of the disc with the cannula anchored inside the anulus. The cannula was advanced past the anulus and remained there under fluoroscopic control. Matthews' transforaminal approach for microdiscectomy allowed for routine visualization of the epidural space and greater access to the traversing nerve root.[39]

The development of a working channel scope and use of the transforaminal approach utilizing beveled and slotted cannulas enhanced endoscopic lumbar surgery. Using this approach, surgeons are able to operate under full visualization throughout most of the procedure and follow the neural structures into the epidural space. The specialized cannulas provide greater access to pathology; and they help protect and retract sensitive anatomy such as the exiting nerve and dorsal root ganglion. The working channel also allowed the passage of high-speed burrs for bone removal and direct foraminal enlargement and decompression of foraminal stenosis (foraminoplasty) (**Fig. 10.3**).

■ Indications and Contraindications

Current indications for the use of an endoscopic posterolateral approach to the lumbar spine include foraminal and far-lateral disc herniations, contained central and paracentral disc herniations, small nonsequestered extruded disc herniations, recurrent herniations, symptomatic annular tears, synovial cysts, biopsy and debridement of discitis, decompression of foraminal stenosis with or without spondylolisthesis, visualized total nuclectomy (prior to nucleus replacement), visualized discectomy, and endplate preparation prior to interbody fusion.

Perhaps the ideal lesions for posterolateral selective endoscopic discectomy are the foraminal and extraforaminal disc herniations. The cannula inserts directly at the herniation site and the exiting nerve is routinely visualized and protected. This approach requires less manipulation of the exiting nerve root than the paramedian posterior approach.

Any herniation contiguous with the disc space not sequestered and migrated is amenable to endoscopic disc excision if the bony anatomy permits an unobstructed approach. This utilizes an "inside-out" technique in which the herniation is grasped from its base within the disc space, pulled back into the working intradiscal cavity, and removed via the cannula. The size and types of herniations

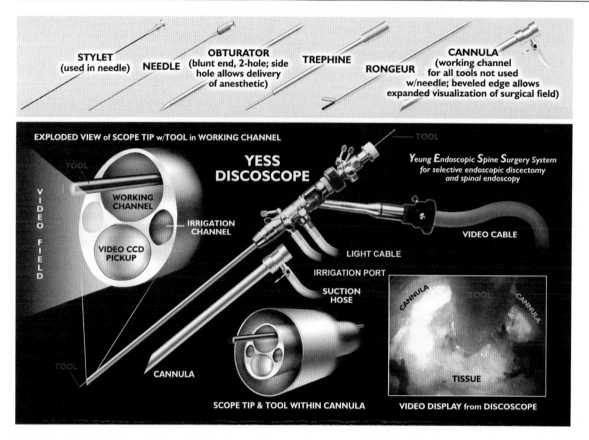

Fig. 10.2 The YESS (Yeung Endoscopic Spine Surgery) system. (Courtesy of Richard Wolf Surgical Instruments, Vernon Hills, IL)

chosen by the surgeon for endoscopic excision will depend on the skill and experience of the surgeon. Certainly, all contained disc herniations are appropriate for endoscopic decompression. With experience, extruded herniations can be routinely addressed. This approach is especially attractive for recurrent herniations after a traditional posterior approach because the surgeon can avoid the scar tissue from the previous surgery.

Radiofrequency energy can be applied to the annular tears under direct visualization to contract the collagen and ablate ingrown granulation tissue, neoangiogenesis, and sensitized nociceptors.[40] Frequently, interpositional nuclear tissue is seen within the fibers of the annular tear preventing the tear from healing. This tissue can then be removed.

Endoscopic foraminoplasty can be readily achieved with bone trephines/rasps, the side-firing Holmium:YAG laser, and endoscopic high-speed drills.[41,42] The roof of the foramen is formed by the undersurface of the superior articular facet. This is easily visualized and accessed via the endoscope and the previously mentioned tools are utilized to remove bone and enlarge the foraminal opening. Synovial cysts can also be visualized and removed.

In cases of discitis the posterolateral endoscopic approach will provide a robust biopsy for culture diagnosis, and the infected/necrotic disc tissue can be thoroughly debrided to reduce the bacterial load and accelerate healing.

Contraindications include any pathology not accessible from the posterolateral endoscopic approach. This may include some extruded sequestered disc herniations, extruded migrated disc herniations (migrated >20% of vertebral body superiorly or inferiorly), recurrent or virgin disc herniations with associated epidural scarring, moderate-severe central canal stenosis, and hard calcified herniations. These contraindications are considered relative contraindications dependent on the surgeons' technical experience and comfort level. More experienced endoscopic surgeons can gain greater access to pathology utilizing advanced techniques for bone removal of osteophytes, stenosis, and the posterolateral corner of the vertebral body prior to addressing the pathology. Other relative contraindications include inadequate support staff or equipment to successfully perform the procedure, and uncooperative patients.

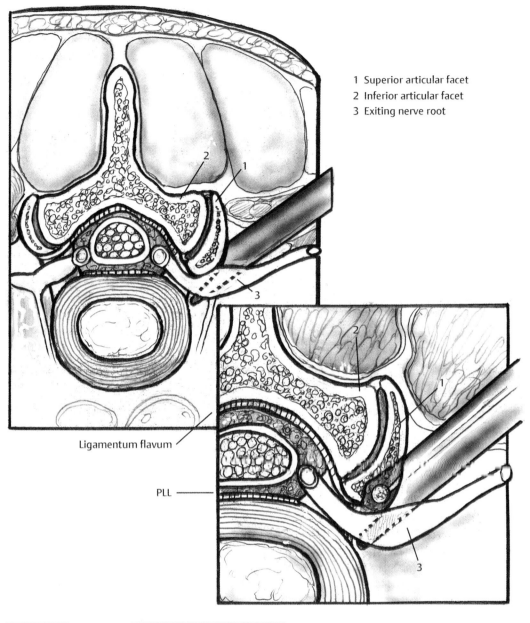

1 Superior articular facet
2 Inferior articular facet
3 Exiting nerve root

Ligamentum flavum

PLL

A

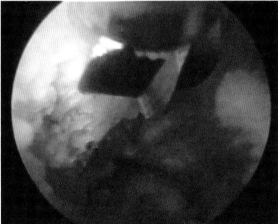

B

Fig. 10.3 Foraminoplasty with a high-speed burr. The beveled cannula is rotated so that the protruding lip is protecting and retracting the exiting nerve root. The opening of the cannula is up against the undersurface of the superior articular facet. The high-speed burr is placed through the working channel to remove this bone and enlarge the foramen. PLL, posterior longitudinal ligament.

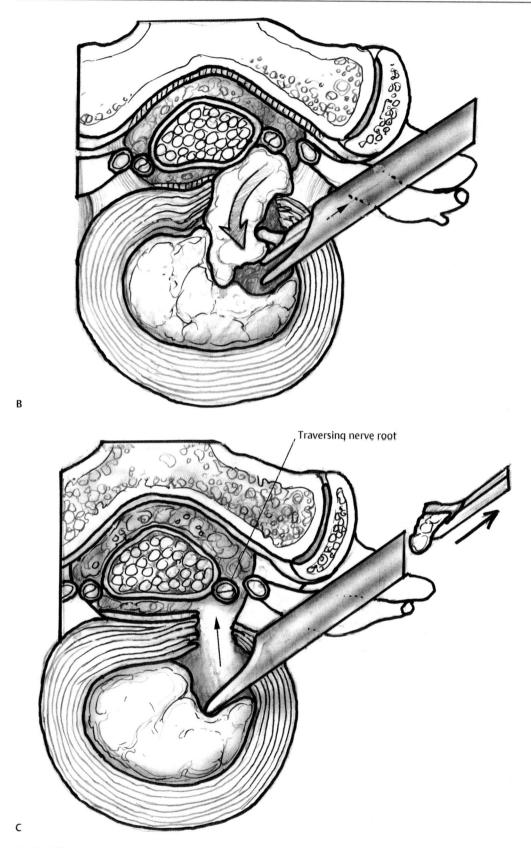

B

Traversing nerve root

C

Fig. 10.4 *(Continued)* The annulotomy is medialized with cutting forceps **(B)** and the side-firing laser to allow the apex of the herniation to be pulled back into the disc and out the cannula with the pituitary rongeurs **(C)**.

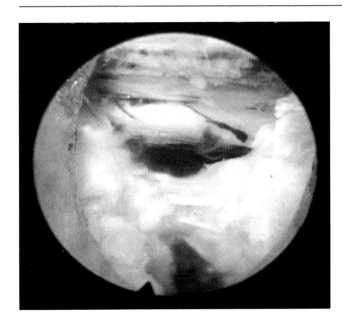

Fig. 10.5 Inspection of the freed traversing nerve root. After successful removal of an extruded paracentral herniation, the traversing nerve root is visualized, confirming complete decompression of the nerve. This is routine in extruded herniations. If it is a contained herniation, the surgeon would visualize the undersurface of the thinned-out posterior annular fibers rather than the traversing nerve root because the herniation did not extrude past the posterior anulus.

the cavity. The flexible radiofrequency bipolar probe is used to contract and thicken the annular collagen at the herniation site. It is also used for hemostasis throughout the case.

The vast majority of herniations can be treated via the uniportal technique. Sometimes, for large central herniations, the disc needs to be approached from both sides, a biportal technique. This allows the use of larger articulating instruments that fit through the contralateral 7-mm access cannula under direct endoscopic vision.

■ Clinical Outcomes

Yeung and Tsou[44] reported their initial results using the YESS system in their first 307 patients with disc herniations that were candidates for open microdiscectomy. The study included intracanal and extracanal herniations. Recurrent herniations and patients with previous surgery at the same level were not excluded. Results were reported with 1-year follow-up. The overall patient satisfaction was 91%. The same percentage of patients said they would undergo the procedure again if faced with the same diagnosis. The overall complication rate was 3.5%.[44] Tsou and Yeung separated out a subgroup of 219 patients with noncontained herniations and reported results at 1 year. Patient

satisfaction was 91%.[45] These initial results demonstrated that endoscopic surgery could provide equivalent results to reported results of open microdiscectomy, even with noncontained herniations. Others have reported 85% satisfactory outcome for transforaminal percutaneous discectomy for far lateral and foraminal disc herniations as well.[46]

There are two reported studies comparing traditional microdiscectomy and percutaneous endoscopic discectomy. Hermantin et al[47] performed a prospective randomized study with 30 patients in each group. The mean duration of follow-up was 31 months. Patient satisfaction was 93% in the open surgical group and 97% in the endoscopic group. The endoscopic group had shorter duration of narcotic use and shorter time out of work compared with open discectomy. Mayer and Brock performed a randomized prospective study in 1993 with 20 patients in each group. They chose return to previous occupation as their measurement of success. This study showed a significant difference in this outcome measure. In the percutaneous group, 95% of patients returned to their previous profession, whereas only 72% of the microdiscectomy group returned to their previous profession.[48]

Kambin et al[49] reported an 82% success rate for the treatment of lateral recess stenosis and foraminal herniations using an oval cannula with two portals and the transforaminal approach. Even though they were working next to the exiting nerve root they reported no neurovascular complications in their series.[49] Knight and Goswami[42] have reported on the use of the endoscope in foraminal decompressions for isthmic spondylolisthesis. In 79% of patients, a good or excellent outcome was obtained with an average follow-up of 34 months. Of the initial group only two went on to have spinal fusion.[42]

The ability to effectively remove pathology using endoscopic surgery has been validated by postprocedure imaging studies. Casey et al[50] looked at a group of patients who had immediate postoperative CT scans. The imaging studies demonstrated 88.9% of patients undergoing biportal endoscopy had significant reduction in the amount of neural compromise. The results of uniportal, extraforaminal, and foraminal herniations showed only mild to moderate change in canal diameter. They concluded that arthroscopic discectomy had a high rate of canal clearance and removal of disc fragments.[50]

■ Complications and Avoidance

The risks of serious complications or injury are low, ~3%. The usual risks of infection, nerve injury, dural tears, bleeding, and scar tissue formation are always present as with any surgery. Because the transforaminal endoscopic approach passes adjacent to the exiting spinal nerve root and dorsal root ganglia, there is potential for nerve irritation

11 Decompressive Surgery for Herniated Nucleus Pulposus (Open, Micro, and Minimally Invasive Approaches)

Christian M. DuBois, Frank M. Phillips, and Kevin T. Foley

Surgery to treat a symptomatic herniated nucleus pulposus (HNP) remains a frequent operation with improvement in symptoms in most patients. The surgery has gone through technical modifications since its introduction in the early 20th century; however, the primary goal remains the same. This principle is to decompress the affected nerve root by removing the HNP with the least damage to the surrounding structures.

■ Historical Perspective

Walter Dandy's report of two patients with cauda equina syndrome associated with rupture of intervertebral disc (IVD) in 1929 may have been the first to successfully identify and surgically treat a ruptured IVD.[1] However, it is Mixter and Barr's 1934 article in the *New England Journal of Medicine* that is widely accepted as the original report popularizing surgical cure for sciatica related to IVD disease.[2] Initial enthusiasm for discectomy was tempered by reports of negative explorations and patients suffering from persistent postoperative back pain.

Despite the lack of contemporary medical technologies such as microscopes and magnetic resonance imaging (MRI), the forefathers of disc operations persevered and performed "open" discectomies with good results. Four decades later, Caspar[3] and Yarsagil[4] reported on the routine use of the microscope to perform lumbar discectomy. The era of "microdiscectomy" was born, emphasizing minimal soft tissue trauma while the microscope improved lighting and visualization. In 1997, Foley and Smith[5] reported a "microendoscopic" technique for discectomy using a sequential tube dilating system in combination with an endoscope. The visual limitations of the two-dimensional (2D) working environment encountered with an endoscope proved to be challenging. This prompted the development of a tubular dilation system that could be used with standard three-dimensional visualization techniques, either the operating microscope or loupe magnification.

■ Relative and Absolute Indications

Surgical indications for treating sciatica associated with herniated IVD are controversial at best, particularly since the Spine Patient Outcomes Research Trial (SPORT) study was published.[6,7] In the study, nonoperative patients fared as well as the surgical patients at long-term follow-up, although the more immediate pain relief provided with surgery did have a positive socioeconomic impact. Unfortunately, there were a significant number of patients that crossed over between their assigned operative or nonoperative group, and the use of the "intent to treat" analysis makes it difficult to provide absolute conclusions to support either nonoperative or operative treatment.[8,9] Nevertheless, lumbar discectomy remains the most frequent spinal procedure in the United States.

Despite the controversy, absolute indications for surgery do exist. Patients demonstrating a progressive neurologic deficit or the development of cauda equina syndrome should be treated with urgent surgical decompression. Patients who experience radicular pain with corresponding radiologic evidence of disc herniation, and who have failed at least 6 weeks of appropriate conservative therapy would also be considered surgical candidates. Other relative indications for surgery would include intractable sciatica or a static motor deficit with positive nerve root tension signs.

As for all surgical procedures, proper patient selection is critical for a successful outcome. Most patients will not meet the absolute criteria discussed. As in every medical decision, the patient should be involved in the decision-making process. The final decision to proceed with surgery should be made only after a patient has had a thorough discussion with the surgeon regarding the risks and benefits of both nonoperative and operative options.

■ Surgical Approaches

Open Discectomy and Microdiscectomy

History

Traditionally, "open" discectomy implied that the surgeons completed a hemilaminotomy through large skin and fascial incisions to access the disc space without magnification. The contemporary open discectomy is typically now performed using magnification with either loupes or microscopes emphasizing microsurgical techniques. The incision is minimized, and an intraoperative x-ray study is introduced early on to locate and verify the correct operative level. A study by Katayama and colleagues[10] prospectively compared the clinical outcomes between traditional open discectomy and microdiscectomy and demonstrated that the outcomes are similar, with microdiscectomy's having a slight benefit in regard to bleeding and hospital stay. Current minimally invasive discectomy techniques imply the use of a specialized retractor system, which minimizes adjacent soft tissue trauma combined with some form of illumination and magnification.

Positioning and Technique

Positioning a patient for lumbar discectomy starts by relieving pressure off the abdominal contents, including the great vessels, to minimize venous bleeding during the dissection. There are a variety of tables and frames available on the market for this purpose (**Fig. 11.1**). In general, a patient is placed in prone position with knees in a flexed, kneeling position. After ensuring that all pressure points are padded properly, the skin is then prepped and draped in the standard fashion. A spinal needle is then advanced through the skin toward the interspinous process space, and a radiograph is taken to confirm the correct operative level. With the open technique, a small skin incision over the spinous process is made and subperiosteal dissection is performed unilaterally to detach the muscle off the lamina on the affected side. Another radiograph is taken at this point to confirm the operative level. Using loupe or microscopic magnification, the bony and soft tissue landmarks of the lamina and ligamentum flavum are then identified (**Fig. 11.2A**). The ligamentum flavum can then be safely separated from the undersurface of the more cephalad lamina using a small curette.

1 Patient in prone-kneeling position
2 C-arm fluoroscopy
3 Jackon frame
4 Knees flexed
5 Padding

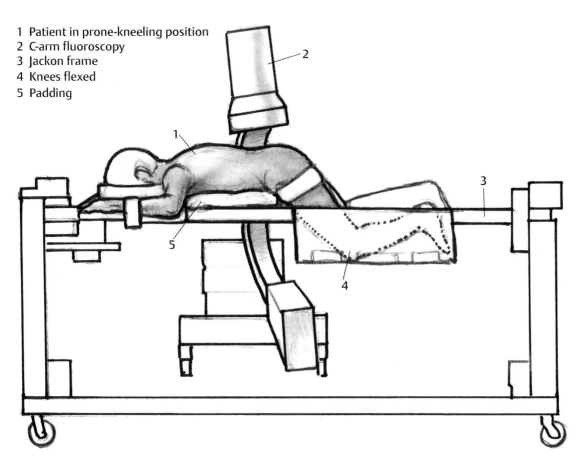

Fig. 11.1   Jackson frame for the proper positioning of a patient for lumbar discectomy.

In cases with a wide enough interlaminar window, the removal of the ligament will provide an adequate working channel to access the disc space to remove the HNP without any bony resection. However, it is usually necessary to perform some degree of laminotomy with limited medial facetectomy to adequately expose the lateral aspect of the nerve root (**Fig. 11.2B**). This is typically performed using rongeurs and Kerrison punches; however, a high-speed burr may be used in the case of a thickened lamina.

The nerve root can be safely retracted toward the midline using a nerve root retractor (**Fig. 11.2C**). It is particularly important to ensure that the entire lateral edge of the nerve root is visualized and that the nerve root and the ventral surface of the thecal sac are free of any adhesions to underlying tissue. Failure to do so may result in an inadvertent durotomy. With safe and gentle retraction medially, the anulus or herniated fragment will be visualized. There

are cases in which large disc fragments may exert dorsal pressure, effectively thinning the nerve roots, which can then mimic the appearance of the anulus. It is imperative that proper identification and differentiation of both the nerve root sleeve and the anulus or disc fragment are performed prior to proceeding with the procedure. After proper identification, the nerve root can be safely retracted and held in place, while the anulus is incised or the extruded fragment is removed (**Fig. 11.2D**). In general, it is safer to make the initial cut into the disc space along the longitudinal direction of the nerve root as this will minimize the risk of potentially cutting the nerve root. Prolonged retraction of the nerve root should be avoided to prevent iatrogenic traction injury, and retraction should be released frequently during the procedure.

Once the disc space is incised, herniated material can be removed with the assistance of a ball-tipped probe and

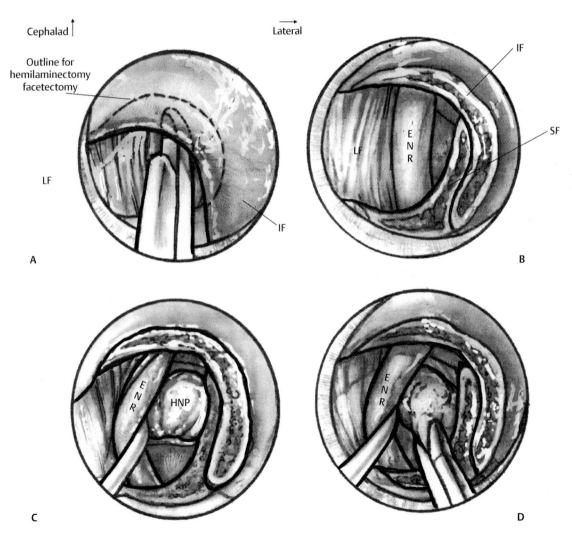

Fig. 11.2 Minimally invasive microdiscectomy technique. HNP, herniated nucleus pulposus; ENR exiting nerve root; LF, ligamentum flavum; IF, inferior facet; SF, superior facet.

pituitary rongeur. If a pituitary rongeur is used, it should not be placed into the disc space any deeper than its jaws to decrease the risk of iatrogenic injury to the great vessels anterior to the spine.

There are two schools of thought on the amount of disc material removed during a discectomy. Some surgeons favor removing a generous amount of disc from the intervertebral space. This is thought to reduce the rate of reherniation at the same operative site. Some hypothesize that the decreased disc height contributes negatively and causes spondylosis and possible failed-back syndrome. With this in mind, other surgeons aim to minimize the amount of disc material removed during surgery and only remove the offending disc material. Recent data would seem to support the latter.[11,12] Barth and colleagues reported on 84 patients who were randomized to either sequestrectomy or traditional microdiscectomy and followed prospectively for 2 years. The technique for those patients who underwent sequestrectomy allowed removal of the offending disc fragment without entering the disc space. Discectomy in those patients in the traditional group involved placing a pituitary rongeur into the disc space "in an attempt to remove as much of the loose intradiscal tissue as possible." Reherniation rates and objective symptoms of neurologic compression were similar between the two groups. However, functional outcome at 2 years postoperatively was worse among those who underwent a traditional microdiscectomy. In addition, radiographic evidence of postoperative disc degeneration such as loss of disc space height, and Modic endplate changes were less pronounced in the

sequestrectomy group. The authors postulate that this may "avert the development of postoperative low back pain."[11,12] These current findings would seem to confirm the findings of Hanley and Shapiro, who postulated that limiting the excision of disc material decreases the incidence of postoperative low back pain.[13]

Minimally Invasive Discectomy

The major advantage of a minimally invasive approach is to limit the damage to the surrounding soft tissue while accessing the disc space (**Fig. 11.3**).[14–16] Muscle is not devascularized nor is it under high-pressure retraction during the case. The common pathway to perform minimally invasive discectomy is via a muscle-splitting technique. The natural tissue plane between the sacrospinalis muscle medially and the longissimus and iliocostalis muscle laterally is typically utilized for access. Once a patient is prepped and draped for the surgery, the midline is marked either by a palpation or under C-arm fluoroscopy. A paramedian incision 1.5 cm off the midline is then made for the initial skin incision. The usual length of the incision is ~1.5 cm. There is not a routine need for separate incision on the fascia. A Kirschner wire is then advanced through the fascia and toward the bony spine. The smallest dilator is passed over the Kirschner wire through the fascia, and the wire is removed. Using the smaller dilators, most of the muscle can be stripped off the lamina using a small, circular motion (**Fig. 11.4**). This maneuver will minimize the amount of soft tissue removed to expose the lamina. A 16- to 22-mm diameter tube is

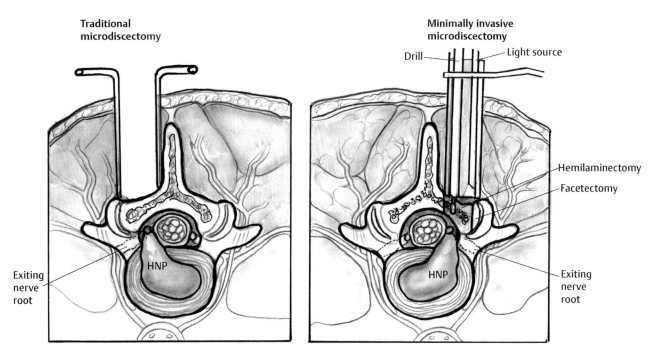

Fig. 11.3 Traditional versus minimally invasive microdiscectomy. HNP, herniated nucleus pulposus.

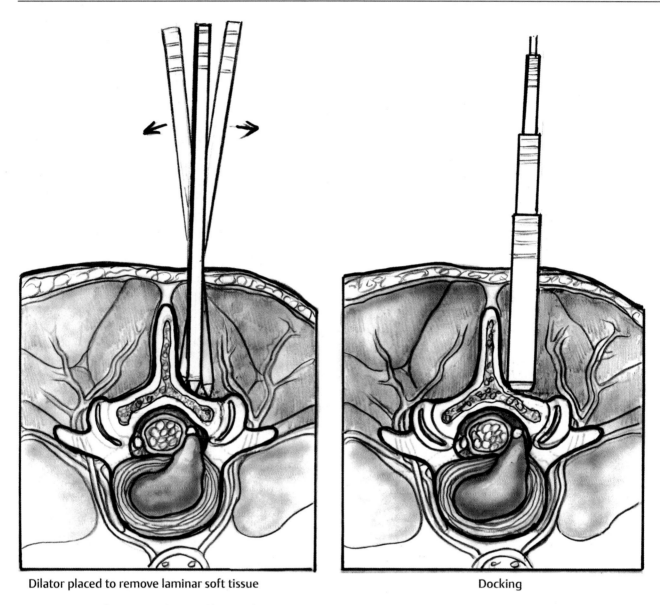

Dilator placed to remove laminar soft tissue   Docking

Fig. 11.4   Minimally invasive soft tissue dilation technique.

routinely used at the appropriate depth for each patient and is positioned over the interlaminar space (**Fig. 11.5**). Bayoneted instruments are utilized to perform the procedure via the tube. Once the exposure is done and tubes are in place, the rest of the procedure utilizes the same technique as a routine microdiscectomy.

There is a learning curve for the surgeons to become familiar with the small circular view through tubular retractors. In addition, 2D working views via endoscopes can make the technique even more difficult. Thirty cases appear to be the minimal number to acquire the necessary skill to perform the operation proficiently.[17] When it is done properly with adequate training, the result of microendoscopic discectomy (MED) is comparable to the

open microdiscectomy.[18] More surgeons are now using the microscope with the minimally invasive surgical approach. This essentially eliminates the need for dealing with the 2D aspect of endoscopes while still getting the full benefit of the muscle-splitting technique.

Minimally invasive techniques are thought to decrease tissue trauma. Recent research supports this claim. A study reported in 2006 by Sasaoka and colleagues[19] analyzed sequential sampling of interleukin-6 (IL-6), interleukin-10 (IL-10), C-reactive protein, and creatine phosphokinase (CPK) following open laminotomy, MED, and microdiscectomy. There was significantly lower level of IL-6 after 24 hours in the MED group compared to the other two groups, indicating that there is potentially less

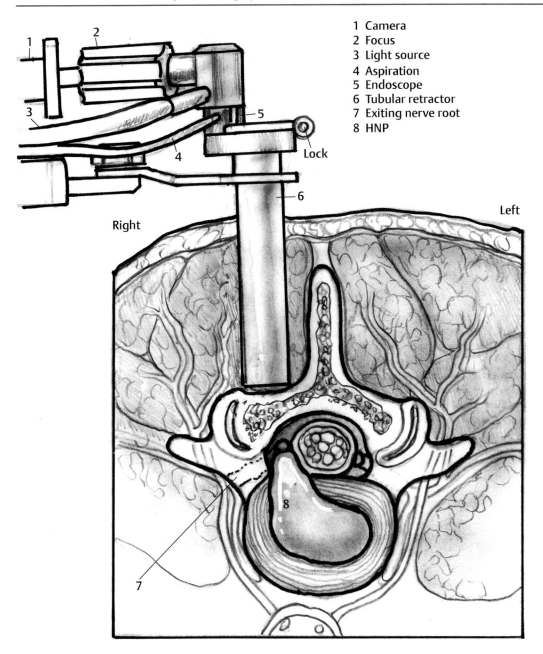

1 Camera
2 Focus
3 Light source
4 Aspiration
5 Endoscope
6 Tubular retractor
7 Exiting nerve root
8 HNP

Fig. 11.5 Minimally invasive retractor configuration. HNP, herniated nucleus pulposus.

tissue inflammation using a minimally invasive approach. The remaining markers failed to show a significant difference between MED and microdiscectomy.[19]

A critical approach should be taken when evaluating any new technique. The newest and latest technology may not necessarily represent the best option for patients. However, exploring new technology and its possible benefit to patients is important to advance any field of medicine. Minimally invasive spinal surgery is still an actively evolving field that will take time and research to fully realize its place in the treatment armamentarium of spinal surgeons.

■ Postoperative Care
Outpatient versus Inpatient

Ambulatory outpatient surgery centers have recently provided an environment for a multitude of surgical procedures to be performed in an outpatient setting. Although some of this is due to technical advances in surgical procedures, there is no debating that evolving financial incentives and regulations have played a large role in this trend as well. The introduction of minimally invasive spinal surgery into the outpatient setting may provide benefits to both patients and surgeons by limiting cost and improving efficiency compared with the in-patient setting.

Gray and colleagues[20] conducted a population-based study investigating multiple national patient databases to find the rate of ambulatory lumbar spine surgery. The National Hospital Discharge Service (NHDS), the National Survey of Ambulatory Surgery (NSAS), and the Healthcare Cost and Utilization Project (HCUP) for four geographically diverse states showed an increasing trend in the proportion of discectomies being done as an outpatient (4% in 1994 versus 26% in 2000). Because it is rare for outpatient fusions or decompressive laminectomies to be performed, discectomy was found to make up 70 to 90% of all the outpatient lumbar procedures.[20]

Best and Sasso[21] reported on their series of 1377 microdiscectomies performed from 1992 to 2001 as intended outpatient procedures and found only a 4% conversion to an inpatient stay. Those converted were due to either a surgical complication or secondary to the patient's request. The overall complication rate was 8%, which included a recurrent disc herniation rate of 6.4%. The authors concluded that outpatient microdiscectomy could be performed safely and with a low complication rate.[21]

Activity Limitation

The fear of reherniation following a discectomy has traditionally forced surgeons to restrict a patient's activity at home and work from a few weeks to months. Although it is generally an accepted practice to release patients to resume work earlier if he or she does less physically demanding work than those patients who perform heavier-duty activity, there is a lack of data supporting the practice.

In contrast, a prospective study by Carragee et al[22] of 152 cohorts with average follow-up time of 4.8 years showed earlier return to work without long-term complications when the patients were not placed under activity restrictions postoperatively by the surgeon. Five years following surgery, the same group reported a radiologic reherniation rate of 11.5% and reoperation rate of 5%, both of which compare favorably to what has been reported in the literature.[21–25] The anecdotal practice of placing limitations on postoperative activity should not be completely ignored based on a single clinical study. But it is noteworthy to acknowledge that there is a different method of treatment that may be as efficacious as the current practice standards.

■ Complications

A survey conducted by the European Spine Society showed that microdiscectomy has a high rate of effectiveness with a negative overall risk value score. This would

Table 11.1 Complications Related to Lumbar Discectomy

Dural tear with cerebrospinal fluid leak
Pseudomeningocele formation
Nerve root injury
Bowel or bladder dysfunction
Bleeding
Abdominal vessel injury
Wrong level operation
Missed fragment
Infection
Epidural hematoma
Compression neuropathy from positioning
Recurrent herniation

seem to indicate that it is a fairly "low risk–high gain" procedure.[26] However, despite this understanding, it is imperative not to become complacent in the treatment of patients. It is critical to understand the possible complications of the procedure and not only how to prevent them but also treat them effectively when they do occur. **Table 11.1** lists complications related to the lumbar discectomy. Every effort should be made to minimize the likelihood of complications, beginning with the initial consultation and patient selection to proper postoperative care. Simple preventative measures such as intraoperative radiographs and proper patient education should be used by all surgeons.

■ Outcome Data

Clinical Outcome

Lumbar discectomy performed for sciatica has a reported improvement rate and success of between 80 and 90%.[18,27,28] The primary purpose of a lumbar discectomy is to relieve the radicular symptoms associated with the herniated disc. Some patients will complain of persistent low back pain postoperatively, which many surgeons consider a separate disease process, rather than classifying it as a component of poor surgical outcome. Patients should be counseled of this possibility prior to the procedure.

Recurrence

The rate of reherniation at the same side and level of previous discectomy has been reported between 1 and 11%.[23–25] Surgeons have tried variations in the amount of herniated disc material removed in an attempt to reduce the rate of recurrence. Many believe aggressive removal of nucleus pulposus confined within the anulus will prevent future reherniation by reducing the amount of material that can potentially herniate through the defect on the anulus. Some have demonstrated data contradicting this general belief. Thome and colleagues[25] conducted a small prospective, randomized study comparing the microdiscectomy and sequestrectomy. The clinical outcome among 84 patients favored sequestrectomy after at least 12 months of follow-up.[25] In a recent report by the same group, there were no differences in reherniation found between the two groups at 2 years of follow-up.[10,11]

Reoperation for recurrent disc herniation is more technically challenging and carries higher surgical complication risk. Successful outcome with symptomatic relief following reoperation is less likely and is reported to be near 50%, although there are smaller series that report a successful outcome in up to 90% of cases.[24] Recently, Wera and colleagues[23] retrospectively evaluated 1320 patients who underwent a primary subtotal discectomy. Among this cohort, there were 14 symptomatic reherniations within the first year of their index procedure. These patients all had a subsequent reexploration and discectomy and were followed for an average of 52.6 months. Despite their multiple procedures, there were no significant outcome differences between those patients who underwent a single subtotal discectomy and those who had a second operation for reherniation. Papadopoulos et al found similar results when comparing primary and revision microdiscectomy patients and concluded that "the results of microdiscectomy for treatment of a recurrent lumbar disc herniation at the same location were comparable with those of primary discectomy."[29]

References

1. Dandy WE. Loose cartilage from intervertebral disc simulating tumor of the spinal cord. Arch Surg 1929;19:660–672
2. Mixter WJ, Barr JS. Rupture of the intervertebral disc with involvement of the spinal canal. N Engl J Med 1934;211:210–215
3. Caspar W. A new surgical procedure for lumbar disc herniation causing less tissue damage through a microsurgical approach. Adv Neurosurg 1977;4:74–77
4. Yasargil MG. Microsurgical operation of herniated lumbar disc. Adv Neurosurg 1977;4:81–83
5. Foley KT, Smith MM. Microendoscopic discectomy. Tech Neurosurg 1997;3:301–307
6. Weinstein JN, Tosteson TD, Lurie JD, et al. Surgical vs nonoperative treatment for lumbar disk herniation: the Spine Patient Outcomes Research Trial (SPORT): a randomized trial. JAMA 2006;296(20):2441–2450
7. Weinstein JN, Lurie JD, Tosteson TD, et al. Surgical vs nonoperative treatment for lumbar disk herniation: the Spine Patient Outcomes Research Trial (SPORT) observational cohort. JAMA 2006;296(20):2451–2459
8. Flum DR. Interpreting surgical trials with subjective outcomes: avoiding unSPORTsmanlike conduct. JAMA 2006;296:2483–2485
9. Carragee E. Surgical treatment of lumbar disk disorders. JAMA 2006;296:2485–2487
10. Katayama Y, Matsuyama Y, Yoshihara H, et al. Comparison of surgical outcomes between macro discectomy and micro discectomy for lumbar disc herniation: a prospective randomized study with surgery performed by the same spine surgeon. J Spinal Disord Tech 2006;19(5):344–347
11. Barth M, Diepers M, Weiss C, Thome C. Two-year outcome after lumbar microdiscectomy versus microscopic sequestrectomy. Part 2. Radiographic evaluation and correlation with clinical outcome. Spine 2008;33(3):273–279
12. Barth M, Weiss C, Thome C. Two-year outcome after lumbar microdiscectomy versus microscopic discectomy. Part 1. Evaluation of clinical outcome. Spine 2008;33(3):265–272
13. Hanley EN, Shapiro DE. The development of low-back pain after excision of a lumbar disc. J Bone Joint Surg Am 1989;71:719–721
14. Schick U, Doehnert J, Richter A, et al. Microendoscopic lumbar discectomy versus open surgery: an intraoperative EMG study. Eur Spine J 2002;11:20–26
15. Parke WW. The significance of venous return in ischemic radiculopathy and myelopathy. Orthop Clin North Am 1991;22:213–220
16. Weber BR, Grob D, Dvorak J, et al. Posterior surgical approach to the lumbar spine and its effect on the multifidus muscle. Spine 1997;22:1765–1772
17. Nowitzke AM. Assessment of the learning curve for lumbar microendoscopic discectomy. Neurosurgery 2005;56(4):755–762
18. Wu X, Zhuang S, Mao Z, Chen H. Microendoscopic discectomy for lumbar disc herniation: surgical technique and outcome in 873 consecutive cases. Spine 2006;31(23):2689–2694
19. Sasaoka R, Nakamura H, Konishi S, et al. Objective assessment of reduced invasiveness in MED: compared with conventional one-level laminotomy. Eur Spine J 2006;15(5):577–582
20. Gray DT, Deyo RA, Kreuter W, et al. Population-based trends in volumes and rates of ambulatory lumbar spine surgery. Spine 2006;31(17):1957–1963
21. Best NM, Sasso RC. Success and safety in outpatient microlumbar discectomy. J Spinal Disord Tech 2006;19(5):334–337
22. Carragee EJ, Han MY, Yang B, Kim DH, Kraemer H, Billys J. Activity restrictions after posterior lumbar discectomy: a prospective study of outcomes in 152 cases with no postoperative restrictions. Spine 1999;24(22):2346–2351
23. Wera GD, Marcus RE, Ghanayem AJ, Bohlman HH. Failure within one year following subtotal lumbar discectomy. J Bone Joint Surg Am 2008;90:10–15
24. Isaacs RE, Podichetty V, Fessler RG. Microendoscopic discectomy for recurrent disc herniations. Neurosurg Focus 2003;15(3):E11
25. Thome C, Barth M, Scharf J, Schmiedek P. Outcome after lumbar sequestrectomy compared with microdiscectomy: a prospective randomized study. J Neurosurg Spine 2005;2(3):271–278

26. Kraemer R, Wild A, Haak H, Herdmann J, Krauspe R, Kraemer J. Classification and management of early complications in open lumbar microdiscectomy. Eur Spine J 2003;12(3):239–246 Epub 2002 Dec 19.

27. Fisher C, Noonan V, Bishop P, et al. Outcome evaluation of the operative management of lumbar disc herniation causing sciatica. J Neurosurg 2004;100:317–324

28. Errico TJ, Fardon DF, Lowell TD. Open discectomy as treatment for herniated nucleus pulposus of the lumbar spine. Spine J 2003;3 (3 suppl)45S–49S

29. Papadopoulos EC, Girardi FP, Sandhu HS, et al. Outcome of revision discectomies following recurrent lumbar disc herniation. Spine 2006;31:1473–1476

12 Annular Repair and Barrier Technologies

Pablo R. Pazmiño and Carl Lauryssen

The intervertebral disc (IVD) serves as the core dynamic stabilizer to the complex spinal system. Injuries to the disc alter its intrinsic biomechanics and result in adverse load transfers toward the secondary surrounding structures, primarily the facet joints. This premise has garnered interest in annular repair and barrier technologies, which promise to provide a more biomechanically stable motion segment while diminishing the risks of recurrent disc herniations.

Since Fedor Krause's first discectomy in 1909, management of disc herniations has been primarily directed toward excision.[1] Annular repair, however, is not a new concept; the first known repair was performed in 1967 by Professor MG Yasargil using 7.0 suture in efforts to decrease adhesions.[2] Despite this report, this procedure attracted little or no attention, and initially clinical management was directed toward nucleotomy, in which a central portion of the disc was widely excised to prevent reherniation of disc material. Symptomatic reherniation rates after lumbar discectomies still range from 3 to 27%.[3,4] Outcome analysis after repeat surgical management to address these reherniations has shown diminished success rates compared with those of the index procedure.[3–5] Until recently, annular repair attracted little or no attention as the anulus was believed to be of little importance and largely incapable of healing. Advances in cell biology have demonstrated the crucial role of the nucleus pulposus (NP) in the development and establishment of the anulus fibrosus (AF).[6] These studies have resulted in a renewed interest in the basic science of the NP and the AF in terms of their structure, physiology, and function.

New biologic techniques and advances in engineering may address annular deficiencies on a cellular, genetic, or mechanical level. These novel measures may lead to clinical applications using annular repair or the establishment of barrier technologies to preserve disc biology and function.

■ Anulus Structure and Function

The AF makes up the peripheral border of each disc as a thick, convex attachment along the inner surface of the anterior and posterior longitudinal ligaments. The medial and lateral borders of the AF taper to a thin, free edge.[7] The AF is made of both type I and type II collagen fiber bundles arranged circumferentially into distinct lamellar layers with varying thickness around the disc. Depending on the patient age, level, and location these laminates can range anywhere from 15 to 25 layers thick.[8] There is a corresponding transition area along the posterolateral junction of the disc that represents an intersection of the maximum and minimum concentration of these laminate layers. This posterolateral quadrant also represents a change in the inclination of the fiber bundles themselves, which vary from 0 degrees and parallel to as much as 90 degrees of inclination along the interface.[8] These inherent structural irregularities may help explain the frequency of herniations from the posterolateral quadrant, where circumferential tensile strains are highest in bending and extension modes.[9]

First described in the 1970s, the Kirkaldy-Willis "degenerative cascade" of disc disease has set the framework for the biochemical and structural changes associated with disc pathology.[10] Essentially, degenerative changes begin as recurrent strains that lead to small circumferential tears in the AF. These tears then coalesce and form radial annular tears giving the NP a path toward the outer innervated annular lamellae.[10,11] Throughout this process, there is a series of complex structural, physiologic, morphologic, and biochemical changes leading to mechanical dysfunction, and ultimately pain. Histologically dehydration, decreased cellularity, disorganization, and annular disruption have been described throughout the disc and its extracellular matrix.[7–9,11] IVD cells exhibit both anabolic and catabolic responses to different types of mechanical stimuli, depending on the loading type, magnitude, duration, and anatomic zone of cell origin. In response to these stimuli, the chondrocytes regulate expression of cytokines, proteases, and matrix metalloproteinases, which subsequently remodel the extracellular matrix.[12,13] This modification of the matrix subsequently alters disc height, elasticity, and hydrostatic and interstitial pressures. With time, the disc loses its basic morphology through a loss of proteoglycans, fibrosis, calcification, and ankylosis. Progression through the cascade ultimately results in stress redistribution as demonstrated by ligamentum flavum hypertrophy, foraminal stenosis, vertebral endplate edema, and facet damage.

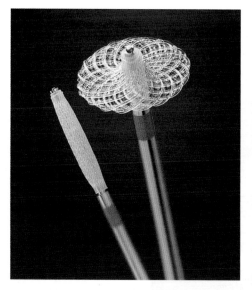

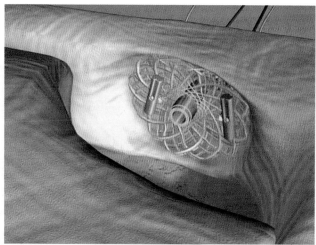

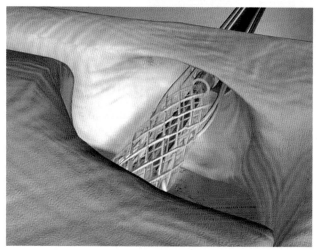

Fig. 12.3 The Inclose Surgical Mesh System. **(A)** Device. **(B)** Mesh implant. **(C)** Mesh implant insertion. (Courtesy of Anulex Technologies Inc.)

scaffolds for AF and chondrocyte seeding. Polymer scaffolds, hydrogels, and hyaluronan-gelatin composite sponges have all served as substrates.[26,27] Materials such as Gelfoam are also being investigated as a carrier for adult mesenchymal stem cells as a means of regeneration therapies.[27] Recently, Wang et al[28] demonstrated establishment of a zonal architecture as seen in native cartilage using a porous silk scaffold.[29] Sato et al[30] allografted cells of the AF both in vitro and in vivo using an atelocollagen honeycomb-shaped scaffold with a membrane seal (**Fig. 12.5**). The cultured anulus cells retained the ability to express and deposit type II collagen. Using this scaffold, they were able to prevent narrowing of the IVD space in vivo, which may allow for disc regeneration through allografting of AF cells. The capacity of the annular and chondrocyte cells to replicate the matrix production of the nucleus cells through scaffolds suggests a potential avenue for repairing and ultimately restoring the normal structure and function of the disc.

■ Summary

Advancements in barrier technologies, primary surgical repair, and gene therapy may provide surgeons with alternative options to add to their therapeutic cache. As these methods and devices are evaluated, several issues should be addressed. The indications for annular repair should be clear. The theoretical benefits of each implant or device as well as the mechanism through which it is effective should be demonstrated through cadaveric preclinical analysis. Subsequent clinical trials should clearly demonstrate efficacy, safety, and benefits that outweigh the risks of the implant

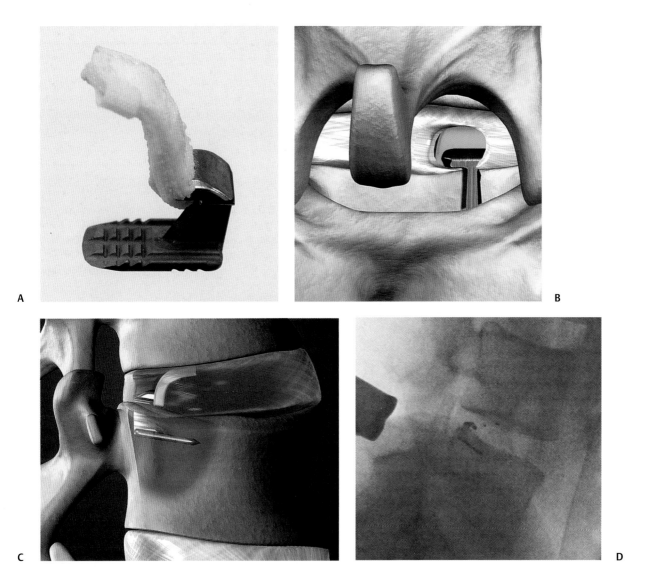

Fig. 12.4 **(A)** The Barricaid annular reconstruction device (ARD). **(B)** Implantation of the ARD through an annular defect after a limited discectomy procedure. **(C,D)** The titanium bone anchor. (Courtesy of Intrinsic Therapeutics Inc.)

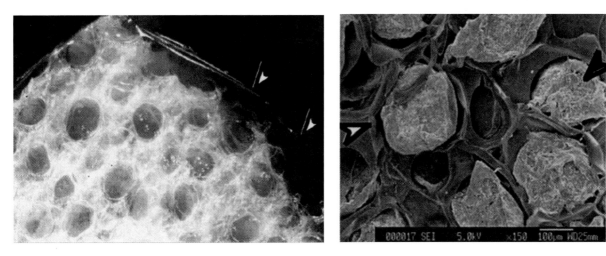

Fig. 12.5 **(A)** An atelocollagen honeycomb-shaped scaffold with a membrane seal. **(B)** Scanning electron microphotograph of the scaffold cultured anulus fibrosus cells after 21 days. (From Sato M, Kikuchi M, Ishihara M, et al. Tissue engineering of the intervertebral disc with cultured annulus fibrosus cells using atelocollagen honeycomb-shaped scaffold with a membrane seal [ACHMS scaffold]. Med Biol Eng Comput 2003;41:365–371. Reprinted with permission.)

and the requisite surgical procedure. Clinically meaningful improvements should be demonstrated through validated outcome scores compared with those of control populations undergoing the current gold standard. The potential for intraspinal scarring induced by these products as well as their effect on the disk over time must be studied. Because of great strides being made through cell transplantation, molecular biology, and bioengineering, the goal of annular repair and restoration of disc function holds promise for the future.

References

1. Castro I, Santos DP, Christoph DH, et al. The history of spinal surgery for disc disease: an illustrated timeline. Arq Neuropsiquiatr 2005;63:701–706
2. Yasargil MG. Microsurgical operation of herniated lumbar disc. Neurosurgery 1977;4:22–24
3. Carragee EJ, Han MY, Suen PW, Kim D. Clinical outcomes after lumbar discectomy for sciatica: the effects of fragment type and anular competence. J Bone Joint Surg Am 2007;85(1):102–108
4. Ebeling U, Kalbarcyk H, Reulen HJ. Microsurgical reoperation following lumbar disc surgery: timing, surgical findings, and outcome in 92 patients. J Neurosurg 2007;1989(70):397–404
5. Herron L. Recurrent lumbar disc herniation: results of repeat laminectomy and discectomy. J Spinal Disord 1994;7:161–166
6. Kim KW, Lim TH, Kim JG, et al. The origin of chondrocytes in the nucleus pulposus and histologic findings associated with the transition of a notochordal nucleus pulposus to a fibrocartilaginous nucleus pulposus in intact rabbit intervertebral discs. Spine 2003;28:982–990
7. Coventry M. The intervertebral disc its microscopic anatomy and pathology: Part I. Anatomy, development, and physiology. J Bone Joint Surg Am 1945;27:105–112
8. Marchand F, Ahmed AM. Investigation of the laminate structure of lumbar disc anulus fibrosus. Spine 1990;15:402–410
9. Tsantrizos A, Ito K, Aebi M, et al. Internal strains in healthy and degenerated lumbar intervertebral discs. Spine 2005;30:2129–2137
10. Kirkaldy-Willis W. Managing Low Back Pain. 4th ed. Churchill Livingstone; 1970
11. Kim Y. Prediction of peripheral tears in the anulus of the intervertebral disc. Spine 2000;25:1771–1774
12. Olmarker K, Blomquist J, Stromberg J, et al. Inflammatogenic properties of nucleus pulposus. Spine 1995;20:665–669
13. Setton LA, Chen J. Cell mechanics and mechanobiology in the intervertebral disc. Spine 2004;29:2710–2723
14. Ahlgren BD, Vasavada A, Brower RS, et al. Anular incision technique on the strength and multidirectional flexibility of the healing intervertebral disc. Spine 1994;19:948–954
15. Ahlgren BD, Lui W, Herkowitz HN, et al. Effect of anular repair on the healing strength of the intervertebral disc: a sheep model. Spine 2000;25:2165–2170
16. Bourgeault C, Beaubien B, Griffith S. Biomechanical Assessment of Anulus Fibrosus Repair with Suture Tethered Anchors. Berlin: Spine Arthroplasty Society; 2007
17. Yorimitsu E, Chiba K, Toyama Y, et al. Long-term outcomes of standard discectomy for lumbar disc herniation: a follow-up study of more than 10 years. Spine 2001;26:652–657
18. Kamaric E, Gorensek M, Eustacchio S, et al. Surgical factors affecting reherniation rate after lumbar discectomy: the need for an annular closure device. Woburn, MA: Intrinsic Therapeutics, Inc.; 2007.
19. Gorensek M, Vilendecic M, Eustacchio S, et al. Clinical investigation of intrinsic therapeutics Barricaid, a novel device for closing defects in the anulus. Spine J 2007;8(suppl):144S.
20. Yeh O, Chowa S, Smalla M, Einhorna J, Lambrechta G. Pressure: implications for expulsion testing of intra-discal devices. Spine J 2007;6(suppl)146S–147S.
21. Sherman J, Cauthen J, Griffith S. Pre-clinical evaluation of a mesh device for repairing the anulus fibrosus. 7th Annual Spine Arthroplasty Society Global Symposium on Motion Preservation Technology, May 5–7, 2007, Berlin, Germany.
22. Bajares G, Perez A, Diaz M, et al. One year follow up of discectomy patients who received a mesh to repair the anulus fibrosus. 7th Annual Spine Arthroplasty Society Global Symposium on Motion Preservation Technology, May 5–7, 2007, Berlin, Germany
23. Taylor W. Biologic collagen PMMA injection (Artefill) repairs: mid-anular concentric defects in the ovine model. Spine J 2007;6(5):48S–49S
24. Guo JF, Jourdian GW, MacCallum DK. Culture and growth characteristics of chondrocytes encapsulated in alginate beads. Connect Tissue Res 1989;19:277–297
25. Saadeh PB, Brent B, Mehrara BJ, et al. Human cartilage engineering: chondrocyte extraction, proliferation, and characterization for construct development. Ann Plast Surg 1999;42:509–513
26. Williams CG, Kim TK, Taboas A, et al. In vitro chondrogenesis of bone marrow-derived mesenchymal stem cells in a photopolymerizing hydrogel. Tissue Eng 2003;9:679–688
27. Ponticiello MS, Schinagl RM, Kadiyala S, et al. Gelatin-based resorbable sponge as a carrier matrix for human mesenchymal stem cells in cartilage regeneration therapy. J Biomed Mater Res 2000;52:246–255
28. Wang Y, Kim UJ, Blasioli DJ, et al. In vitro cartilage tissue engineering with 3D porous aqueous-derived silk scaffolds and mesenchymal stem cells. Biomaterials 2005;26:7082–7094
29. Chang G, Kim HJ, Kaplan D, Vunjak-Novakovic G, Kandel RA. Porous silk scaffolds can be used for tissue engineering annulus fibrosus. Eur Spine J 2007;16(11):1848–1857
30. Sato M, Kikuchi M, Ishihara M, et al. Tissue engineering of the intervertebral disc with cultured annulus fibrosus cells using atelocollagen honeycomb-shaped scaffold with a membrane seal (ACHMS scaffold). Med Biol Eng Comput 2003;41:365–371

III Degenerative Disc Disease

13 Clinical Presentation of Disc Degeneration

Andrew P. White, Eric L. Grossman, and Alan S. Hilibrand

The intervertebral disc (IVD) is a vital and dynamic component of spinal architecture (**Fig. 13.1**). It assists in the distribution of loads and allows for stable yet complex motion. Over time, the disc undergoes a characteristic aging process that is manifested by consistent radiographic changes. In some patients, certain clinical signs and symptoms associated with disc degeneration may also be present.

With advanced degeneration, the disc becomes less competent in appropriately distributing loads, and an alteration of normal spinal biomechanics may result. Increased strain on related structures, including the paired facet joints, can occur and can be associated with varied pathology. Regardless of the underlying physiologic process, the most common symptom seen with degenerative disc disease (DDD) is low back pain (LBP), which in a minority of patients may also be accompanied by neurologic symptoms.[1]

■ Pathophysiology of Disc Degeneration

Repetitive mechanical loading may be related to the characteristic physiologic aging of the spine. Other factors may also be related, including the diminished porosity of the lamina cribrosa, resulting in decreased diffusion of nutrients and waste products. Over time, the IVD undergoes a characteristic degenerative process, with associated signs and symptoms often incident in the third decade. Early degeneration, including disc desiccation and loss of viscoelastic properties, leads to an alteration of spinal biomechanics. This can accelerate the degenerative process and ultimately cause pathologic conditions.[1]

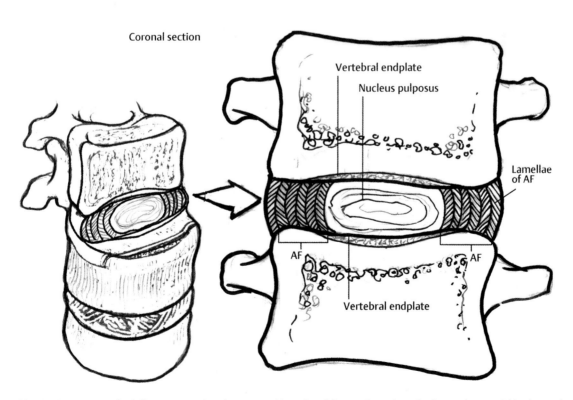

Fig. 13.1 Intervertebral disc cross-sectional anatomy. Note the oblique orientation of adjacent layers within the anulus. AF, anulus fibrosus.

With degeneration, the inner anulus fibrosus (AF) and the outer AF lose their nascent organization and differentiation; they take on a fibrocartilaginous character with indistinct boundaries. In particular, as degeneration occurs, the inner AF and the nucleus pulposus (NP) become virtually indistinguishable. As this occurs, the weakened lamellar structure of the outer AF becomes less resilient to applied forces and may develop defects that can predispose the disc both to herniations of inner disc material and to disc bulging.[1]

The NP in the younger IVD is composed of a high concentration of proteoglycan that helps maintain adequate water content and preserve viscoelastic properties. As aging occurs, maintenance of disc hydration becomes compromised secondary to the tenuous blood supply and decreasing nutritional diffusion. Furthermore, there typically is a decrease in overall proteoglycan content, which leads to an inability to maintain hydration. The IVD's water content may decrease by ~20%. These changes ultimately alter disc structure, volume, and height. This change is associated with an alteration in spinal biomechanics.[2] Immunohistochemical studies have demonstrated deeper penetration of the inner and outer AF by nerve endings in the diseased disc. Additionally, these nerve fibers have tested positive for substance P.[3]

Desiccation of the NP is seen with normal physiologic aging of the lumbar spine. This loss of water content and NP volume causes the "dark disc" phenomenon commonly seen on T2-weighted magnetic resonance imaging (MRI) sequences (**Fig. 13.2**). It is often associated with buckling of the AF. Subsequently, the balance between the breakdown and anabolic repair of trivalent pyridinoline cross-links, responsible for tissue cohesiveness, may be lost. This leads to apoptosis and degeneration of arterioles supplying both the disc and the vertebral endplates. Resultant loss of nutrient and oxygen supply causes excessive lactic acid production, more apoptosis, and additional degenerative changes.[4]

■ Clinical Presentation

The most common clinical symptom thought to be directly associated with lumbar DDD is LBP. Neurologic symptoms such as radicular pain and neurogenic claudication may occur secondary to neural compression. Degeneration of intervertebral structures can be related to the development of neurological symptoms when loss of disc height, bulging of AF and ligamentum flavum, hypertrophy of facet joints, and other degenerative changes limit the space available for neural structures.

Low Back Pain and Degenerative Disc Disease

LBP is the second most common reason that patients seek medical attention and is the fifth most common reason for

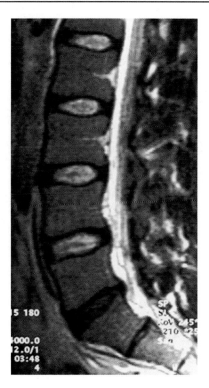

Fig. 13.2 Sagittal T2-weighted magnetic resonance image of the lumbar spine demonstrating an L5–S1 "black disc."

all orthopaedic physician visits. It is common in industrialized countries, with prevalence estimates between 60 and 80%. The etiology of LBP is often related and or exacerbated by socioeconomic, psychological, biochemical, biomechanical, and other factors. LBP is a primary cause of physical disability and has an important socioeconomic impact.

LBP may be caused by injury as well as the degenerative processes and may be affected by poor muscle conditioning or obesity. It may also be a presenting symptom of more serious conditions, such as tumor or infection. As such, evaluating physicians should consider "red flag" signs and symptoms that may motivate a more aggressive evaluation of patients with LBP (**Table 13.1**).

Patients with LBP related to DDD typically present with nonspecific symptoms and without radiculopathy. Pain associated with DDD may arise from the paraspinal musculature, ligaments and tendons, facet joints, discs, and vertebrae. A distinct etiology is rarely identified, however. Degenerative anatomic changes in the spine that have been associated with painful disc degeneration include annular tears, herniated NP, and degenerative instability, including spondylolisthesis, lateral listhesis, and scoliosis. Patients with social and psychological stressors, depression, substance abuse, pending or past litigation or disability compensation, low socioeconomic status, work dissatisfaction, and a history of previous back pain are more likely to have persistent LBP.

Table 13.1 Medical Conditions Associated with Acute Low Back Pain

Category	Symptoms/Risk Factors	Physical Findings
Cancer	History of cancer Unexplained weight loss >10 kg within 6 months Age >50 years or <17 years Failure to improve with therapy Pain persists >4–6 weeks Night pain or pain at rest	Tenderness over the spinous process Range of motion is decreased due to protective muscle spasm
Infection	Persistent fever (>100 4°F) History of intravenous drug abuse Recent bacterial infection, urinary tract infection, or pyelonephritis Cellulitis Pneumonia immunocompromised states Systemic corticosteroids organ transplant Diabetes mellitus Human immunodeficiency virus Rest pain	Tenderness over spinous processes Decreased range of motion Vitals signs consistent with systemic infection Tachycardia, tachypnea, hypotension Elevated temperature Pelvic or abdominal mass or tenderness
Vertebral fracture	Corticosteroids Mild trauma in patients >50 years Osteoporosis in patients >70 years Recent significant trauma at any age Ejection from motor vehicle Fall from substantial height	Findings related to the site of fracture
Herniated nucleus pulposus	Muscle weakness (strength 3 of 5 or less) Foot drop	Significant progression of weakness Significant increased sensory loss New motor weakness Radicular signs
Acute abdominal aneurysm	Abdominal mass Atherosclerotic vascular disease Pain at rest or nocturnal pain Age >60 years	Pulsatile midline abdominal mass
Renal colic	Excruciating pain at costovertebral angle radiating to testis History of urolithiasis	Possible tenderness at costovertebral angle
Pelvic Inflammatory disease	Vaginal discharge Pelvic pain Prior episodes of pelvic inflammatory disease	Uterine tenderness Pelvic mass Cervical discharge
Urinary tract infection	Dysuria History of urinary tract infections	Suprapubic tenderness
Retrocecal appendix	Subacute onset without inciting event Constipation	Low-grade fever

Source: From Bratton RL. Assessment and management of acute low back pain. Am Fam Physician 1999;60:2299–2308.

It is typically difficult to categorize patients with DDD as to the specific cause of their LBP. Diagnostic imaging findings consistent with lumbar disc degeneration are common and can be found in 34% of people between 20 and 39 years old, 59% of people between 40 and 59 years old, and 93% of people between 60 and 80 years old.[5] Disc degeneration, however, is not ubiquitously associated with LBP. Additionally, LBP is not always associated with findings of degeneration on imaging studies. Indeed, it has been reported that 30% of asymptomatic subjects will have a major abnormality on an MRI of the lumbar spine.[5] Regardless of these confounding observations, it is likely that a combination of disc degeneration and the biochemical mediators released during the degenerative process are a component of the nerve sensitization mechanism related to LBP.

14 Degenerative Disc Imaging

Troy Hutchins and M. Marcel Maya

Essential to radiographic evaluation of lumbar degenerative disc disease are appropriate patient selection and thorough clinical evaluation. A significant overlap of radiographic findings between symptomatic and asymptomatic individuals can lead to misdiagnosis or mistreatment. One study of 98 asymptomatic patients showed 64% of patients had at least one disc abnormality on lumbar spine magnetic resonance imaging (MRI),[1] findings supported by numerous additional studies.[2–4] It is therefore crucial to carefully interpret imaging findings with respect to specific clinical signs and symptoms.

In this chapter we review the current concepts in degenerative disc imaging, focusing on the findings that are most important in affecting patient outcome or clinical research.

■ Imaging Findings

Disc Morphology

Plain films have a low sensitivity for detecting early degenerative disc disease (DDD). Late findings of disc space narrowing, sclerotic endplate changes, and gas centrally within the disc (vacuum clefts) are common in the elderly and correlate poorly to symptoms.[5] Although computed tomography (CT) provides better bony detail and soft tissue contrast than plain films, MRI is best suited for the evaluation of disc morphology and content, as well as marrow changes in the adjacent vertebral endplates, and will be the focus of discussion. Provocative testing (discography) is covered in Chapter 15.

Typical MRI protocols consist of sagittal T1-, T2-, and axial T2-weighted images. Contrast-enhanced images are usually reserved for patients with previous disc surgery[6] or suspected infection.[7] Sagittal T2-weighted MRI is best for demonstrating degenerative changes of the disc, thought to be secondary to loss of proteoglycan and fluid content. Pfirrmann et al[8] developed a five-level grading system for disc degeneration to standardize disc assessment for research and clinical applications.[9]

A normal adolescent disc (grade I) has white signal equal to that of cerebral spinal fluid, a homogeneous contour, no loss of height, and clear distinction between the anulus fibrosus (AF) and nucleus pulposus (NP). A normal adult disc (grade II) shows similar features but has an inhomogeneous contour and may have horizontal gray bands. A mildly degenerated disc (grade III) will be gray in signal with indistinct AF–NP border and may have normal to slight loss of height. A moderately degenerated disc (grade IV) will show complete loss of AF–NP distinction, will be gray or black, and may have normal to moderate loss of height. A severely degenerated disc (grade V) will be black with a collapsed disc space (**Table 14.1; Fig. 14.1**).[8]

The importance of such a standardized grading system is illustrated by a study that evaluated risk factors for recurrent disc herniation after microdiscectomy. Lower-grade discs showed higher rates of recurrence, with a 6.8-fold increased risk in grade II (normal adult) versus grade IV (moderately degenerated) discs, a finding with meaningful implications in preoperative patient counseling.[10]

Table 14.1 Pfirrmann Classification of Disc Degeneration

Grade	Degree of Degeneration	T2 Brightness	Nucleus/Anulus Distinction	Disc Height
I	None (normal adolescent)	Bright white	Clear	Normal
II	None (normal adult)	White (may have gray bands)	Clear	Normal
III	Mild	Gray	Unclear	Normal to slightly decreased
IV	Moderate	Gray or black	Lost	Normal to moderately decreased
V	Severe	Black	Lost	Collapsed

Source: Adapted from Pfirrmann CW, Metzdorf A, Zanetti M, Hodler J, Boos N. Magnetic resonance classification of lumbar intervertebral disc degeneration. Spine 2001;26:1873–1878, with permission.

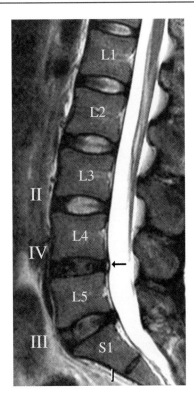
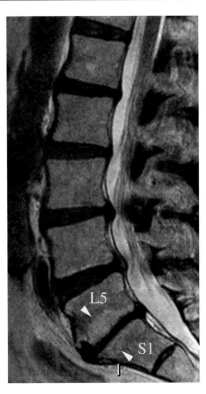

A   B

Fig. 14.1 T2-weighted magnetic resonance images. **(A)** Grade II discs (normal adult) are noted from L1–L2 to L3–L4, grade IV (moderate degeneration) at L4–L5, and grade III (mild degeneration) at L5–S1. Note differences in nucleus pulposus/anulus fibrosus distinction from distinct (grade II) to indistinct (grade III) to absent (grade IV). An annular fissure high-intensity zone is noted at L4–L5 (*arrow*). **(B)** Grade V disc (severe degeneration) is noted at L5–S1, with associated endplate changes (*arrowheads*). T1-weighted imagess are needed to determine if they are Modic type I (low T1-weighted) or II (high T1-weighted).

Vertebral Endplate/Marrow Changes (Modic)

Since their first description by Modic et al in 1988,[11] our understanding of the three types of vertebral endplate and marrow changes associated with degenerated discs in the lumbar spine and how they relate to segmental instability and low back pain has evolved.

Modic type I changes represent vertebral endplate fissuring with infiltrative vascularized fibrous tissue, reflected on MRI as an edema pattern of decreased T1- and increased T2-weighted signal. Type II changes represent postischemic yellow marrow infiltration, with MRI findings of increased T1-weighted, and normal to increased T2-weighted signal reflecting fatty content. Type III changes are those of sclerotic, woven bone, demonstrated by T1- and T2-weighted hypointensity (**Fig. 14.2**).[11,12]

Modic type I changes are the most important to recognize on imaging, as they may best correlate to segmental instability, discogenic low back pain, and positive response to lumbar fusion.[12–18] Their MRI signal characteristics are easy to remember as those of inflammation or edema found in other parts of the body (low T1-, high T2-weighted). Type II changes are generally believed to represent the evolution of type I changes to a more stable state: less associated with pain and less responsive to surgical fusion.[13,19] However, some recent studies have questioned this concept, suggesting that type II changes can reconvert to or develop superimposed type I changes.[13,20] To date, little is known of the clinical significance of type III changes (**Table 14.2**).[13]

Modic changes can be further classified as mild (<25% vertebral body height), moderate (25 to 50%), or severe (>50%), using the vertebral body most severely affected. A correlation between severity of endplate changes (types I and II) with concordant pain on discography has been suggested although not conclusively proven.[12]

Disk Infection

Disc infection with adjacent vertebral body osteomyelitis (spondylodiscitis) needs to be differentiated from Modic type I changes, as both create a marrow edema pattern on MRI (T1-weighted hypointense, T2-weighted hyperintense, T1-weighted post–contrast enhancement).[7,21] The combination of high T2-weighted disc signal, vertebral endplate irregularity, and epidural or paraspinous inflammation should lead to a diagnosis of spondylodiscitis.[7,21] High T2-weighted signal in the disc alone should be interpreted with caution, as degenerated discs with vacuum clefts can accumulate T2-weighted hyperintense fluid after prolonged supine positioning.[22] In questionable cases, C-reactive protein is a sensitive marker for infection and is nearly always elevated in spondylodiscitis.[23]

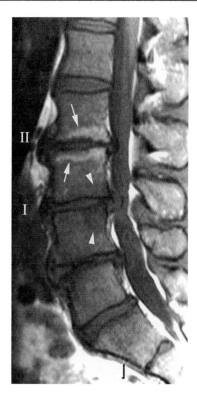
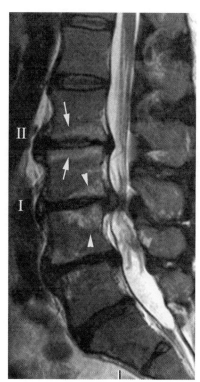

Fig. 14.2 Modic type I changes (*arrowheads*) show decreased T1-weighted **(A)** and increased T2-weighted **(B)** magnetic resonance (MR) signal. Modic type II changes (*arrows*) show increased T1-weighted **(A)** and intermediate or increased T2-weighted **(B)** MR signal. Modic type III changes (not shown) have low T1- and T2-weighted MR signal.

Annular Fissure or Tear

Annular fissure is a synonym for annular tear and the two terms can be used interchangeably, provided it is understood that neither term implies a traumatic etiology.[24] There is some debate over the clinical significance of finding an annular tear or fissure on MRI. It can cause pain by stimulation of the peripheral annular nociceptive fibers. However, a significant number of annular fissures or tears are found in asymptomatic individuals.[24] They are identified on MRI as foci of high T2-weighted signal with possible enhancement on the disc periphery, referred to as high-intensity zones

(**Fig. 14.1A**). There is no correlation between T2-weighted signal/enhancement and acuity of lesion,[25] and their locations poorly correlate to side of pain.[26] They should be identified and interpreted with care.

■ Future Directions

Although MRI of the lumbar spine demonstrates the morphologic changes of aging and disc degeneration in exquisite detail, it often fails to identify the cause of pain.[1] Functional

Table 14.2 Degenerative Vertebral Endplate/Marrow Changes (Modic)

Type	MR Signal	Pattern	Clinical	Pathophysiology
I	T1: Low T2: High	Edema	Most associated with segmental instability, pain, positive response to fusion	Fibrovascular proliferation
II	T1: High T2: Intermediate to high	Fat	Thought to be more stable, less associated with pain, less responsive to fusion than type I	Postischemic yellow marrow infiltration
III	T1: Low T2: Low	Sclerosis	Unknown	Sclerotic woven bone

Source: Data from Modic MT, Steinberg PM, Ross JS, Masaryk TJ, Carter JR. Degenerative disk disease: assessment of changes in vertebral body marrow with MR imaging. Radiology 1988;166:193–199; and Rahme R, Moussa R. The Modic vertebral endplate and marrow changes: pathologic significance and relation to low back pain and segmental instability of the lumbar spine. AJNR Am J Neuroradiol 2008;29:838–842.

Abbreviation: MR, magnetic resonance.

MRI techniques have been applied to lumbar disc evaluation, with promising results. At the forefront, for their potential clinical relevance, are dynamic imaging and T2 relaxometry.[27]

Dynamic imaging aims to identify regions of segmental instability or motion that may be sources of pain, and thus be amenable to surgical fusion.[28,29] Strategies employed in attempts to simulate axial loading include upright MR scanners and radiostereometric analysis. Drawbacks of such techniques include decreased image quality in upright scanners and the invasive nature of radiostereometry, which relies on radiographic measurements after placement of markers on spinous or transverse processes.[28,30]

A recently developed noninvasive technique uses a special table to apply standardized axial torque to the hips during CT or MRI, with degree of axial rotation measured at each level by an automated program.[28,31] Degenerated discs show increased degree of rotation when compared with normal discs. One study defined the average degree of rotation in normal discs (0.5 degrees) versus that in degenerated discs with concordant pain on discography (1.8 degrees).[32]

T2 relaxometry is an MR technique that quantitatively analyzes the T2-weighted value of the disc to determine the degree of degeneration as a function of relative water content. This technique uses a modified three-dimensional (3D) fast spin echo sequence to calculate T2-weighted relaxation times from multiple echoes in the echo train.[27,28] Using these values, 3D color plots can be created for each disc (**Fig. 14.3**).

There are many potential advantages over the previously described qualitative grading system by Pfirrmann. There is decreased intraobserver and interobserver variability. It provides normative values useful for research on aging, degenerative, and traumatic alterations of the disc. Also, with increased sensitivity to disc changes not appreciated with visual classification systems, T2 relaxometry may be useful to precisely measure outcomes of experimental genetic or surgical treatments.[27,28]

■ Summary

Imaging for DDD should be ordered based on specific clinical questions, as there is significant overlap of findings in symptomatic and asymptomatic individuals. MRI is best suited for evaluation of the degenerated lumbar disc and the adjacent vertebral body endplates. A five-level grading system for disc morphology has been proposed to help standardize clinical and research reporting of disc degeneration.

Modic type degenerative endplate changes may help guide therapy in symptomatic patients. Modic type I changes (low T1-, high T2-weighted MRI signal) are most likely to correspond to segmental instability, discogenic pain, and positive response to surgery. Modic type II changes (high T1-, intermediate to high T2-weighted MRI signal) probably represent a more stable evolution of type I changes less associated with pain. High T2-weighted MRI disc signal, irregular endplates, and paraspinal or epidural inflammatory changes help differentiate infectious spondylodiscitis from Modic type I changes.

Dynamic CT/MR imaging and T2 relaxometry are promising functional imaging techniques that may play a future role in DDD evaluation.

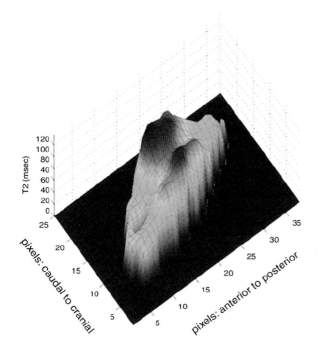
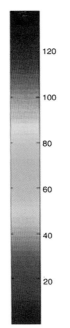

Fig. 14.3 T2 relaxometry three-dimensional color plot of a normal adult disc (grade II). For orientation, anterior is to the reader's left and superior toward the top of the page. Relatively decreased T2-weighted magnetic resonance values are noted centrally representing the intranuclear cleft. (From Haughton VM. Imaging intervertebral disc degeneration. J Bone Joint Surg Am 2006;88[Suppl 2]: 15–20. Reprinted with permission.)

included the exclusion of 23% of injected discs as they were judged invalid due to technical difficulties in performing the procedure. All the subjects were prisoners—Holt performed a significant number of annular injections known to be painful, and he used a highly irritating contrast medium. He did not include positive pain response as a criterion for positive injections, and the criteria for a positive test were based primarily on radiologic images.[16,17]

At the same time of Holt's study, Wiley et al[18] reported on a large series and believed that discography was most valuable in the evaluation of patients with pain and no definite herniation. The concept of an internal disc disruption syndrome with back pain as its primary symptom was introduced by Crock in 1970.[19] The introduction of newer, safer contrast material developed for myelography occurred around the same time,[20] which allowed for safer imaging. In 1984 the introduction of computed tomographic (CT) discography enabled the imaging of intradiscal architecture.[21] Bernard demonstrated that plain discography combined with postdiscography CT gives structural information not attainable by other means of that period.[22]

The more frequent use of manometry has recently been of interest. Manometry allows for the measurement and correlation of incremental injectable pressure with the pain response. The concept of measuring intradiscal pressure is not a new one; Nachemson as early as 1959 attempted to record intradiscal pressure.[23] It has been hypothesized that this technique may permit more specific interpretation and diagnosis and therefore may guide treatment with a higher degree of accuracy.[24,25]

Despite the increasing technical sophistication surrounding the clinical use of discography, it has also been the subject of ongoing uncertainty and controversy.

■ Indications and Guidelines

Some clinicians believe discography is of clinical value and recommend its use in certain indications. Others believe that unless the clinical accuracy and utility of the test can be established using conventional evidence-based medicine methodology, the test should remain investigational.

On the one hand, indications for discography in the management of LBP have been suggested by the Executive Committee of the North American Spine Society Diagnostic and Therapeutic Committee.[26] In this paradigm, discography should be performed only when a patient has failed an adequate course of nonoperative treatment, and other noninterventional tests (e.g., magnetic resonance imaging [MRI]) have failed to provide sufficient diagnostic information. These guidelines give wide latitude

for clinical application and define general uses for discography to include but not be limited to the following[26]:

1. Further evaluation of demonstrably abnormal discs to help assess the extent of abnormality or correlation of the abnormality with clinical symptoms. Such may include recurrent pain from a previously operated disc and lateral disc herniation.
2. Patients with persistent, severe symptoms in whom other diagnostic tests have failed to reveal clear confirmation of a suspected disc as the source of pain
3. Assessment of patients who have failed to respond to surgical procedures to determine if there is a painful pseudarthrosis or a symptomatic disc in a posteriorly fused segment, or to evaluate possible recurrent disc herniation
4. Assessment of discs before fusion to determine if the discs within the proposed fusion segment are symptomatic and to determine if discs adjacent to this segment are normal
5. Assessment of minimally invasive surgical candidates to confirm a contained disc herniation or to investigate dye distribution pattern before chemonucleolysis or other intradiscal procedures

The Guidelines of the American Association of Neurological Surgeons/Congress of Neurological Surgeons (AANS/CNS) recommend that discography not be used as a "stand-alone test" and that positive discography with normal MRI findings should be considered a contraindication to surgical or other invasive interventions. These recommendations suggest a negative test may be most accurate and helpful in limiting fusion length and further caution against diagnosing multiple positive discs with this method.[27]

On the other hand, the AHCPR Guidelines recommend against any use of discography for the evaluation of acute LBP syndromes. Similarly, the European Cost Guidelines recommend against the use of discography in chronic LBP syndromes as being without demonstrable utility of validity. Finally, the Bone and Joint Decade Task Force on Neck Pain and Associative Disorder found there was no evidence to support provocative discography of the cervical spine in patients with neck pain. This group also noted that pain response to provocative discography cannot accurately distinguish between subjects with and without neck pain.[28]

■ Technique for Provocative Lumbar Discography

Patient Evaluation

Most authors of the numerous review articles on discography recommend taking a preliminary history to ascertain that there is no systemic infection, or local infection at the surgical site, no underlying bleeding diathesis, and no inappropriate psychological status of the patient.[29–36] These would all be considered contraindications to the procedure. Note should also be taken of any prior back or disc surgery. Prior imaging studies need to be carefully assessed to exclude other pathology and guide the number and order of the discs to be injected.

The patient's pain should be evaluated, including:

1. The location of the pain (may include a pain diagram)
2. The amount of back pain versus buttock or leg pain
3. Patients assessment of the pain (Visual Analog Scale [VAS])
4. Aggravating and relieving factors

The patient's history of allergies, especially to local anesthetic or contrast media, needs to be assessed, as should the need for prophylactic medication. The patient should have full informed consent prior to the procedure, which should include discussion of the discography-associated risks (see Complications section below).

Anesthesia

Provocative discography requires the patient to be awake and coherent enough to answer questions about the reproduction of pain. Therefore, it is imperative to use sufficient local anesthetic and as little general sedation to keep the patient comfortable, yet avoid disorientation, uncooperative behavior, or somnolence. The patient should ideally be able to recall the procedure well, as the referring surgeon will often ask procedure-related questions at follow-up.

Antibiotics

The use of antibiotics in discography has been of some debate. The administration of a broad-spectrum antibiotic, such as cefazolin, clindamycin, or ciprofloxacin, has been advocated by some authors. This can either be administered intravenously or added to the intradiscal suspension.[37]

Positioning

Care should be taken with positioning to optimize visualization and reducing the difficulty of the procedure. Several discographers prefer to place the patient in a prone or lateral position. Others have described a position in which the patient's body is slightly oblique and at a 45-degree angle to the bed and rotated forward.[38] This position allows for less movement during the procedure, obviates the need for restraints, and improves visualization of the lumbosacral junction, thereby reducing the risk of abutting the iliac crest when inserting the needle.[38] The fluoroscope should then be moved into position. The technique of preliminarily tilting the C-arm to visualize the optimal route into the disc, particularly at the lumbosacral junction, was emphasized by Schellhas.[33]

Approach

Standard sterile preparation of the back should be performed. Local anesthetic should be infiltrated into the skin and possibly underlying musculature. The superior articular pillar (SAP) should not be anesthetized as this may spread anesthetic to the foramen and margin of the disc, increasing the likelihood of a false-negative response. An oblique extradural approach is used through the safe zone lateral to the SAP following the adjacent endplate, using a coaxial two-needle approach. The use of a curved distal needle tip has been advocated to circumvent the SAP and allow positioning of the tip into the mid disc.[39] The placement of needles on the contralateral side to the patient's habitual pain has also been recommended by some authors to avoid interfering with the pain response by inadvertently anesthetizing the spinal nerve to the adjacent disc.[29,33] This concern has not been confirmed.[40] Placement of the needle in the center of the disc is confirmed by biplanar fluoroscopy. Needles are usually placed in at least three consecutive levels.

Assessment

A low osmolar, nonionic contrast has been recommended for discography. The patient should be unaware of the precise moment of injection, the level or levels injected, and the amount injected. The following should be monitored:

- *Pain response.* Anderson[29] recommended an initial injection of a morphologically normal disc (by MRI) to improve the rate of valid pain responses. In this strategy, the suspected painful disc should be injected last, and as each level is injected the patient should be questioned about whether pain was provoked and if so to compare this with the usual symptoms in terms of both quality and distribution. Pain responses are recorded at each level as none or pressure alone, similar or exact pain, termed concordant, and dissimilar or discordant pain. Pain is usually rated on a scale of 0 to 10. It is also important to note the patient's pain mannerisms. Videotaping the patient's face during the procedure may be helpful in eliminating false-positive results but has only been reported in experimental settings.

- *Injection pressure.* The use of a digital manometry has been advocated to obtain information regarding the opening pressure, pressure at the onset of pain, and maximum pressure. The hydraulic integrity of the disc can be determined by assessing the pressure that the disc will hold with a defined injection volume. Pressure may rapidly dissipate in an incompetent disc secondary to leakage through the anulus or endplate. An intact disc/anulus and endplate complex can usually hold a pressure up to 90 mmHg.[38] It is important to avoid pressures that are too high to avoid false-positive results due to endplate deflection, facet distraction, or frank injury to the disc.[25]

pain generator. Various anatomic sites have been implicated, briefly enjoyed popularity, and then discredited, including common osteophytes, facet sclerosis, minor lumbar scoliosis, etc. The concept of the disc as being the pain generator has persisted and the pathognomonic finding in a degenerative disc, which can be definitively and reliably linked to serious axial pain, is the Holy Grail that many investigators seek.

The opposing view holds that the pain generator approach is misplaced after serious underlying diseases have been excluded. These researchers point to the epidemiologic trends and poor results of treatments directed at the spine per se. As imaging studies show similar pathology in those suffering mild discomfort or no LBP at all and those with severe pain, the difference in clinical manifestation must be due to other nonstructural factors. Treatment should then be directed at the other causes, such as central pain processes, psychological factors, social disincentives, poor coping strategies, etc., and aim at restoring function and supporting adaptive techniques.

Anatomic Basis

The concept of the disc being an intrinsic source of pain assumes that common disc abnormalities and internal architectural changes of the anulus also innervated. The innervation of the disc, has of itself, been a source of controversy and whether the cause of the pain is biomechanical or chemical. In discography, the injected substance exerts a mechanical strain on some annular fibers[41] the pain that is generated is believed to arise when these annular fissures or nuclear herniations extend into the outer third of the anulus.[52] In adult degenerative discs, nerve endings from branches of the sinuvertebral nerves, the gray rami communicantes, and the lumbar vertebral rami consistently innervate the outer third of the dorsal, lateral, and ventral aspects of the anulus, respectively.[53] Neurotransmitters associated with nociception have been detected in the posterior longitudinal ligament and anulus. Therefore, a reasonable anatomical basis exists for the disc to be a pain generator.

Confounding Factors in Spinal Pain Perception

The pain reported with disc injection can be influenced by multiple local and generalized factors. Although pain may come from several local sources, several common factors have the potential to suppress or amplify pain perception. These factors need to be carefully considered when evaluating a patient's history, examination, and responses during provocative disc injections.[54]

- *Adjacent tissue injury.* This effect occurs when damage to tissues causes an amplification of pain perception by increasing the local inflammatory and nociceptive processes, resulting in secondary neurologic sensitization of the local nondamaged area. This hyperalgesic effect is especially relevant in patients with LBP with serious structural disease at one or more levels (e.g., unstable spondylolisthesis or disc herniation with root compression) that may sensitize adjacent levels to provocative testing.[55]

- *Tissue injury in same or adjacent sclerotome.* Lower spinal elements that have the same or adjacent afferents shared with a sclerotome that has sustained injury may increase the sensitivity of the spinal elements on which provocative testing is performed. This confounding effect is important when considering the specificity of discography at sites of similar embryonic origin to a known pathologic structure.

- *Local anesthetic.* Perception of pain may be decreased at a local site by local anesthetic injection. This may be the source of false-negative results in provocative discography if the careful placement of the anesthetic is not well controlled.

- *Chronic pain syndromes.* Chronic pain from sites near the lumbar spine (chronic pelvic pain, failed hip arthroplasty, etc.), or distant from the lumbar spine (chronic headache, neckpain, etc.) may increase pain sensitivity and complicate LBP syndromes. The effect on the neural axis may be reflected either globally or locally. Furthermore, chronic pain syndromes are associated with depression and narcotic use habituation, which of themselves affect pain perception, and have been demonstrated to affect pain intensity with discography in experimental subjects.[55]

- *Narcotic analgesia.* The effect of narcotics occurs at multiple levels to decrease the pain thresholds, intensity, and affective response, and may act as a confounder in provocative discography in the perception of pain.[55-57]

- *Narcotic habituation.* Chronic narcotic habituation in the absence of increased narcotic intake may act to decrease pain tolerance in the absence of accustomed opioid intake. It can also be associated with depression and sleep disturbances.

- *Psychological stressors.* Psychological distress from any etiology may increase pain perception. The threshold to a painful response with disc injection may be decreased and the perceived pain intensity and affective response can be increased.[56,58,59] In this situation, discography may erroneously identify otherwise minor structural processes, contributing little to the overall chronic pain illness, as the cause of an extremely painful and gravely disabling condition.

- *Social/cultural factors.* A depressed pain perception or a dissociation of pain perception and functional loss may result from overriding social or cultural factors. Certain cultural groups are less expressive or emotional when describing their chronic pain,[60] and this may decrease the specificity of provocative discography.

- *Secondary gain.* There are common clinical situations in which an exaggerated pain response will result in a real or perceived social benefit or monetary compensation. This may have direct effects on reporting during provocative discography. Patients may have conflicting incentives in reporting pain intensity rating or degree of pain concordance, particularly if large economic fortunes are perceived to be at stake.

In summary, the subjective pain response and quality reported with provocative discography must be evaluated in context of the patient's clinical, psychological, and social circumstance.

■ Diagnostic Accuracy

For a diagnostic test to be of use it has to be reliable and valid and have good utility. The following section will examine the reliability, validity, and utility of provocative discography as a diagnostic test by current methodology standards used in evidence-based medicine.

Reliability

Reliability is the extent to which repeated application of the same test in the same circumstance will produce the same result (i.e., precision or reproducibility).[61] It refers to the capacity of a test to give the same result on repeated application. Although reliability does not imply nor guarantee validity (i.e., high sensitivity and specificity), unreliability will probably make a test insufficiently sensitive or specific to be valid.[62]

Reliability of Discogram Images

Walsh et al[17] used five raters to evaluate the discograms initially into a three-point scale (normal, degenerate, or degenerated and herniated), but later a two-point scale was used. Using a consensus rating the adjusted percent agreement was 96%.[17] Adams et al[41] introduced the fluoroscopic classification of discogram images on cadavers in 1986 and reported 87% reproduction of their results when repeated 6 months later. Later studies have looked at the interobserver and intraobserver agreement in the clinical setting. In the clinical setting, the kappa value for the paired interobserver agreement is excellent at 0.77.[63] Absolute interobserver and intraobserver agreement occurred in 82 levels (62%).[63]

Reliability of Pain Interpretation

Walsh and colleagues in their 1990 work used a two-camera technique to videotape the fluoroscopic image of the discogram as well as the patient's reactions to the injection and the responses to postinjection interview.[17] Pain was evaluated by two of the authors who assessed the patient's pain-related behavior as well as the patient's pain intensity as measured on a pain thermometer. Interobserver reliability was good for the intensity of pain and pain-related behavior (Pearson correlations, 0.986 and 0.926, respectively).[17] Regarding the similarity of the pain, this was in agreement 88% of the time between the two observers.[17] Similar agreement on image interpretation was found in several experimentally designed discography studies.[64,65]

Reliability of Results after Repeated Injections

There are no good reliability data on the pain response or concordancy reporting by patients undergoing discography. It is not clear that repeated testing after a short interval (several hours) or with another set of needle placements on another day would yield the same pain intensity response or concordancy assessment.

Validity

Provocative discography aims to diagnose the presence or absence of a disc lesion as the sole or primary pain generator responsible for an individual's LBP illness. The problem remains that there is no commonly accepted pathoanatomic gold standard for confirming the diagnosis of primary discogenic pain. Sackett and Haynes[1] have described the criteria for the evidence-based evaluation of the validity for diagnostic tests. The four phases of scrutiny are shown in **Table 15.2**. Several clinical and experimental studies have been done to examine the validity of provocative discography.

Table 15.2 Sackett and Haynes Criteria for the Evidence-Based Evaluation of the Validity for Diagnostic Tests

1. Do test results in patients with the target disorder differ from those in normal people?

2. Are patients with certain test results more likely to have the target disorder than patients with other test results?

3. Does the test result distinguish patients with and without the target disorder among patients in whom it is clinically reasonable to suspect that the disease is present?

4. Do patients who undergo this diagnostic test fare better (in their ultimate health outcomes) than similar patients who are not tested?

Evaluation of Pain Response in Asymptomatic Subjects

Psychological Factors in Patients Undergoing Discography

A few studies have investigated the potential impact of psychological factors on discographic pain provocation in clinical practice. Block et al[66] found that patients with elevated scores on the hysteria and hypochondriasis scale of the Minnesota Multiphasic Personality Inventory were significantly more likely to report pain during injection than those without elevated scores. Similarly, patients who indicated unusual patterns on pain drawings were more likely to report pain provocation during injection of a nondisrupted disc than those without unusual pain patterns.[67]

Validity of the Concordancy Response

Whether patients can accurately identify the source of LBP by the quality of sensation when a disc is injected is not clear. Carragee et al performed discography in a group of 8 patients asymptomatic for LBP who had undergone posterior iliac crest bone graft for reasons other than thoracolumbar surgery.[65]Most of these patients experienced low back and buttock pain for some months following the procedure, which is of a similar distribution to what is normally considered typical lumbar discogenic pain. When discography was performed in these subjects, each was asked to compare the quality and location of the injection pain to the usual iliac crest bone graft site pain. In 9 of the 24 discs (37.5%) injected, the pain produced was similar or exact pain, and three of the eight patients (37.5%) would have met the criteria for a positive discogram.

In clinical practice, "positive" concordant lumbar discography has been reported in subjects with known nondiscogenic pain syndromes. Pain from spinal neoplasm (osteoid osteoma), pelvic pathology, and fracture has been confused with the pain of disc injection.[68]

In summary, the validity of the concordancy rating as confirming the source of axial pain has not been proven. Anecdotal reports and small experimental studies indicate the finding of a similar pain perception with disc injection cannot be used with a high degree of confidence to confirm a discogenic source of back pain.

Discography in Subjects with Minimal Low Back Pain

Critical to the validity of provocative discography as a test is the ability to distinguish between a clinically relevant pain generator as the cause of serious disabling back pain as opposed to a disc that may be associated with minimal or inconsequential pain. Derby and colleagues[24] performed discography in a group of 16 subjects with minimal or occasional LBP, which did not require medical care or were experiencing disability. In this group, 5 of 16 (31%) subjects

had a pain response equal to 5/10, and 2 of 16 (12.5%) had a response of 6/10.

In another study, 25 subjects with mild persistent LBP with no functional limitation, who were not seeking medical attention for their problem, underwent provocative discography.[69] Nine of the 25 patients (36%) had discographic injections of one or more discs, which were both significantly painful and concordant. All positive discs had annular disruption, and all had negative control discs. By the usual proposed criteria, these were fully positive disc injections for clinically serious discogenic pain illness.

These findings indicate that even if a disc is correctly identified as being capable of producing some perception of pain with injection, this disc may actually contribute only minimally to the overall pain illness. Consequently, aggressive treatment (e.g., fusion) of a minimally painful disc, although "positive" with discography, will be unlikely to be highly effective.

Utility

For any diagnostic test to be useful (i.e., have clinical utility), the use of the test should be shown to improve outcomes of relevant clinical features. The question remains whether discography appears to have demonstrable utility in the management of patients with chronic LBP. To date, no randomized controlled trial of discography has tested this hypothesis. The data from less rigorous studies are mixed.

Colhoun et al[70] studied 195 patients in whom discography was performed and who later underwent surgery, generally fusion. This retrospective study compared two groups, with and without positive preoperative provocative discography, in whom surgery was technically successful. The group with a positive image and pain provocation had an 88% success rate, whereas in the group with a positive image but negative pain provocation the success rate was only 52%. However, the two groups were not similar at baseline. Furthermore, systematic biases causing some patients to be examined with discography and others to proceed directly to surgery were unexamined.

Madan and colleagues[71] recently studied the outcomes of 73 consecutive patients following spinal fusion who had been evaluated with and without preoperative discography. The authors performed all fusions with discography for a set time interval, then without discography for a matching time interval. The patients were well matched in terms of demographic data and psychometric and radiographic features. At a minimum of 2 years follow-up, there was no significant outcome difference. These authors concluded provocative discography as an additional screening tool was not very helpful in improving patient outcome after circumferential fusion for discogenic back pain.

Finally, Cohen et al[72] compared the outcomes literature for fusion when performed in studies using discography and compared these to studies in which fusion was performed for presumed discogenic pain on the basis of MRI or CT alone. They found no systematically improved outcomes in the studies using discography as a selection criterion. The authors concluded that the use of discography had not been proved to improve the outcome of surgical treatment for degenerative disc disease.

Outcome as Gold Standard

The diagnostic validity of positive discography was assessed by Carragee et al[73] in a highly selected and controlled cohort where positive results were compared against a gold standard of substantial clinical improvement after removal of the supposed pain generator (disc and posterior anulus) and successful interbody arthrodesis. Thirty-two patients with LBP and a positive single-level low-pressure provocative discogram underwent spinal fusion. Generic surgical limitations/morbidity were controlled by comparison to the clinical outcomes of a strictly matched cohort of 34 patients having a well-accepted single-level lumbar pathology (unstable grade I or II isthmic spondylolisthesis). The proportion of patients who met the minimal acceptable outcome was 29 of 32 (91%) in the spondylolisthesis group and 13 of 30 (43%) in the presumed discogenic pain group. This study demonstrated that positive discography was not highly predictive in identifying bona fide isolated intradiscal lesions primarily causing chronic LBP illness. Despite removal of the pain generator as diagnosed by discography, approximately half the patients continued with significant pain and impairment. This is the first study to apply an external gold standard evaluation of the diagnostic validity of discography in any manner.

Other Studies

Moneta et al[52] demonstrated that in clinical practice discs with annular disruption were more likely to be painful with injection than those with disc degeneration alone. There was considerable overlap, however, between these two groups, and it is unclear whether there were more or less false-positive or false-negative injections in those patients with extensive annular disruption.

Laslett et al[74] found that patients coming to discography who had more persistent pain between LBP episodes, a greater feeling of "vulnerability" in the neutral zone, and a centralization phenomenon with lumbar posturing, tended to have more painful disc injections than those without these findings. This group as a whole had longstanding chronic pain, severe psychological distress, and chronic opioid use. Again, which if any of these injections correlated with either true "discogenic pain" or a positive response to proposed treatment was not reported.

Many authors have noted a correlation between bright signal annular fissures (high-intensity zone [HIZ]) seen on MRI and a painful response to disc injection. Aprill and Bogduk[75] reported that an HIZ was "pathognomonic" of severe symptomatic discogenic pain. Further investigation, however, found that HIZ are commonly found in completely asymptomatic subjects and that injection of discs with HIZ in asymptomatic subjects was frequently very painful at low pressures.[76,77]

Summary

It is clear that standard methods to assess the reliability, validity, and utility of provocative discography do not strongly support this test. Test reliability is poorly or inadequately documented. Validity testing in asymptomatic subjects indicates few false-positive results in the subset of persons with no chronic pain processes, no psychological distress, no litigation history, and less annular disruption. Although sometimes meeting this profile, this is not the typical patient coming to discographic evaluation for chronic disabling LBP illness with otherwise age-appropriate studies. The best-case scenario of subjects without these comorbidities and a positive low pressure, single-level disc injection still only found a 50% positive predictive value of "treatable" discogenic pain syndrome. The utility of discography, even in the best-case setting, has not been proved. Data from one well-matched controlled study showed no utility.

Table 15.3 Recommendations for Provocative Discography

Best case for a valid and useful test result

1. Negative discogram (next to other pathology—e.g., spondylolisthesis)
2. Positive single level, normal psychological status, normal social profile (no worker's compensation)

Unclear or doubtful validity or usefulness

1. Two-level positive, normal psychological status, normal social profile
2. Postoperative discs, normal psychological status, normal social profile
3. Intermediate (at risk) psychometrics, equivocal pain behavior, single-level

Poor validity, usefulness, and serious risk of misdirecting care

1. Spine with multilevel pathology
2. Abnormal or chronic behavior
3. Abnormal psychometric findings
4. Disputed compensation cases

Source: Adapted from Carragee EJ, Hannibal M. Diagnostic evaluation of low back pain. Orthop Clin North Am 2004;35:7–16, with permission.

preoperative cessation of smoking.[17,18] Certainly, the longer a patient is abstinent from smoking preoperatively, the more likely he or she will be able to stay abstinent during the lengthy and often-stressful postoperative recovery period.

Alcohol and Substance Abuse

It is difficult to accurately assess alcohol or substance abuse in spine surgery candidates because many patients are reluctant to reveal this type of information.[1] As a result, few studies have directly examined the effect of alcohol or substance abuse on spine surgery outcome. Excessive alcohol use has the potential to negatively impact a patient's recovery from spine surgery in several ways, including slower wound healing, sleep disruption, increased depression and anxiety, increased likelihood of smoking due to lowered impulse control, poor nutrition, amplified endocrine changes in response to surgery, and synergistic interactions with medications.[1,19,20]

Substance abuse in spine surgery candidates might include use of illicit drugs (current or history) or abuse of prescription medications. With the increased acceptance of long-term opioid treatment in the management of chronic pain conditions, evaluation of the possible abuse of prescription medications becomes more difficult. As part of the BPSS, the surgeon should be aware of the following questions: what is the overall level of pain medication use, is the patient showing a need for escalating dosages, has the medication actually improved patient function, is the patient taking the medications as prescribed (compliance or noncompliance), is there any evidence of abuse of prescription medications (e.g., doctor shopping, frequent emergency room visits, getting medication from illegitimate sources), are all the patient's medications related to the chronic pain problem being managed by one physician, and is the patient under an opioid treatment contract? If there is any evidence of alcohol or substance abuse, or if the patient has been on high doses of opioids for quite some time, it is most prudent to address these issues prior to surgery.

Obesity

Body weight has not emerged as a consistent predictor of spine surgery outcome,[9] but recent studies have demonstrated an increased risk for surgical site infection in spinal surgery patients who were morbidly obese.[21,22] Obesity has been found to contribute significantly to several variables predictive of poor outcome to spine surgery.[23] In a workers' compensation population, it has been correlated with greater compensation costs but not medical costs.[24] Elderly obese patients undergoing decompressive laminectomy and/or discectomy (fusion cases excluded), have demonstrated a greater level of being "very dissatisfied" with the

surgery outcome, higher pain ratings, and lower activities of daily living relative to the nonobese comparison group.[25] Interestingly, studies have generally found no differences between obese and nonobese spine surgery groups in terms of duration of surgery, blood loss, duration of hospitalization, and most clinical outcomes.[25,26]

The inconsistent findings of these studies are likely due to the marked differences in patient population variables (age, work status, etc.), definitions of obesity, and type of spine surgery being investigated (fusion versus nonfusion procedures). As a predictor of poor spine surgery outcome, obesity probably interacts with these other factors. As such, it is conceptualized as a variable to be assessed within the context of other more powerful predictors (e.g., disability, litigation, psychological distress).

Work-Related Variables

Work-related variables, as a group, demonstrate some of the strongest correlations with poor spine surgery outcome. Those variables amenable to a BPSS include workers' compensation, litigation, and extended disability duration.

Workers' Compensation

A great number of studies have demonstrated that involvement in the workers' compensation system predicts a poorer outcome to spinal surgery.[1,9] Although it might be concluded that this is related to financial incentives for staying disabled, it is more likely due to the various difficulties experienced by the disabled worker, including such things as financial distress, loss of identity related to the job, an adversarial relationship with the employer and insurance carrier, delays in treatment, having to "prove" one is injured, among other things. The longer the patient is off of work, the more time a "system-induced functional disability syndrome" has to develop.[27] Although workers' compensation status is a significant predictor of spine surgery outcome, studies suggest that this effect is mediated by other variables such as time off of work, legal representation, job satisfaction, and so forth.[1,9,27] For the patient who loves his job and is undergoing a spine surgery for a disc herniation that occurred at work just 2 months prior, workers' compensation status will rarely be a predictor of poor outcome.

Litigation

Another predictor variable that has consistently been linked to poorer spine surgery outcome is litigation status (related to workers' compensation, personal injury, or disability benefits).[1,5,7,9,24] Although one might surmise that this is due to symptom exaggeration for secondary gain, it must be assumed that the spine surgery is being recommended because some evidence of pathophysiology has been identified.[5] The litigious patient might very well do poorly because of increased somatic sensitivity to pain as a consequence of financial incentives and social-contextual variables.[5,9]

Duration of Sick Leave

Lengthy preoperative sick leave is a consistent predictor of diminished response to spine surgery including global outcome, overall satisfaction, back-specific function, and return to work.[1,3,9,28,29] Longer duration of sick leave allows for development of the functional disability or chronic pain syndrome, which is probably the reason for the poorer spine surgery outcomes.[1,27]

Psychological Factors

Psychological factors are among the most frequently investigated predictive variables for spine surgery outcome. Some of the common psychological variables assessed include pain sensitivity, depression, anxiety, anger, fear avoidance, severe psychopathology, and various personality disorders or features.[1,9] Psychological predictive variables are often assessed through the use of psychometric testing, and the most commonly researched test has been the Minnesota Multiphasic Personality Inventory (MMPI/MMPI-2).[30,31] It is beyond the scope of a brief initial presurgical screening to include an MMPI-2 (567 questions and 1.5 hours to complete), although it is often used as a component of a comprehensive presurgical screening.[1] Ideally, a BPSS would include some very brief questionnaires that assess the same predictive psychological variables captured by the MMPI-2 and other more comprehensive tests. Although many psychological variables have been identified as predictive of poor spine surgery outcome, pain sensitivity and depression have received the most attention.

Pain Sensitivity

Of all the psychological factors investigated, those falling under the rubric of "pain sensitivity" have shown the most consistent predictive power.[1,9] Pain sensitivity might be defined as a patient's propensity to display pain behaviors beyond what would be expected due to nociceptive input and objective findings. Pain sensitivity also encompasses the idea of how much the patient is "suffering" due to the pain; or, the emotional contribution to the patient's perception of pain and level of disability. Pain sensitivity includes such concepts as heightened somatic awareness, fear of movement (kinesophobia), somatic anxiety, and general psychological distress (but not necessarily depression). Given this conceptualization of pain sensitivity, it is not surprising that any test that assesses some component of this construct might predict poor spine surgery outcome. This is probably why many tests (aside from the MMPI-2) have been shown to correlate with spine surgery outcome, including the Distress Risk and Assessment Method (DRAM),[29,32] the Dallas

Pain Questionnaire,[33] the Mental Component Score of the SF-36,[12] and the Waddell Non-Organic Signs,[1,34] among others.

The pain drawing is another purported assessment of pain sensitivity. Pain drawings are hypothesized to identify the psychological contribution to a patient's pain and are scored in several ways.[35] Pain drawings that are deemed "abnormal" or "nonorganic" (unexplainable pain distribution) are thought to identify patients with a greater psychological component to their pain, although this conclusion has been contested in a recent review.[35] The pain drawing has been investigated as a predictor variable for spine surgery outcome but the results are inconsistent.[36] Even so, the pain drawing is easily administered; when it is grossly abnormal, it might be a useful piece of information to incorporate with other screening variables.[1]

Assessing pain sensitivity as part of a BPSS might be done in several ways. Certainly, the pain drawing can be used adjunctively, but not as a stand-alone predictive test. The DRAM system was developed as a measure of distress in back pain patients[32] and has been used as a rapid presurgical screening tool.[29] The DRAM consists of a modified version of the Zung Depression Inventory (ZDI; 23 items) and the Modified Somatic Perceptions Questionnaire (MSPQ; 22 somatic items). The DRAM takes ~10 minutes to complete and places patients into one of four categories based upon classification rules for the results of the two tests: Normal (N), at Risk (R), Distressed-Depressive (DD), and Distressed-Somatic (DS). Patients in the distressed groups (DD, DS) have been found to have a diminished response to spine surgery,[29] although results did not always rise to the level of statistical significance.[11,37] Research suggests the DRAM may be most useful in screening of chronic back pain patients rather than more acute conditions.[10,11]

Another instrument that is emerging as a possible choice for quickly assessing pain sensitivity and other predictive variables is the Brief Battery for Health Improvement version 2 (BBHI-2).[37] This 63-item test takes ~10 minutes to complete and was developed for use with medical patients. The BBHI-2 yields scores for six scales covering three content areas: validity (defensiveness), physical symptoms (somatic complaints, pain complaints, functional complaints), and affective symptoms (depression and anxiety). The BBHI-2 assesses many areas that have been found to be predictive of poor outcome to spine surgery (e.g., somatic complaints, pain complaints, depression, anxiety); however, it has not been directly tested in any spine surgery outcome studies.[38]

Depression

Major depression occurs frequently in patients with chronic spine pain[39,40] and has been found to predict poor spine surgery outcome in some studies[5,6,23,29] but not in others.[3,11,41] These inconsistent findings are likely due to several reasons.[1] Patients with protracted depressive symptoms (either antedating a chronic pain problem or associated with it) may be less likely to have their psychological symptoms resolve after surgery than a patient with depression that is more acute and reactive to the pain. This has been substantiated in recent studies suggesting that spine pain patients with shorter duration of symptoms and lack of other psychosocial risk factors might show preoperative depression in response to the pain ("reactive depression") but this resolves after successful surgery.[10,11] If the DRAM or BBHI-2 is used to assess pain sensitivity, a depression score is included in the test. Other rapid measures of depression are the Beck Depression Inventory-II (BDI-II) and the BDI-PC (BDI for primary care).[42]

Medical Variables

Few studies have identified medical factors that are consistent and unequivocal predictors of poor spine surgery outcome. Of the predictive variables investigated (**Table 16.1**), duration of symptoms, number of previous spine surgeries, and associated medical problems have reasonable support in the outcome studies and are most amenable to a BPSS.

Duration of Symptoms

Duration of symptoms has been measured directly and as a component of other predictor variables (e.g., length of disability, workers' compensation, sick leave).[1,9] Consistent with theories on the development of the chronic pain syndrome,[27] the longer duration of symptoms allows for other psychosocial issues to emerge that adversely impact spine surgery outcome (e.g., physical deconditioning, psychological distress).

Number of Previous Spine Surgeries

It is estimated that the failed back surgery syndrome occurs in 10 to 40% of all spine surgeries,[43] and the probability of good surgical outcome decreases with each successive surgical intervention.[1,9] However, there is evidence that patients who have responded well to a previous spine surgery are more likely to do better with additional surgery, assuming a clear pain generator has been identified and is amenable to surgical intervention.[1,9]

Associated Medical Problems

This predictive variable category is assessed by evaluating prior medical utilization and comorbid health conditions. A myriad of studies have demonstrated diminished spine surgery outcomes in patients with a history of many prior illnesses and nonspine surgeries. This may be due to the fact that prior medical utilization reflects sensitivity not only to pain, but also to physical symptoms in general.[1] Comorbid medical conditions and poor general health might impact spine surgery outcome due to such things as problems with wound healing (e.g., with diabetes) or postoperative rehabilitation (e.g., with other joint problems or systemic issues such as fibromyalgia).

■ The Brief Presurgical Screening

As part of the surgery decision-making process, the BPSS can help avoid the creation of a failed back surgery syndrome case. **Table 16.2** summarizes those variables that are amenable to rapid screening and have, as a group, been shown to have reasonable predictive power. There are no empirical guidelines or scoring criteria for the checklist; however, the research suggests that the greater the number of risk factors the more likely the spine surgery outcome will be diminished. There are some risk factors that the surgeon might want to "weight" more heavily than others. For instance, according to the research, a patient who is in the workers' compensation system, represented by an attorney, has been on disability for 4 years, and is facing a third surgery is at high risk for failure regardless of any other variables.

Disposition of patients identified as high risk for clinical failure might include (1) referring the patient to a qualified psychologist for more extensive screening, and possibly pain management or preparation for surgery treatment[1,44]; (2) helping the patient successfully address the risk factors and then reassessing for surgery at a later date (e.g., detoxification, quitting smoking, weight loss, treating a clinical depression, etc.); and (3) avoiding spine surgery and referring the patient to an appropriate functional restoration program.[3,45]

References

1. Block AR, Gatchel RJ, Deardorff WW, Guyer RD. The Psychology of Spine Surgery. Washington, DC: American Psychological Association; 2003
2. Fritzell P, Hagg O, Wessberg P, Nordwall, A; Swedish Lumbar Spine Study Group. A 2001 Volvo Award Winner in Clinical Studies. Lumbar fusion versus nonsurgical treatment for chronic low back pain: a multicenter randomized controlled trial from the Swedish Lumbar Spine Study Group. Spine 2001;26:2521–2532
3. Hagg O, Fritzell P, Ekselius L, Nordwall A. Predictors of outcome in fusion surgery for chronic low back pain: a report from the Swedish Lumbar Spine Study. Eur Spine J 2003;12:22–33
4. Turner JA, Ersek M, Herron L, et al. Patient outcomes after lumbar spinal fusions. JAMA 1992;268:907–911
5. LaCaille RA, DeBerard MS, Masters KS, Colledge AL, Bacon W. Presurgical biopsychosocial factors predict multidimensional patient outcomes of interbody cage lumbar fusion. Spine J 2005;5:71–78

6. Franklin GM, Haug J, Heyer NJ, et al. Outcome of lumbar fusion in Washington state workers' compensation. Spine 1994;17:1897–1903

7. DeBerard MS, Masters KS, Colledge AL, Schleusener RL, Schlegel JD. Outcomes of posterolateral lumbar fusion in Utah patients receiving workers' compensation. Spine 2001;26:738–747

8. Peolsson A, Hedlund R, Vavruch L, Oberg B. Predictive factors for the outcome of anterior cervical decompression and fusion. Eur Spine J 2003;12:274–280

9. Mannion AF, Elfering A. Predictors of surgical outcome and their assessment. Eur Spine J 2005;15(suppl 1):S93–S108

10. Carragee EJ. Psychological screening in the surgical treatment of lumbar disc herniation. Clin J Pain 2001;17:215–219

11. Hobby JL, Lutchman LN, Powell JM, Sharp DJ. The distress and risk assessment method (DRAM): failure to predict the outcome of lumbar discectomy. J Bone Joint Surg Br 2001;83:19–21

12. Trief PM, Ploutz-Snyder R, Fredrickson BE. Emotional health predicts pain and function after fusion: a prospective multicenter study. Spine 2006;31:823–830

13. Andersen T, Christensen FB, Laursen M, Hoy K, Hansen ES, Bunger C. Smoking as a predictor of negative outcome in lumbar spinal fusion. Spine 2001;26:2623–2628

14. Glassman SD, Anagnost SC, Parker A, Burke D, Johnson JR, Dimar JR. The effect of cigarette smoking and smoking cessation on spinal fusion. Spine 2000;25:2608–2615

15. Droomers M, Schrijvers CTM, Mackenbach JP. Why do lower educated people continue smoking? Explanations from the longitudinal GLOBE study. Health Psychol 2002;21:263–272

16. Vogt MT, Hanscom B, Lauerman WC, Kang JD. Influence of smoking on the health status of spinal patients. Spine 2002;27:313–319

17. Fardon DF, Whitesides TE. The smoking patient: to fuse or not to fuse. Spineline 2002;Sept/Oct:10–12

18. Porter SE, Hanley EN. The musculoskeletal effects of smoking. J Am Acad Orthop Surg 2001;9:9–17

19. Kehlet H. Multimodal approach to control postoperative pathophysiology and rehabilitation. Br J Anaesth 1997;78:606–617

20. Uomoto JM, Turner JA, Herron LD. Use of the MMPI and MCMI in predicting outcome of lumbar laminectomy. J Clin Psychol 1988;44:191–197

21. Olsen MA, Mayfield J, Lauryssen C, et al. Risk factors for surgical site infection in spinal surgery. J Neurosurg 2003;98:149–155

22. Telfeian AE, Reiter GT, Durham SR, Marcotte P. Spine surgery in morbidly obese patients. J Neurosurg 2002;97:20–24

23. Block AR, Ohnmeiss DD, Guyer RD, Rashbaum RF, Hochschuler SH. The use of presurgical psychological screening to predict the outcome of spine surgery. Spine J 2001;1:274–282

24. LaCaille RA, DeBerard MS, LaCaille LJ, Masters KS, Colledge AL. Obesity and litigation predict workers compensation costs associated with interbody cage lumbar fusion. Spine J 2007;7:266–272

25. Gepstein R, Shabat S, Arinzon ZH, Berner Y, Catz A, Folman Y. Does obesity affect the results of lumbar decompressive spinal surgery in the elderly? Clin Orthop Relat Res 2004;426:138–144

26. Andreshak TG, An HS, Hall J, Stein B. Lumbar spine surgery in the obese patient. J Spinal Disord 1997;10:376–379

27. Gatchel RJ, Turk DC. Psychosocial Factors in Pain: Critical Perspectives. New York: Guilford Press; 1999

28. Nygaard OP, Kloster R, Solberg T. Duration of leg pain as a predictor of outcome after surgery for lumbar disc herniation: a prospective cohort study with 1-year follow up. J Neurosurg 2000;92:131–134

29. Trief PM, Grant W, Frederickson B. A prospective study of psychological predictors of lumbar surgery outcome. Spine 2000;25:2616–2621

30. Deardorff WW. The MMPI-2 and chronic pain. In: Gatchel RJ, Wiesber JN, eds. Personality Characteristics of Pain Patients: Recent Advances and Future Directions. Washington, DC: APA Books; 2000:109–125

31. Butcher JN, Dahlstom WG, Graham JR, Tellegen A, Kaemmer B. Manual for Administration and Scoring of the MMPI-2. Minneapolis: University of Minnesota Press; 1989

32. Main CJ, Wood PLR, Hollis S, Spanswick CC, Waddell G. The distress assessment methods: a simple patient classification to identify distress and evaluate risk of poor outcome. Spine 1992;17:42–50

33. Andersen T, Christensen FB, Bunger C. Evaluation of a Dallas Pain Questionnaire classification in relation to outcome in lumbar spinal fusion. Eur Spine J 2006;15:1671–1685

34. Spratt KF, Keller TS, Szpalski M, Vandeputte K, Gunzburg R. A predictive model for outcome after conservative decompression surgery for lumbar spinal stenosis. Eur Spine J 2004;13:14–21

35. Carnes D, Ashby D, Underwood M. A systematic review of pain drawing literature: Should pain drawings be used for psychologic screening? Clin J Pain 2006;22:449–457

36. Hagg O, Fritzell P, Hedlund R, Moller H, Ekselius L, Nordwall A. Pain-drawing does not predict the outcome of fusion surgery for chronic low-back pain: a report from the Swedish Lumbar Spine Study. Eur Spine J 2003;12:2–11

37. Disorbio JM, Bruns D. Brief Battery for Health Improvement-2 Manual. Minneapolis: NCS Pearson Assessments; 2003

38. Deardorff WW. Review of the Brief Battery for Health Improvement-2. In: Gatchel RJ, ed. Compendium of Outcome Instruments for Assessment and Research of Spinal Disorders. 2nd ed. La Grange, IL: North American Spine Society; 2006:26–27

39. Currie SR, Wang J. Chronic back pain and major depression in the general Canadian population. Pain 2004;107:54–60

40. Sullivan MJ, Reesor K, Mikail S, Fisher R. The treatment of depression in chronic low back pain: review and recommendations. Pain 1992;52:249–255

41. Tandon V, Campbell F, Ross ERS. Posterior lumbar interbody fusion: association between disability and psychological disturbance in non compensated patients. Spine 1999;24:1833–1838

42. Deardorff WW. Review of the Beck Depression Inventory-2. In Gatchel RJ, ed. Compendium of Outcome Instruments for Assessment and Research of Spinal Disorders. 2nd ed. La Grange, IL: North American Spine Society; 2006:25

43. Oaklander AL, North RB. Failed back surgery syndrome. In: Loeser JD, Butler SH, Chapman CR, Turk DC, eds. Bonica's Management of Pain. 3rd ed. Philadelphia: Lippincott, Williams & Wilkins; 2001; 1540–1549

44. Deardorff WW, Reeves JL. Preparing for Surgery. Oakland: New Harbinger Press; 1997

45. Sørensen R, Friis A, Nygaard Ø, et al. Randomized clinical trial of lumbar instrumented fusion and cognitive intervention and exercises in patient with chronic low back pain and disc degeneration. Spine 2003;28:1913–1921

IV Treatment of Degenerative Disc Disease

17 Mechanical Diagnosis and Therapy

Ronald Donelson

Selecting the appropriate nonoperative treatment for low back pain (LBP), with or without sciatica, or selecting appropriate patients for lumbar disc surgery are two critical decision points in the management of this common and expensive health care challenge. The lack of reliable correlation between clinical signs and imaging complicate these decisions as well as contribute to the high variability in the meaning of the phrase "exhausting conservative care," a routinely stated prerequisite to considering surgical intervention. This is all reflected in the 8-fold difference in the rate of lumbar discectomies and the 20-fold difference in fusion surgeries across the United States.[1]

This chapter serves as an important bridge between the preceding section dealing with assessment methods for degenerative disc disease (DDD) and the chapters that follow targeting the treatment of DDD. The important assessment phase of mechanical diagnosis and therapy (MDT), though often misunderstood and certainly underutilized, enables clinicians to first determine the presence or absence of an absolutely unique feature of LBP disorders, whether or not the pain of DDD and herniated discs is rapidly reversible or not (a topic well covered in a recently published book).[2] For individuals with a rapidly reversible condition, this assessment also identifies the means to eliminate these reversible symptoms, correct and stabilize the pain-generating reversible pathology, and then prevent its recurrence.

Over the past two decades, multiple studies have demonstrated the reliability and validity of this MDT approach in producing superior outcomes as well as in identifying the presence or absence of symptomatic discs *and their reversibility,* a dynamic quality that even our most advanced imaging technologies are unable to evaluate.

■ Current Criteria for Surgery and Outcomes

Diagnosis of herniated, compressive disc pathology is precise and consists of a history of radicular pain, positive straight-leg-raising, positive nerve root findings based on neural deficits, and objective demonstration of concordant pathology (e.g., computed tomography [CT] or magnetic resonance imaging [MRI] findings of herniated nucleus pulposus [HNP]). Surgical treatment then carries a high rate of success.[3–7]

Nevertheless, in light of good long-term outcomes with nonoperative treatment in this group[6–8] the decision of whether to operate on this compressive form of lumbar disc disease carries its own challenges in the context of patients' preferences for surgical versus nonsurgical care.[9]

The picture is far less clear in the setting of disc disease producing axial pain only. Based on the inability of conventional imaging techniques to identify such symptomatic levels,[10,11] lumbar discography has become prevalent. Although many studies have reported discographic utility,[12–20] more recent articles emphasize the importance of proper technique and recognition of confounding variables of psychological or occupational distress.[21] Meanwhile, with highly variable rates of success reported following surgery for DDD,[13,22–27] surgical selection criteria are obviously in need of refinement.

■ Mechanical Diagnosis and Therapy Assessment

The MDT form of assessment was brought to our attention by Robin McKenzie, a physiotherapist from New Zealand, in 1981.[28] It is widely recognized that disc pain is commonly aggravated by positions and movements requiring lumbar flexion, but there are at least four randomized controlled trials (RCTs) that have actually reported on the interesting relationship between the direction of spinal loading and the distal extent and/or intensity of low back and leg pain.[29–32] The authors of these articles related specific lumbar directional symptom responses directly to disc pathology[29,30] or the extent of the distal spread of leg pain to the severity of that disc pathology.

The MDT assessment also focuses on monitoring patients' patterns of pain response (changes in pain intensity and location) first to positions, movements, and activities as reported in patients' histories, but then also during each patient's performance of a standardized sequence of repeated end-range spinal test movements and positions to the extent their pain permits (**Fig. 17.1**).

It is as a result of performing these test movements that so many patients report that a specific direction of spinal movement promptly *centralizes* their referred or radiating pain, that is promptly decreases the extent of its distal radiation to a more proximal or central location, even fully abolishing the pain. This centralization pain response was

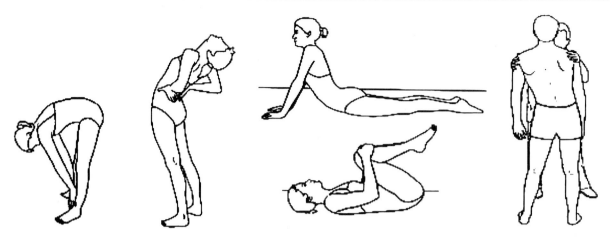

Fig. 17.1   Most common forms of end-range lumbar testing included within the MDT physical examination process: standing flexion, standing extension, supine flexion, supine extension, and standing lateral-gliding. Lateral testing is also conducted with the subject lying prone by manually shifting the hips laterally maximally to the right or left. The test movements themselves are performed repetitively while monitoring the patient's report of a pain response. Sitting flexion or recumbent extension or lateral loading are also commonly tested and informative test positions when monitoring pain response.

first described by McKenzie in 1981 (**Fig. 17.2**).[28,33,34] What is particularly intriguing is that centralization often persists after these test movements have been concluded, as though the pain generator has somehow been altered in some beneficial way. Particularly revealing are the many with pain radiating to the calf or foot with neural deficits where a single direction of end-range lumbar testing is found that promptly centralizes and then even eliminates their pain, revealing the means to a rapid and full recovery. Such rapid reversibility of patients with sciatica and neural deficits was documented in 32 patients in a 1986 cohort study that will be discussed later.[35]

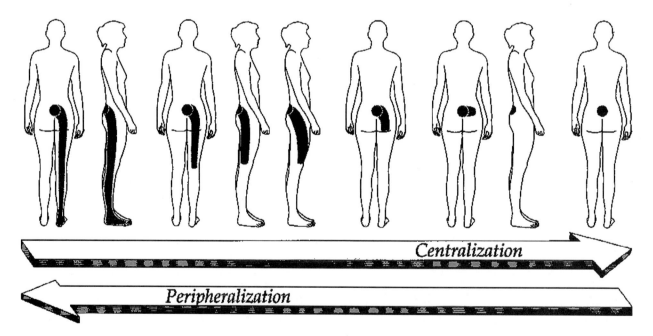

Fig. 17.2   A decrease or abolition of the most distal extent of a patient's pain is the first sign of centralization. If centralization continues with more repetitions of the beneficial direction of testing and all but midline pain is abolished, the pain is said to have fully centralized. When only midline pain is present, it too can often be intentionally abolished using either repeated flexion or extension testing, with the opposite direction of repeated testing typically making it worse or even "peripheralizing" the pain. (From McKenzie R. The Lumbar Spine: Mechanical Diagnosis and Therapy. Waikanae, New Zealand: Spinal Publications New Zealand Ltd; 1981; reprinted with permission.)

Another attractive feature of MDT care is that this rapid improvement is routinely achieved by patients themselves using directional end-range movements or exercises, along with postural modifications also identified during the assessment. The value increases greatly when these same exercises and posture strategies also quickly eliminate any recurring symptoms.

Such a centralizing pain response indicates the likely presence of a discrete mechanical pathology and, more importantly, one that is rapidly reversible when addressed using a single direction of patient-generated repeated end-range spinal loading forces.

This MDT assessment is well described.[34] So let us now focus on the growing body of scientific literature that supports the widespread use of this MDT assessment.

Scientific Evidence for Efficacy

Over the past two decades, centralization and directional preference have been widely investigated, with most studies falling into three distinct and useful study designs.

Interexaminer Reliability

The value of any clinical test is fundamentally based on its interexaminer reliability. There can be no validity without this reliability. Spratt et al[36] were the first to report strong reliability for conducting repeated end-range test movements, concluding that this assessment provided useful diagnostic information and was helpful in identifying the most efficacious form of physical therapy for patients with nonspecific LBP. Many more studies have since similarly reported high reliability of well-trained examiners in determining the presence or absence of the centralization pain response and in categorizing patients into the MDT classification scheme.[37–41] One study supported the importance of examiner training by showing that those with little formal MDT training had poor interexaminer reliability.[42]

Observational Cohorts

Multiple cohort studies have reported on the high prevalence of centralization, elicited in 73 to 89% of acute LBP patients[41,43–45] and in 45 to 52% of *chronic* LBP patients.[46,47] One RCT studied acute, subacute, and mostly chronic patients reporting a directional preference prevalence of 74%.[48] Even patients with sciatica and neural deficits often have a directional preference (DP).[35,48]

In each of these cohort studies, centralizing patients with a DP reported significantly better outcomes than those of noncentralizing patients. Indeed, all patients in the sciatica cohort with neural deficits and a DP recovered full lumbar motion and eliminated all their pain within 5 days of commencing directional exercises as directed by their lumbar testing.[35]

One acute LBP cohort ($N = 223$) reported that the presence or absence of centralization during the baseline assessment was far superior in predicting one-year outcomes than 23 other baseline variables, including psychosocial factors often reported as outcome predictors.[49] Specifically, both good and poor one-year outcomes were much better predicted by the presence or absence of centralization than by psychosocial factors.

Randomized Clinical Trials

Four RCTs have so far investigated this large subgroup whose pain centralizes with a DP at baseline.[48,50–52] All four reported superior outcomes when treatment was matched to baseline findings versus other forms of treatment. One study specifically showed superiority in treating this subgroup with MDT principles rather than by current LBP clinical guidelines' treatment.[48]

Although contradicting our conventional thinking about LBP, but of great importance, when pain centralizes and/or abolishes with a directional preference, one still-to-be-published study confirms other cohort reports that it does not matter whether pain is acute or chronic, or whether axial or sciatica with neural deficits, these patients, properly treated, do very well.[48] In terms of predicting outcomes, the evidence so far is that LBP with a DP usually trumps pain duration, pain location, neural status,[48] as well as psychosocial factors[49] by routinely recovering rapidly.

A Dynamic Internal Disc Model for Rapidly Reversible Lower Back Pain

No single clinical finding or physical sign has been shown to be pathognomonic of discogenic pain. However, a growing number of studies suggest that centralizing pain strongly correlates with symptomatic disc pathology,[41,43–47,49] helping to document the significant usefulness of the MDT assessment in clinical decision making.[35,46]

Directional Nuclear Movement

Numerous cadaveric,[53–55] discographic,[56] and MRI[57,58] studies document the posterior migration of nuclear content in response to anterior disc loading that occurs with lumbar flexion and the resulting anteroposterior pressure gradient across the disc. The direction of this gradient can then be intentionally reversed with posterior loading that occurs with lumbar extension creating anterior nuclear migration (**Fig. 17.3**).[59] With nociceptors in the outer third of the anulus as a common source of pain,[60–62] it is then quite plausible that flexion may create tension and fissuring of the posterior anulus coupled with the posterior migration of nuclear contents down a fissure enabling the stimulation of mechanoreceptors in the outer anulus.[2,34,46,58,63]

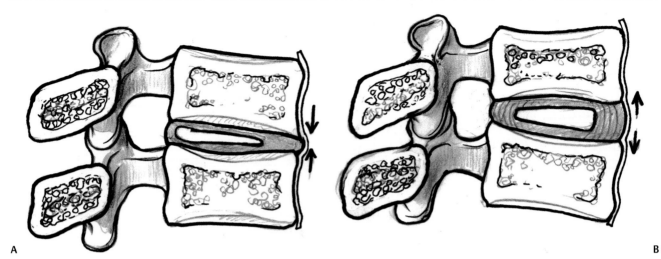

A

B

Fig. 17.3 **(A)** The anterior loading that occurs with prolonged or repeated lumbar flexion causes an internal pressure gradient resulting in posterior migration of nuclear content. **(B)** The direction of this gradient can then be reversed with prolonged or repetitive posterior disc loading using lumbar extension that causes a reversal of the internal pressure gradient across the disc.

Kopp et al[35] reported that many patients with sciatica, even with neural deficits, can rapidly reverse compressive disc pathology using repeated end-range extension loading. No other explanation for these rapid and lasting changes seems plausible than that the extension exercises likely created a pressure gradient across the symptomatic disc that reduced posteriorly displaced nuclear content, decompressing the pain-generating herniation and adjacent nerve root. This disc model, named a dynamic internal disc model (DIDM), has been described elsewhere.[2,46,63]

Degenerative Disk Disease and Diskography Studies

In those with noncompressive internal disc pain, two studies support this DIDM model by showing a strong correlation between discography and MDT assessments' findings.[46,64] The first reported that 31 patients whose pain *centralized* during their mechanical assessment reported immediate positive discography results including a competent anulus, consistent with centralizing pain being discogenic with an intact hydrostatic mechanism.[46] In contrast, 16 patients in that same study whose pain only *peripheralized* during their MDT testing also had positive discography but tended to have an incompetent anulus consistent with a malfunctioning hydrostatic mechanism. Finally, nearly all of another 16 patients whose pain location or intensity was not affected during their MDT testing reported negative discography consistent with their nonchanging pain with end-range loading tests being nondiscogenic.

The second study of 107 lumbar patients also used discography as a reference standard and reported that centralization had a specificity of 89% in identifying positive discograms,[64] which went to 100% in those without severe disability or distress. Sensitivity was only moderate, however (35 to 40%). This all suggests that in nondistressed and not severely disabled chronic LBP patients, discography may be delayed or even avoided if an MDT assessment and treatment program elicits centralization because there is such a good prognosis with MDT care for centralizing patients.

Both discography and the MDT exam may well stimulate the symptomatic disc while monitoring patients' symptom response. The MDT exam mechanically and repetitively loads isolated areas around the disc's margin while discography fills and internally loads it. Both assessments create a mechanical and even a chemical stimulus to the innervated outer anulus.

Considering the strong evidence of good outcomes for centralizers using MDT self-care,[41,43–45,47] disc surgery in those whose pain centralizes during this form of mechanical assessment would be at least temporarily contraindicated, independent of symptom duration or the number of other failed forms of conservative care. Again, centralizing pain, by indicating that the pain-generating lesion remains "reversible" or recoverable, has such a good prognosis with proper treatment that the MDT assessment should fast become a routine part of exhausting conservative care preoperatively.

Mechanical Diagnosis and Therapy Assessment and Treatment of Sciatica and Neural Loss

Although diagnosing compressive disc pathology is far easier, only MDT assessment can evaluate the presence or absence of any reversibility of this pathology and its related symptoms and loss of range-of-motion. The high prevalence of rapid centralization and elimination of pain, accompanied by the simultaneous restoration of full lumbar motion,[35,48] strongly suggests that both the generated pain and the movement inhibition are related to a single, reversible lesion, in most cases being posterior or posterolateral nuclear displacement of the symptomatic disc.[35,65]

Again, Kopp et al[35] reported that of 67 patients with sciatica and neural deficits who were on the verge of undergoing disc excision but were evaluated at the 11th hour with lumbar extension testing, 34 had signs of rapidly reversible pain with 100% then eliminating their symptoms and restoring full range of lumbar motion within 5 days using sets of extension exercises. They consequently all avoided what would have been unnecessary surgery. Of the other 33 patients whose pain was aggravated during their initial extension testing, 91% went on to disc surgery.[35]

The authors postulated that this extension treatment was in keeping with the DIDM. They also pointed out that for a large percentage of patients with compelling clinical evidence of nonrecovering compressive disc disease, there is a means of discovering who might still have a rapidly reversible disc problem. Further, other patients' disc disorders may have been reversible if testing had not been limited to extension. Testing other directions may have elicited the same beneficial centralizing response and is routinely evaluated by fully trained MDT clinicians.

Treatment

Treatment for this large centralizing/DP subgroup is self-evident: the performance of sets of 8 to 10 simple, direction-specific, end-range exercises throughout the day, along with appropriate symptom-specific posture strategies when not exercising. Flexion routinely worsens symptoms and prolongs a LBP episode for those with an extension or lateral DP. Rapid recovery therefore requires a temporary avoidance of flexion in keeping with the four RCTs described earlier.[29-32]

One RCT found that 74% of a wide spectrum of LBP patients had a DP.[48] Within just 2 weeks, significant improvement or complete resolution was reported by 100% of back pain-only patients, 83% with sciatica and neural deficits, 100% of the acute pain patients, and 91% of the chronic pain patients. Patients also reported significant drops in medication use, activity interference, and depression, while significantly improving patient-reported function and satisfaction.

The final goal of treatment is always to restore all directions of lumbar movement without the return of symptoms, including lumbar flexion in those with an extension preference. Those patients are routinely progressed to a flexion recovery phase of care once their extension emphasis and temporary prohibition of flexion have abolished their pain and stabilized their underlying pathology. This is akin to progressively adding weight-bearing and motion to

a sufficiently healed fractured leg to help restore its full function.

A final note of caution must be sounded. Although the lumbar intervertebral disc is a very common symptom generator in patients with acute and chronic LBP, it is not the only one. Pain provocation and relief have been reported with diagnostic injections of both sacroiliac and facet joints and, occasionally, in more than one of these locations.[66-69] In the context of the MDT examination, it has been shown that pain produced by facet and sacroiliac pathologies neither centralizes nor peripheralizes, although other response patterns may occur during the assessment.[70-74]

Selecting Surgical Candidates Using Mechanical Diagnosis and Therapy Assessment

Given the high prevalence of centralization, its strongly favorable prognosis with nonoperative care, and the low cost of providing an MDT assessment, it is appropriate for all LBP care providers to provide this form of MDT assessment as a routine part of "exhausting conservative care" prior to considering an invasive procedure or even an expensive imaging study. Regardless of the patient's pain duration, its location, the diagnostic label(s), or prior treatments provided by other caretakers, patients often still have a reversible problem. If not provided the opportunity to be properly assessed, they remain undiscovered and often undergo unnecessary and expensive interventions.

A much smaller MDT subgroup also has assessment findings consistent with disc pain, but there is no sign of reversibility; that is, they do not centralize or have a directional preference, and therefore these individuals are often the ones who are candidates for lumbar epidural injections or even a disc surgical procedure. This is an important subgroup to reliably identify given the high stakes of undergoing disc surgery and the limitations of MRI and discography imaging. These patients are discussed more extensively elsewhere.[2]

There are several other even smaller MDT syndromes and subgroups for which space does not permit a discussion and in whom disc pathology is unlikely.

Training and Expertise

Reliability in performing the MDT methods has been shown to require formal training consisting of four basic courses provided by The McKenzie Institute and then at least one level of training verification and examination, called the credentialed level. A more advanced level of training leads to the Diploma in MDT. Both recognitions are granted by The McKenzie Institute upon passing the appropriate examination. The published reliability data alone show the benefits of this advanced training.[36-41] Patient outcomes not surprisingly also substantially improve with

64. Laslett M, Oberg B, Aprill CN, McDonald B. Centralization as a predictor of provocation discography results in chronic low back pain, and the influence of disability and distress on diagnostic power. Spine J 2005;5:370–380

65. Van Helvoirt H, Donelson R, Aprill C. Rapid non-surgical recovery of chronic sciatica and neurologic deficit: a case report. Int J Mech Diag Ther 2007;2:47–53

66. Dreyfuss P, Michaelsen M, Pauza K, McLarty J, Bogduk N. The value of history and physical examination in diagnosing sacroiliac joint pain. Spine 1996;21:2594–2602

67. Schwarzer AC, Aprill CN, Bogduk N. The sacroiliac joint in chronic low back pain. Spine 1995;20(1):31–37

68. Schwarzer AC, Aprill CN, Derby R, Fortin J, Kine G, Bogduk N. Clinical features of patients with pain stemming from the lumbar zygapophysial joints: is the lumbar facet syndrome a clinical entity? Spine 1994;19(10):1132–1137

69. Schwarzer AC, Aprill CN, Derby R, Fortin J, Kine G, Bogduk N. The relative contributions of the disc and zygapophyseal joint in chronic low back pain. Spine 1994;19(7):801–806

70. Young S, Laslett M, Aprill C, Donelson R, Kelly C. The sacroiliac joint: a study comparing physical examination and contrast enhanced pain provocation/anesthetic block arthrography. Paper presented at the North American McKenzie Conference; August 21–23, 1998; New Orleans, LA

71. Laslett M, McDonald B, Aprill CN, Tropp H, Oberg B. Clinical predictors of screening lumbar zygapophyseal joing blocks: development of clinical prediction rules. Spine J 2006;6(4):370–379

72. Young S, Aprill C, Laslett M. Correlation of clinical examination characteristics with three sources of chronic low back pain. Spine J 2003;3:460–465

73. Laslett M, Oberg B, Aprill CN, McDonald B. Zygapophysial joint blocks in chronic low back pain: a test of Revel's model as a screening test. BMC Musculoskelet Disord 2004;5:43

74. Laslett M, Aprill CN, McDonald B, Young SB. Diagnosis of sacroiliac joint pain: validity of individual provocation tests and composites of tests. Man Ther 2005;10:207–218

18 The Role of Education and Back Schools

Gunnar B. J. Andersson

All physicians should be educators. Our patients deserve to know about their health and diseases, diagnosis, treatments, and prevention. Medical school generally does not prepare us well in this respect. Mostly we learn by observing. For time and cost-related reasons the education of patients has changed from a one-to-one approach to other methods such as books, pamphlets, videos, Internet, and group education often provided by nonphysician health care providers. The success of these approaches can be measured by two yardsticks; how much did the patient learn and retain? And what effect did the education have on the individual's health? Learning and retaining are measured by simple memory tests or by monitoring the intended results of the education. For example, how well treatment advice was followed. The health effect of education is ideally measured in prospective randomized controlled trials.

■ Educational Environments

For a variety of reasons the education environment in the physician's office is less than optimal. It is not designed for education. The patient is not in an optimal state for education (nervous, undressed, and often uncomfortable or in pain). The physician is hurried by other waiting patients and the cost of education per patient is high. Many physician offices have a separate room for education purposes often with exhibits, models, videos, and computers. Teaching in that environment is clearly better. Still the patient may not be optimally ready and the one-on-one education is costly even when performed by an allied health care provider.

Group education has several positives. It can be done in a good learning environment, it allows for discussion with and between patients suffering from the same problems and it is cost-effective. Although the home environment (video, DVD, Internet) has the benefit of comfort and individual choice of time as well as the possibility to easily repeat, it is more difficult to ask questions (but not impossible with a computer), and other patients are not there to ask questions and share their experiences.

■ Back Schools

The first back school was developed in Sweden in 1969 by Zachrisson-Forsell, a physical therapist.[1] The intended purposes were to reduce symptoms and prevent chronicity and recurrence of back pain by education. It was formally structured to teach anatomy, biomechanics, body postures, ergonomics, and exercises. It was delivered in the physical therapy setting as four group sessions over a 2-week period. It was widely embraced and adopted worldwide. Although the content and schedule have since changed, many of the features of the early back schools are still used today with great variation.

Effectiveness

A large number of randomized controlled trials have been performed over the years. Some of these involve primarily acute or subacute patients; others are chronic patients. Some of the trials have been specific to an occupational setting. Most published studies compare back schools to other treatments. Some use placebo interventions. Outcomes are typically pain and functional status, but in some instances, return to work is also measured. Because of the significant variation in study populations, content, type of control intervention, and outcome measurements, it is difficult to combine these studies for the purposes of a meta-analysis. Several systematic reviews have been published, including two by the Cochrane Collaboration Back Review Group.[2-5] Generally, it is reported that the methodologic quality of most studies is low. Heyman et al found 19 studies worthy of inclusion in a systematic review.[2] The conclusions of the reviews are that there is moderate evidence suggesting that back schools have better short- and intermediate-term effects on pain and functional status than other treatments for patients with recurrent and chronic low back pain (LBP). Moderate evidence also suggests that back schools for chronic LBP in an occupational setting are more effective than other treatments, including placebo or waiting list controls, with respect to pain and functional status and return to work in the short- and intermediate-term follow-up.[2] Although none of the studies in the reviews specifically addresses the issue of the painful intervertebral disc, many patients enrolled likely have pain originating from the disc. A few of the studies warrant closer inspection.

Several studies have tried to determine the efficacy of back schools compared with other treatments (medical, manual therapy, and orthotics) in patients with acute LBP.[6-9] Indahl et al report superior results for the back school group; however, other studies report no differences.[8,9] The efficacy of back schools compared with exercises, manual therapy, myofascial therapy, and medication in patients with chronic LBP (which probably includes most patients with discogenic pain) has also been studied by several groups.[9–11] Although there is moderate evidence in support of back schools in the short- and intermediate-term perspective there is no long-term benefit. When compared with no treatment or placebo, one study reports positive outcomes[12,13]; two studies found no benefit.[11,14]

Cost-effectiveness

Given the methodologic weakness of published RCTs, and the limited evidence suggesting a small effect if any, it is not surprising that few studies have been published on cost-effectiveness. The cost of a back school depends on its curriculum, place of education, and class size—all of which vary significantly. Brown et al[15] and Versloot et al[16] found no significant differences in favor of back schools compared with other treatment approaches.

Discussion

Given the mixed (mostly poor) quality of RCTs comparing back schools to alternatives, it would be compelling to discard this alternative. However, it would be a mistake to equate this with a notion that education is not important. Although we need to improve on the quality of studies to explore the benefits of back schools, it may be even more important to reconsider their content, delivery, and educational settings. Taking advantage of modern teaching delivery systems and the moderate evidence that back schools conducted in the occupational setting is more effective may provide benefits particularly to patients with recurrent and chronic back pain.[2]

There is general agreement that shared decision making about treatment is beneficial. This requires a well-educated patient with realistic expectations and the ability to engage in discussions about treatment alternatives and outcomes.

References

1. Zachrisson-Forsell M. The back school. Spine 1981;6:104–106
2. Heymans MW, van Tulder MW, Esmail R, Bombardier C, Koes BW. Back schools for nonspecific low back pain. Spine 2005;30: 2153–2163
3. van Tulder M, Furlan A, Bombardier C, et al. Updated method guidelines for systematic reviews in the Cochrane Collaboration Back Review Group. Spine 2003;28:1290–1299
4. Cohen JE, Goel V, Frank JW, et al. Group educational interventions for people with low back pain. Spine 1994;19:1214–1222
5. Koes BW, van Tulder MW, van der Windt DAWM, et al. The efficacy of back schools: a review of randomized clinical trials. J Clin Epidemiol 1994;47:851–862
6. Bergquist-Ullman M, Larsson U. Acute low-back pain in industry. Acta Orthop Scand 1977;170(suppl):1–117
7. Leclaire R, Esdaile JM, Suissa S, et al. Back school in a first episode of compensated acute low back pain: a clinical trial to assess efficacy and prevent relapse. Arch Phys Med Rehabil 1996;77:673–679
8. Indahl A, Velund L, Reikeraas O. Good prognosis for low back pain when left untampered: a randomized clinical trial. Spine 1995; 20:473–477
9. Indahl A, Haldorsen EH, Holm S, et al. Five-year follow-up study of a controlled clinical trial using light mobilization and an informative approach to low back pain. Spine 1998;23:2625–2630
10. Linton SJ, Bradley LA, Jensen I, et al. The secondary prevention of low back pain: a controlled study with follow-up. Pain 1989;36: 197–207
11. Donchin M, Woolf O, Kaplan L, et al. Secondary prevention of low-back pain: a clinical trial. Spine 1990;15:1317–1320
12. Lønn JH, Glomsrød B, Soukup MG, et al. Active back school. Prophylactic management for low back pain: a randomized controlled 1-year follow-up study. Spine 1999;24:865–871
13. Glomsrød B, Lønn JH, Soukup MG, et al. Active back school, prophylactic management for low back pain: three-year follow-up of a randomized controlled trial. J Rehabil Med 2001;33:26–30
14. Lankhorst GJ, van der Stadt RJ, Vogelaar TW, et al. The effect of the Swedish back school in chronic idiopathic low-back pain. Scand J Rehabil Med 1983;15:141–145
15. Brown KC, Sirles AT, Hilyer JC, et al. Cost-effectiveness of a back school intervention for municipal employees. Spine 1992;17: 1224–1228
16. Versloot JM, Rozeman A, van Son AM, et al. The cost-effectiveness of a back school program in industry: a longitudinal controlled field study. Spine 1992;17:22–27

19 Cognitive Therapy for Symptomatic Disc Degeneration

Donna D. Ohnmeiss

The importance of psychological factors in chronic back pain patients has been consistently well documented for many years. They affect not only treatment outcomes but also diagnostic evaluations requiring effort or feedback from the patient. It is reasonable to think that by addressing psychological factors, a patient's condition can be improved in general and possibly the effects of other treatment interventions, such as active rehabilitation, injections, and surgery, enhanced. In this chapter, overviews of the following will be provided: some of the behavioral factors associated with chronic back pain, the potential role of cognitive intervention in the treatment of back pain, psychological issues that impact diagnosing symptomatic disc degeneration, a review of studies dealing with cognitive intervention for the treatment of symptomatic disc degeneration, and comments on the difficulties of performing such studies.

■ Acute versus Chronic Pain

The experience of acute pain is different from chronic pain. Acute musculoskeletal pain is generally related to a specific event or activity and pain gradually subsides over a reasonable period while healing of the injured tissue takes place. Some people experiencing back pain do not recover in this reasonable time frame and continue to have symptoms. Physiologically, this may be attributable to an ongoing or recurrent acute injury or to changes in the patient's bodily system that increase pain sensitivity to the extent that stimuli that typically would not be painful now are. Although there may be a physiological component to the unresolving pain, however, the progression from acute to chronic pain has a psychological component. It should also be clearly understood that the psychological component to pain is real.

Through life experiences, we have all been taught that when an injury or illness occurs, we should "take it easy" to allow healing and avoid doing further damage to the tissues in the injured area. This is a good philosophy, so long as the period of limited activity is reasonable to accomplish the goal of tissue healing. After some back injuries, patients are reluctant to return to activity even after a reasonable time. One of the forces in play may be fear of reinjury. Considering the severity of pain onset with some acute back injuries, this is understandable, but it is not beneficial.

Factors predicting which acute pain patients will become chronic pain sufferers have been identified. In a working population, the fear of reinjury or increased pain and an expectation of nonrecovery were predictive of nonrecovery of work-related back pain at 6 months after the initial injury.[1]

In a simplistic model, one may expect the extent of injury to be related to the severity of pain, and the severity of pain to the degree of disability. This is not necessarily the case with chronic back pain. Some patients report pain or disability of severity greater than one may anticipate based on the degree of tissue injury that can be identified. In the past, this was often attributed to the patient being a malingerer and faking or exaggerating symptoms to get disability and/or sympathy and attention. In reality, the problem is often not malingering but is behaviorally based. There may be a cycle of a nonsevere injury, the patient responding by being fearful of movement, decreasing activity, general deconditioning, and possibly increased pain sensitivity. With brain imaging, primarily functional magnetic resonance imaging (MRI), there is now strong evidence that pain, including chronic back pain, is associated with structural and/or functional changes in the human brain.[2–5] Among the changes are decreased size of portions of the brain. Such studies support that there are physiological differences present among chronic pain sufferers. The clinical implications for these findings have not yet been identified, but the studies do provide evidence of the strong impact of ongoing pain and that there is more to chronic back pain than what can be identified by radiographic images of the spine or the behavior of malingering.

■ Behavioral Factors Associated with Chronic Back Pain

Waddell et al[6] introduced the fear-avoidance concept in back pain patients. The work was based on the idea that pain is only one contributor to the patient's functional level. They found that fear-avoidance contributed to disability beyond pain severity. The term *kinesophobia* (fear of movement) was later coined. Waddell and colleagues' work suggested the concept that the fear of pain may be as limiting, if not more so, than the actual pain being experienced. This sets the stage for the potential role of cognitive therapy for back pain. Fear-avoidance behavior suggests that patients select their activity, or lack thereof, based on their fear of pain rather than on the actual experience of pain itself. This behavior severely limits the patient's life. Due to the fear of pain, they do not engage in physical activity, which leads to overall deconditioning. Additionally, they will not participate in active rehabilitation for their pain, which greatly reduces their chances of recovery from their back problems. These patients tend to cope with their pain in a passive rather than active fashion and have a negative outlook concerning the outcome of treatment.

There have been numerous studies performed during the last two decades that support the existence of a strong psychological and behavioral component to back pain. In a large population-based study, it was found that catastrophizing and kinesophobia, identified by the administration of a questionnaire, was associated with significantly greater risk of developing back pain and related disability.[7]

Woby et al[8] investigated factors related to pain and disability in patients attending physical therapy for the treatment of chronic low back pain (LBP). They found that after adjusting for demographic variables, cognitive factors accounted for an additional 30% of the variance in pain intensity. Additionally, cognitive factors accounted for 32% of the variance in disability after adjusting for demographic variable and pain intensity. Functional self-efficacy was strongly related to both pain and disability. In another study by the same authors, it was found that reductions in fear-avoidance of activity and increased perceived pain control were significantly related to lower levels of disability, even after the effects of pain intensity, age, and gender were accounted for.[9] This work reinforces the differentiation of the severity of disability related to pain intensity from pain beliefs.

In a study involving a large population of workers, it was reported that pain intensity was significantly related to function and social disability.[10] Regression analyses revealed that fear of reinjury associated with movement added significantly to the predictive value of the models for function and disability beyond the variance explained by pain intensity. These results supported that fear of further injury and pain is significantly related to function and cannot be accounted for by pain intensity.

■ Cognitive Therapy

When working with back pain patients, cognitive therapy involves dealing with beliefs, fears, expectations, self-efficacy, coping skills, and other issues related to how the patients interpret and deal with their symptoms. Understanding these issues and developing a strategy to teach the patient

how to address them forms the basis of cognitive therapy. One of the basic premises of cognitive therapy in relation to the treatment of back pain is primarily built around the concept of the patient's behavior being greatly affected by the fear of pain and not just the experience of pain itself. Although two patients may have similar pain complaints and similar MRI scans of a disc problem, they may deal with the problem very differently. Much of how they deal with it may be shaped by past experiences and personality. To some patients the pain and abnormal images may be interpreted as a significant debilitating problem that creates high levels of fear, anxiety, and helplessness. Other patients may acknowledge the abnormal disc as a problem but are willing to accept it and actively engage in rehabilitation to address it, while altering their routine only as dictated by the actual pain level and advice from care providers. For the group of patients who do not cope well with the injury, there is a major place for education and support—thus the role for cognitive intervention. It is extremely important for patients to understand that activity is good, even after an injury. Traditionally, most people thought that when an injury occurred, the best thing to do was to not use the injured body part for a while. This may have reduced pain due to the lack of tissue loading or movement and allowed healing. Then a gradual return to activity follows as pain, inflammation, and swelling subside. This model is appropriate for many injuries such as sprains and strains. However, patients need to understand that extended lack of activity is detrimental—not moderate activity. In a comprehensive review involving acute, subacute, and chronic back pain patients, Rainville et al found that there was no evidence to support that exercise is related to increased back pain or disability.[11] In fact, just the opposite was true. Exercise was related to increased flexibility and strength, decreased pain, and negative behavior and beliefs about pain. Arming patents with this type of information through education is one of the basic concepts of cognitive therapy; that is, to change the patient's concepts of how to deal with pain. Rather than intentionally avoiding activity and feeling helpless, they can feel confident and empowered to take on an active role in dealing with their pain, and by doing so they can engage in activities without increasing symptoms.

One of the questions that may arise is whether cognitive factors can be altered in pain patients, particularly considering these factors may have been developed over the course of years and are part of the patient's personality. It has been found that cognitive factors can be changed with education and rehabilitation in back pain patients.[12,13] The changes in cognitive factors were also associated with significant improvement in function. Moseley[12] reported a significant relationship between cognitive changes after intervention and the physical measures of straight leg raise and forward bending and attributed the results primarily to changes in the patients' beliefs that pain suggested tissue damage and, in turn, this reduced catastrophizing.

Potential Role of Cognitive Therapy in the Treatment of Back Pain

Considering the strong impact of psychological factors in back pain, it is logical to think that cognitive intervention should be a part of the treatment. By teaching patients that they can function and be active without significantly increasing pain or causing significant injury to themselves, their confidence increases, the fear of additional pain or injury subsides, and overall function and well-being are enhanced. One of the roles of cognitive intervention may be in improving patient participation in exercise therapy. Among a group of subacute back pain patients, it was reported that adding a cognitive–behavioral component to an exercise program enhanced self-efficacy and other parameters as well as improving the frequency of exercise long-term.[14] However, there was no difference in pain intensity.

Linton et al[15] compared the results of minimal care, minimal care with cognitive intervention, and cognitive intervention with physical therapy in the treatment of back or neck pain. They found that the addition of cognitive therapy significantly improved outcomes in terms of reduced health care visits, work absenteeism, and taking long-term sick leave disability. The addition of physical therapy to the cognitive intervention did not further improve the results of cognitive intervention. This same group of patients was assessed 5 years later.[16] At the long-term follow-up the cognitive intervention group had less pain and better overall quality of life and health than did the minimal care group. There was no difference in health care utilization, but in the cognitive group, costs related to lost work and disability were only one third of that in the minimal care group. These studies demonstrate that the benefits of cognitive intervention in the treatment of back and neck pain are significantly maintained long term.

■ Issues Involved with Diagnosing Symptomatic Disc Degeneration

One of the issues of great importance when addressing the role of any intervention, including cognitive therapy, in the treatment of symptomatic disc degeneration is the diagnostic accuracy. Disc degeneration is a naturally occurring phenomenon. However, degeneration as an occurrence of natural history should not be confused with that which is related to injury or premature changes in the intervertebral disc, which is the target of treatment when painful. It is unknown how many people have painful disc degeneration or the percentage of back pain for which it is responsible. The primary diagnostic tool to identify painful disc degeneration

is discography. This is an invasive procedure and is typically not performed until after the patient has failed nonoperative attempts to gain symptom relief. Therefore, the percentage of patients with disc-related pain that resolves with nonoperative care is elusive. Trying to diagnose disc-related pain without discography is not supported in the literature. Although dehydrated discs may be seen on MRI, there is no means by which to determine if such changes are related to symptoms. The false-positive rate of MRI in showing disc degeneration in asymptomatic subjects has been reported to be as high as 85% in a population that was age, gender, and occupation matched to a back pain population.[17] Such studies verify the importance of the pain provocation portion of the discographic assessment. One must also keep in mind, however, that not all discograms are equal; that is, the technique and interpretation employed by the discographer may have a significant impact on the results of the evaluation.

Discography results are also impacted by psychological factors. With respect to disc-related pain, a strong relationship was found between the hypochondriasis and hysteria scales of the MMPI (Minnesota Multiphasic Personality Inventory) and the number of levels at which discographic injection of contrast into a normal disc provoked pain.[18] The influence of psychological factors on discography has been described by others as well.[19] When confirming the diagnosis of lumbar disc-related pain, the benefit of pressure-controlled manometric injection has been reported.[20] The relationship of this discographic technique to treatment outcome has been described.[21] Together these works suggest that psychological factors play a significant role in diagnostic discography. However, performing and interpreting the evaluation based on a precise protocol including pressure-controlled manometry will typically provide reliable results in at least 90% of patients.[22]

■ Impact of Psychological Factors on Surgery

In a group of patients undergoing discectomy, it was found that imaging studies correlated with surgical findings; however, psychological factors were more strongly related to surgical outcome than were imaging studies.[23] This was a very strong finding and although published almost 20 years ago, the role of presurgical psychological testing is still underappreciated. A surgeon would not perform spine surgery without an MRI or computed tomography (CT); nonetheless, although psychological factors are more strongly related to outcome, it remains acceptable in some practices to not perform formal psychological screening on a routine basis. Den Boer et al[24] reported that increased levels of cognitive–behavioral factors, such as fear of movement, passive coping skills, and negative expectations, identified preoperatively were related to greater pain and disability at postoperative follow-up. Block et al have described a presurgical screening tool that has been used on a variety of lumbar and cervical surgical candidates, including those with painful disc degeneration, that had a predictive value of 82% based on clinical outcome.[25,26] The screening instrument was developed based on a comprehensive review of the literature on factors related to surgical outcome.

■ Literature Review of Studies of Cognitive Therapy for the Treatment of Symptomatic Disc Degeneration

There has been very little investigation on the nonoperative treatment of symptomatic disc degeneration, particularly that confirmed by discography. One of the difficulties with this type of study is that a patient is typically not considered a candidate for discography, due to the invasive nature of the procedure, until they have already failed nonoperative care. Thus, the diagnosis of painful disc degeneration is usually verified after failure of nonoperative treatment. It may be unlikely that patients would be willing to participate in a study providing them with a course of treatment that they have already failed prior to the discogram.

Cognitive Therapy in Conjunction with Nonoperative Treatment

Fairbank et al[27] described a study comparing results of fusion to comprehensive nonoperative care incorporating a cognitive component. They found that the fusion group had significantly greater improvement in Oswestry scores; however, they commented that it was only at the threshold of reaching clinical relevance. The authors also noted that in this group of patients who were considered possible surgical candidates, 72% were able to avoid surgery during 24-month follow-up after participation in a cognitive-based nonoperative treatment program. However, the patient population included in the study was not well described (~10% spondylolisthesis, 8% postlaminectomy, and 81% described only as chronic LBP).

In the prospective randomized study by Brox et al[28] surgery was compared with nonoperative treatment. They found no difference in outcomes between the two treatment groups. However, although the authors commented that the patients were being treated for chronic LBP and disc degeneration, how the diagnosis of disc degeneration was formulated was not clear. The only inclusion criterion dealing with the determination of disc degeneration was

"degeneration at L4–L5 and/or L5–S1 (spondylosis) on plain radiographs" and there was also a comment that all patients had plain radiographs, CT, and/or MRI. There is no evidence that painful disc degeneration can be accurately diagnosed from plain radiographs. As stated earlier, MRI has been found to have a high false-positive rate for disc degeneration.[17] Although this study found that nonoperative care and instrumented surgery produced similar results, the context of these findings with respect to painful disc degeneration remains to be verified. Brox et al performed a study comparing lumbar fusion to cognitive intervention and exercise in a group of patients who had previously undergone surgery for disc herniation.[29] The nonoperative treatment group received a lecture emphasizing that ordinary activity would not harm their back and were encouraged to use their spines. This was followed by three daily exercise sessions for 3 weeks. There was no difference in the outcomes of the two treatments, with ~50% of patients in both groups having a successful result. In the cognitive group, their mean Oswestry scores improved significantly from 45 to 32. Further study was done in this group of patients with respect to muscle area and muscle performance.[30] Patients in the cognitive therapy and exercise group increased muscle strength and density. This change was maintained at 12-month follow-up, which led the authors to suggest that the patients had overcome psychological inhibitors and became, as well as remained, more active. In the fusion group, muscle density decreased and function did not increase. This may be due to the muscle damage done during operative intervention and/or lack of structured physical rehabilitation following the surgery.

One significant methodologic factor arises in all studies comparing surgery with nonoperative care. That is, one of the primary indications for elective surgery is a failure of nonoperative treatment. In the randomized studies, should the patients really be considered surgical candidates if adequate attempts of nonoperative care have not been undertaken, such as the treatments delivered in the control group? Or are these patients repeating nonoperative treatment that did not produce the desired result the first time?

Cognitive Therapy in Conjunction with Surgical Treatment

One area yet to be investigated adequately is that of combining cognitive therapy with surgical intervention for symptomatic disc degeneration. The results of fusion in patients with painful disc degeneration are good but seem to have stabilized over the past several years despite the development of materials such as bone morphogenetic protein that increases the rate of bony fusion.[31-33] Some surgeons, although not many, refer patients for formal psychological screening before surgical intervention, but this is not a widely standardized practice. Even with the screening, some patients may have had improved surgical results if they had received cognitive support along with surgical intervention. Ostelo et al reported that patients with some ongoing pain following first-time disc surgery randomized to a behavioral activity group did not have better results than did patients receiving usual care.[34] However, it must be noted that the behavioral therapy was provided by physical therapists who had received training in this area only for purposes of executing the study. Their understanding of behavioral therapy and skills in delivering such may not have been adequate or at the same level as a trained psychologist with experience in working with back pain patients.

■ Summary

There is strong and consistent evidence that psychological factors play a significant role in back pain patients. This may play a role in evaluating patients with any tests that require activity or interpretation from patients such as functional physical testing or discography. Despite the literature, it is doubtful that most back pain patients receive adequate education and treatment involving cognitive intervention. There have been several studies reporting on the clinical results of cognitive intervention in chronic back pain patients, with favorable results. More recently, randomized trials comparing nonoperative treatment, including cognitive therapy, to surgical intervention have been conducted. The results have generally been supportive of surgery; however, not overwhelmingly so. Some of

these studies do not provide an adequate description of the diagnostic evaluation of the patients enrolled including psychological evaluation. Also, some of these studies indicate that patients were treated for discogenic pain; however, the diagnostic work-up did not include discography and thus the diagnosis of painful disc degeneration was not verified. Therefore, the results of such studies cannot be used to evaluate the role of cognitive therapy for disc-related pain. To perform such a study adequately may be difficult. Typically, discography is not indicated until nonoperative treatment has failed and surgery is being considered. The willingness of patients to forgo surgery for more nonoperative treatment, in the form of a cognitive program with physical activity, is questionable.

The role of cognitive intervention specifically for the treatment of disc-related pain has yet to be defined. Considering that many of the studies evaluating this treatment included a mix of chronic back pain patients, however, it is likely that there were several disc pain patients involved. Another consideration is the role of cognitive intervention combined with surgery. Although surgery can address the tissue-based source of the patient's pain, it cannot address the patient's beliefs about pain that result in undesirable behavior such as fear-avoidance beliefs deterring patients from engaging in physical activity. It appears reasonable that outcome may be optimized by evaluating surgical patients, identifying those with a significant psychological component to dealing with their pain and providing a formal cognitive therapy-based postoperative active rehabilitation program.

References

1. Turner JA, Franklin G, Fulton-Kehoe D, et al. Worker recovery expectations and fear-avoidance predict work disability in a population-based workers' compensation back pain sample. Spine 2006; 31:682–689
2. Apkarian AV, Sosa Y, Sonty S, et al. Chronic back pain is associated with decreased prefrontal and thalamic gray matter density. J Neurosci 2004;24:10410–10415
3. Giesecke T, Gracely RH, Grant MA, et al. Evidence of augmented central pain processing in idiopathic chronic low back pain. Arthritis Rheum 2004;50:613–623
4. Schmidt-Wilcke T, Leinisch E, Gansbauer S, et al. Affective components and intensity of pain correlate with structural differences in gray matter in chronic back pain patients. Pain 2006; 125:89–97
5. Baliki MN, Chialvo DR, Geha PY, et al. Chronic pain and the emotional brain: specific brain activity associated with spontaneous fluctuations of intensity of chronic back pain. J Neurosci 2006;26: 12165–12173
6. Waddell G, Newton M, Henderson I, Somerville D, Main CJA. Fear-Avoidance Beliefs Questionnaire (FABQ) and the role of fear-avoidance beliefs in chronic low back pain and disability. Pain 1993;52:157–168

7. Picavet HS, Vlaeyen JW, Schouten JS. Pain catastrophizing and kinesiophobia: predictors of chronic low back pain. Am J Epidemiol 2002;156:1028–1034
8. Woby SR, Roach NK, Urmston M, Watson PJ. The relation between cognitive factors and levels of pain and disability in chronic low back pain patients presenting for physiotherapy. Eur J Pain 2007; 11:869–877
9. Woby SR, Watson PJ, Roach NK, Urmston M. Are changes in fear-avoidance beliefs, catastrophizing, and appraisals of control, predictive of changes in chronic low back pain and disability? Eur J Pain 2004;8:201–210
10. Gheldof EL, Vinck J, Van den Bussche E, et al. Pain and pain-related fear are associated with functional and social disability in an occupational setting: evidence of mediation by pain-related fear. Eur J Pain 2006;10:513–525
11. Rainville J, Hartigan C, Martinez E, et al. Exercise as a treatment for chronic low back pain. Spine J 2004;4:106–115
12. Moseley GL. Evidence for a direct relationship between cognitive and physical change during an education intervention in people with chronic low back pain. Eur J Pain 2004;8:39–45
13. Walsh DA, Radcliffe JC. Pain beliefs and perceived physical disability of patients with chronic low back pain. Pain 2002;97:23–31

14. Gohner W, Schlicht W. Preventing chronic back pain: evaluation of a theory-based cognitive-behavioural training programme for patients with subacute back pain. Patient Educ Couns 2006; 64:87–95

15. Linton SJ, Boersma K, Jansson M, Svard L, Botvalde M. The effects of cognitive-behavioral and physical therapy preventive interventions on pain-related sick leave: a randomized controlled trial. Clin J Pain 2005;21:109–119

16. Linton SJ, Nordin E. A 5-year follow-up evaluation of the health and economic consequences of an early cognitive behavioral intervention for back pain: a randomized, controlled trial. Spine 2006;31:853–858

17. Boos N, Rieder R, Schade V, et al. 1995 Volvo Award in Clinical Sciences. The diagnostic accuracy of magnetic resonance imaging, work perception, and psychosocial factors in identifying symptomatic disc herniations. Spine 1995;20:2613–2625

18. Block AR, Vanharanta H, Ohnmeiss DD, Guyer RD. Discographic pain report: influence of psychological factors. Spine 1996;21: 334–338

19. Carragee EJ, Tanner CM, Khurana S, et al. The rates of false-positive lumbar discography in select patients without low back symptoms. Spine 2000;25:1373–1380

20. Derby R, Kim BJ, Lee SH, et al. Comparison of discographic findings in asymptomatic subject discs and the negative discs of chronic LBP patients: can discography distinguish asymptomatic discs among morphologically abnormal discs? Spine J 2005;5:389–394

21. Derby R, Howard MW, Grant JM, et al. The ability of pressure-controlled discography to predict surgical and nonsurgical outcomes. Spine 1999;24:364–371

22. Derby R, Lee SH, Kim BJ, et al. Pressure-controlled lumbar discography in volunteers without low back symptoms. Pain Med 2005; 6:213–221

23. Spengler DM, Ouellette EA, Battie M, Zeh J. Elective discectomy for herniation of a lumbar disc: additional experience with an objective method. J Bone Joint Surg Am 1990;72:230–237

24. den Boer JJ, Oostendorp RA, Beems T, Munneke M, Evers AW. Continued disability and pain after lumbar disc surgery: the role of cognitive-behavioral factors. Pain 2006;123:45–52

25. Block AR, Ohnmeiss DD, Guyer RD, Rashbaum RF, Hochschuler SH. The use of presurgical psychological screening to predict the outcome of spine surgery. Spine J 2001;1:274–282

26. Block AR, Gatchel RJ, Deardorff WW, Guyer RD. The Psychology of Spine Surgery. Washington, D.C.: American Psychological Association; 2003

27. Fairbank J, Frost H, Wilson-MacDonald J, et al. Randomised controlled trial to compare surgical stabilisation of the lumbar spine with an intensive rehabilitation programme for patients with chronic low back pain: the MRC spine stabilisation trial. BMJ 2005;330:1233

28. Brox JI, Sorensen R, Friis A, et al. Randomized clinical trial of lumbar instrumented fusion and cognitive intervention and exercises in patients with chronic low back pain and disc degeneration. Spine 2003;28:1913–1921

29. Brox JI, Reikeras O, Nygaard O, et al. Lumbar instrumented fusion compared with cognitive intervention and exercises in patients with chronic back pain after previous surgery for disc herniation: a prospective randomized controlled study. Pain 2006;122:145–155

30. Keller A, Brox JI, Gunderson R, et al. Trunk muscle strength, cross-sectional area, and density in patients with chronic low back pain randomized to lumbar fusion or cognitive intervention and exercises. Spine 2004;29:3–8

31. Dimar JR, Glassman SD, Burkus KJ, Carreon LY. Clinical outcomes and fusion success at 2 years of single-level instrumented posterolateral fusions with recombinant human bone morphogenetic protein-2/compression resistant matrix versus iliac crest bone graft. Spine 2006;31:2534–2539

32. Haid RW Jr, Branch CL Jr, Alexander JT, Burkus JK. Posterior lumbar interbody fusion using recombinant human bone morphogenetic protein type 2 with cylindrical interbody cages. Spine J 2004; 4:527–538

33. Burkus JK, Sandhu HS, Gornet MF, Longley MC. Use of rhBMP-2 in combination with structural cortical allografts: clinical and radiographic outcomes in anterior lumbar spinal surgery. J Bone Joint Surg Am 2005;87:1205–1212

34. Ostelo RW, de Vet HC, Waddell G, et al. Rehabilitation following first-time lumbar disc surgery: a systematic review within the framework of the Cochrane collaboration. Spine 2003;28:209–218

20 Biologic Therapies for Disc Repair

Corey A. Pacek, Gwendolyn A. Sowa, Nam Vo, and James D. Kang

The lumbar intervertebral disc (IVD) is the most common site of degenerative changes in the adult spine. Although early patient symptoms may sometimes be successfully managed through the use of nonoperative modalities such as medications, physical therapy, and interventional procedures, these treatments have not been shown to alter the natural history of degenerative disc disease (DDD). The final common pathway of these degenerative changes often leads to stenosis and subsequent compression of spinal nerve roots. Typical surgical treatment consists of correcting deformity, decompressing nerve roots, and achieving bony fusion for stability, when unstable. Although surgical treatment of the degenerative lumbar disc is relatively effective in these ways, these modalities are designed to treat the end stages of DDD. Biologic therapies, on the other hand, seek to treat earlier stages of DDD when the spinal architecture is less degenerated.

Though surgical treatments are decompressive and reconstructive, many new avenues of biologic therapy for DDD are reparative in nature. DDD is commonly thought to be the result of an imbalance in the anabolic and catabolic processes within the disc, where the degradative processes overwhelm the synthetic capabilities of the disc. The theory behind many biologic therapies lies in restoring this imbalance back toward normal homeostasis by supporting the anabolic or inhibiting the catabolic pathways.

Several basic approaches exist for achieving this goal. The most straightforward of these approaches is that of directly injecting therapeutic biomolecules within the IVD that will lead to an increase in anabolic activity. Building on this strategy, another approach consists of modifying the disc cells genetically such that synthetic activity remains increased for longer periods of time than can be achieved with a one-time therapeutic intervention. A final tactic involves the transplantation of modified cells to create lasting increases in the synthetic processes of the IVD. These strategies shall be addressed in turn as to their method and ongoing research into optimization of effectiveness.

■ Injection Therapy

The most straightforward approach to biologic therapy for disc repair is the injection of factors that will result in an increase in the synthetic activity of the disc. After injection into the degenerated nucleus pulposus (NP), it is hypothesized

that the stimulatory effect of the injected factor will slow or reverse the degenerative cascade. The appeal of this modality lies in its simplicity of institution. To achieve this goal, several anabolic factors—such as transforming growth factor β-1 (TGF-β1),[1] bone morphogenic protein-2 (BMP-2),[2] bone morphogenic protein-7 (BMP-7),[3] and growth and differentiation factor-5 (GDF-5)[4]—have been identified as possible treatments for injection therapy. However, only BMP-7 and GDF-5 have been researched as to the utility of in vivo injections.

Bone Morphogenic Protein-7 (OP-1)

Significant research has been done exploring the role of BMP-7, or osteogenic protein-1 (OP-1), as a possible therapy for DDD. Injection of BMP-7 into the IVD is hypothesized to stimulate the IVD cells to increase their production of proteoglycans. Increased proteoglycan content, in turn, is thought to increase the tonicity of the NP and thus increase the water content. It is hoped that through this process an IVD with the morphology and biochemistry closer to that of a normal IVD is produced. BMP-7 has been shown in vitro to stimulate the production of proteoglycans in both NP cells as well as anulus fibrosus (AF) cells.[3] An et al[5] reported an increase in disc height in the spines of healthy rabbits after BMP-7 in vivo intradiscal injections. Biochemical analysis following the sacrifice of these animals showed a significant increase in proteoglycan content as compared with control injections of lactose. Following this, Masuda et al[6] performed intradiscal injections of BMP-7 into degenerative rabbit discs, using a stab model of disc degeneration to test the effect of BMP-7 on the degenerating IVD. The subsequent disc space narrowing that is often seen with DDD was restored in the injected discs, and this height was maintained throughout a 24-week period after injection (**Fig. 20.1**). These studies were the first to suggest that a single injection of a growth factor could lead to the repair of disc degeneration.

Growth and Differentiation Factor-5

GDF-5 is another member of the TGF-β superfamily and BMP subfamily that has shown some promise with respect to biologic therapy of the IVD. GDF-5 deficient mice have been shown to undergo accelerated disc degeneration.[7] GDF-5 has been shown to increase proteoglycan content in both NP and AF cells as well as stimulate cell proliferation

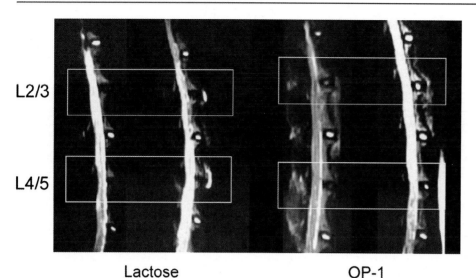

L2/3

L4/5

Lactose   OP-1

Fig. 20.1 Degenerated lumbar discs (L2–L3 and L4–L5) were injected with either lactose or bone morphogenic protein-7 (BMP-7/OP-1). The signal intensity of the BMP-7 injected discs shows increased signal on T2-weighted magnetic resonance imaging as compared with the lactose control. (From Masuda K, et al. Osteogenic protein-1 injection into a degenerated disc induces the restoration of disc height and structural changes in the rabbit annular puncture model. Spine 2006;31:742–754; reprinted with permission.)

as assessed by DNA content analysis in vitro. A single injection of GDF-5 into rabbit NP also has been shown to restore the disc height of degenerated rabbit discs,[4] presumably through the stimulation of proteoglycan synthesis and the reestablishment of water balance.

Summary

The injection of growth factors into the IVD has potential utility for biologic therapy for DDD. Though the effects of several growth factors on NP and AF cells have been studied, only BMP-7 and GDF-5 have been shown in an in vivo model to have promise for repair of degenerated disc tissue. Much more research is needed in this area, as are long-term studies to evaluate the ability for a single injection of these factors to maintain the beneficial changes that it appears to initiate. It is known that single, subcutaneous injections of growth factors have a half-life of approximately 20 minutes.[8] Although injected factors would likely possess a much longer half-life in an avascular structure such as the IVD, it is not known whether multiple injections would be needed throughout the natural history of a patient with DDD. Because of this potential limitation, avenues into other biologic therapies are currently being evaluated as well.

■ Gene Therapy

A second strategy of biologic therapy for IVD repair is that of gene therapy. The main goal of gene therapy is to transfer a gene of interest to the cells of the IVD with the subsequent expression of that gene in large amounts, restoring or upregulating production of a beneficial gene product (**Fig. 20.2**). With efficient and lasting transduction of the NP cells of the disc, a constant supply of the therapeutic

protein would be available to the cells instead of that which would be available from a one-time injection. It is this feature that makes gene therapy an attractive treatment modality.

Transduction can take place in vivo through the direct injection of a vector containing the gene of interest, or the cells can be first transduced in vitro and then injected into the IVD, termed ex vivo gene therapy. Both methods entail their own advantages and limitations, which will be highlighted following a brief discussion of recombinant vectors.

Vectors

A vector is responsible for the transfer of the target gene to the host cell. Two main categories of vectors exist: nonviral and viral. Nonviral vectors, such as liposomes, biolistics or "gene guns" using naked DNA, and DNA–ligand complexes, have not been commonly used for gene therapy for DDD due to their low efficiencies of gene transfer, difficulty of application, and problems with cell death and toxicity.[9–11] Viral vectors commonly used for gene therapy include retroviruses, adenovirus, and adeno-associated virus. They function through the natural protein machinery of the virus to attach to cell membranes and inject DNA. However, the genes necessary for continued viral replication are absent; thus these recombinant viral vectors serve only to deliver the DNA to the host cell. Retroviral vectors, though highly efficient at infecting actively dividing cells, are a less optimal choice for gene therapy of DDD because the cells of the IVD are typically nondividing. Use of adenoviral vectors in gene therapy has shown excellent transduction efficiency. However, their use raises safety concerns due to their immunogenic nature. These limitations have led researchers to focus most recently on adeno-associated virus, a much less immunogenic virus than adenovirus. Although

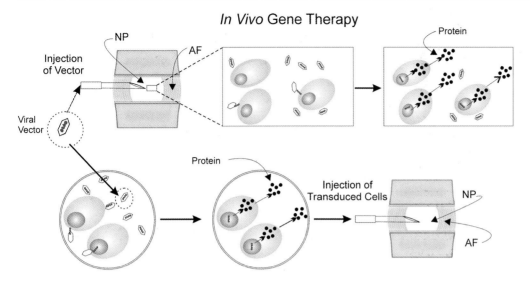

Fig. 20.2 Scheme of gene therapy. In vivo gene therapy involves the direct injection of vector into the nucleus pulposus (NP) of the disc, with subsequent NP cell transduction and protein production. Ex vivo gene therapy involves the transduction of cells in vitro and subsequent injection of cells into the NP of the disc. AF, anulus fibrosus.

the use of adeno-associated virus lessens the risk of host reaction, much lower gene transfer efficiency is observed. Thus, the efficiency of gene transfer must be balanced with the potential immunogenicity of the viral particle.

In vivo Gene Therapy

The potential benefit of in vivo gene therapy is that a single, noninvasive injection is hypothesized to result in consistent, long-term expression of specific growth factor and subsequent increase in extracellular matrix. This method, however, depends on the accuracy of the injection, as well as the efficiency of transduction from this single dose of vector. Additionally, this method requires the host to be exposed to a viral vector, which could lead to an immunogenic reaction. However, such a reaction is less likely in the IVD because it is a relatively avascular and immunogenically isolated organ.

Bone Morphogenic Protein-2

BMP-2 has been shown in the past to stimulate NP cells to increase their production of extracellular matrix proteins.[2] Preliminary evidence by Shimer et al[12] has shown the potential utility of BMP-2. Degeneration of the IVD as assessed by MRI was seen to be slowed significantly through the transduction of NP cells with adenovirus containing the gene for BMP-2. It was thus shown for the first time that gene therapy was able to alter the natural history of DDD.

Transforming Growth Factor β-1

TGF-β1 has also been shown to increase IVD extracellular matrix production,[1] making it an appropriate choice for gene therapy. Nishida et al[13] injected adenovirus containing the gene encoding for TGF-β1 into three adjacent lumbar discs of healthy rabbits. The superior and inferior adjacent discs were used as controls. The injected discs were successfully transduced with the gene through the large increase in TGF-β1 production as compared with the controls (**Fig. 20.3**). The experimental discs also showed an increase in newly synthesized proteoglycans by 200%. Thus, this study showed not only the feasibility of transduction of NP cells, but also the subsequent ability of those cells to produce increased levels of extracellular matrix.

Lim Mineralization Protein-1

Lim mineralization protein-1 (LMP-1) is yet another candidate gene for gene therapy. LMP-1 is a growth factor that stimulates the production of both BMP-2 and BMP-7, both of which have previously shown promise in biologic therapy of the IVD.[2,3,6,12] Yoon et al[14] evaluated this both in vitro as well as in vivo using healthy rabbits. In vitro LMP-1 was found to significantly increase levels of both BMP-2 and BMP-7 expression, as expected. The hypothesized downstream effect of increased proteoglycan production was seen as well. Additionally, the use of a natural BMP inhibitor, noggin, was shown to effectively block these effects, a point of importance when considering the

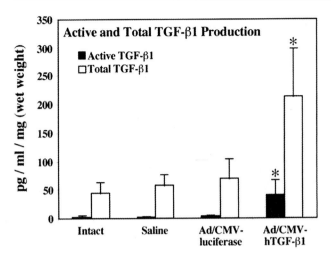

Fig. 20.3 A significant increase in active and total transforming growth factor β-1 (TGF-β1) synthesis in the nucleus pulposus of rabbit discs following in vivo transduction with Ad/CMV-hTGF-β1. Total TGF-β1 = active TGF-β1 + latent TGF-β1. Significant values are indicated by an asterisk. The cytomegalovirus promoter was used in this adenoviral vector. Ad, adenovirus; CMV, cytomegalovirus. (From Nishida K, et al. Modulation of the biologic activity of the rabbit intervertebral disc by gene therapy: an in vivo study of adenovirus-mediated transfer of the human transforming growth factor beta 1 encoding gene. Spine 1999;24:2419–2425; reprinted with permission.)

safety of gene therapy. Finally, rabbit IVD cells were successfully transduced with the LMP-1 gene using an adenoviral vector. Again significant increases in BMP-2, BMP-7, and proteoglycan, specifically aggrecan, were seen as compared with control discs. Although neither the effects of LMP-1 nor TGF-β1 have been tested in vivo using a disc degenerative model, the results suggest that both growth factors could be an additional useful growth factor for gene therapy of DDD.

Ex vivo Gene Therapy

In ex vivo gene therapy, target cells are transduced with the gene of interest in vitro, the transduced cells are cultured, and then injected into the spine of the host. Because the viral vector is only exposed to cells in vitro, rather than directly to the host, the safety of this method of gene therapy is greatly increased. Major limitations of this approach, however, include the availability and difficulty of harvesting cells as well as the viability of the transplanted cells. Although the NP cells are the most physiologically relevant cells, harvesting is a significantly difficult and morbid procedure. Articular chondrocytes, though more readily available and more facile, have the disadvantage of phenotypic distinction from that of NP cells. Additionally, the long-term viability of these cells once transplanted is not certain.

NP/AF Cells

This method of gene therapy has been evaluated by Le Maitre et al[15] using interleukin-1 receptor antagonist (IL-1Ra). Interleukin-1 (IL-1) is a cytokine that is known to upregulate the inflammatory and catabolic pathways of the IVD through the stimulation of various degradative enzymes. The matrix metalloproteinases (MMPs) 3 and 13, which are responsible for disc matrix degeneration, are specifically known to be upregulated with IL-1 stimulation.[16] In vitro testing showed that NP and AF cells could be successfully transduced with IL-1Ra and that subsequent production of the protein led to a significant decrease in the levels of MMP-3 and MMP-13. Human NP and AF cells were then transduced in vitro with the IL-1Ra gene via an adenoviral vector. Next, using human disc explants, these transduced cells were successfully transferred to the NP of the L4–L5 and L5–S1 disc levels. These cells were shown to continue producing IL-1Ra 2 weeks following cell transfer.[15]

Articular Chondrocytes

Zhang et al[17] transduced bovine articular chondrocytes with several subtypes of BMP and cocultured these cells with bovine NP cells. It was shown that BMP-2, 4, 5, and 7 transduced articular chondrocytes stimulated increased proteoglycan and collagen synthesis by the NP cells. Given the greater availability of articular chondrocytes for ex vivo gene therapy and subsequent injection, this study provides an exciting new direction for gene therapy.

Summary

The potential advantage of gene therapy over single injection for the treatment of DDD lies in the potential of the IVD cells to continually produce a factor that would lead to repair and regeneration of the disc. It is hoped that this continual production would lead to greater repair of disc tissue. It is possible, however, that continued exposure to these growth factors could result in as yet unidentified detrimental effects to the spine. Therefore, research into the control of gene expression with gene therapy is needed to improve the safety of gene expression. Ex vivo gene therapy provides some benefits with regard to safety but is limited by problems with cell source and low efficiency. Further research is needed to continue to evaluate the efficacy as well as the safety of gene therapy for the treatment of DDD, but initial work shows great potential.

■ Cellular Therapy

Previously discussed strategies focus on increasing expression of a target protein; however, another line of research is ongoing to investigate the use of entire cells to repopulate

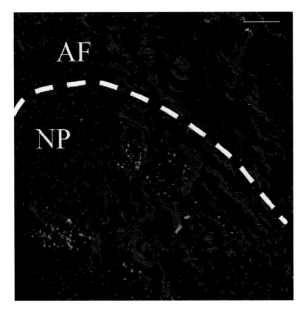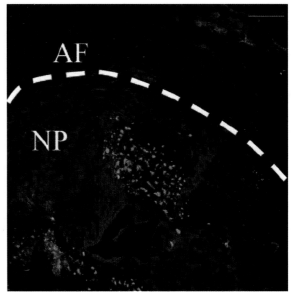

A   B

Fig. 20.4   Green fluorescent protein-labeled MSC are seen at 2 weeks **(A)** and 16 weeks **(B)** after transplantation into the rabbit nucleus pulposus (NP). An increase in cell number is evident. AF, anulus fibrosus. (From Sakai D, et al. Differentiation of mesenchymal stem cells transplanted to a rabbit degenerative disc model: potential and limitations for stem cell therapy in disc regeneration. Spine 2005;30: 2379–2387; reprinted with permission.)

and repair the disc. This strategy of biologic therapy involves transplantation of cells modified in some way into the IVD. The goal is to introduce a healthy population of cells into the disc so that the tissue can be repaired or regenerated. Multiple methods of achieving these goals have been developed and investigated and these will be discussed below.

Mesenchymal Stem Cells

Recently there has been much interest and research into the utility of mesenchymal stem cells (MSC) to regenerate tissues. MSC can be found in bone marrow aspirates and have been shown to possess the ability to differentiate into multiple mesenchymal tissues such as bone, cartilage, muscle, and adipose tissue.[18,19] Thus, the ability of MSC to differentiate into NP and AF cells to reconstitute the IVD has been hypothesized and evaluated. Exposure of MSC to TGF-β1 has been shown to induce a phenotypic change toward that of chondrocyte-like cells, which resemble NP cells more closely than hyaline cartilage based on DNA expression profiles.[19] Additionally, culturing MSC in both the presence of TGF-β1 as well as low oxygen tensions led to the increases in aggrecan and type II collagen,[20] important structural components of the healthy NP.

Sakai et al[18] labeled MSC with green fluorescent protein so that they could be identified following their injection into an aged rabbit IVD. The rabbits were sacrificed at several time points and an increase in cells containing green fluorescence was noted, indicating MSC proliferation within

the IVD (**Fig. 20.4**). Again, these cells were phenotypically similar to NP cells and did not show signs of histologic differentiation into either adipose or osseous tissue.

The availability of MSC through bone marrow aspiration as well as the simple injection into a degenerated IVD represents an exciting avenue of potential cell-based therapy. However, more research is needed to further characterize the nature of these cells and the long-term effects before such a therapy would be available.

Coculture

Another cellular therapy for the repair of DDD makes use of a coculture system. In this scheme, cells that are to be transplanted into the IVD are first cultured alongside cells from the target tissue so that the resulting paracrine interaction would alter and optimize the cells for transplantation. This method has been evaluated using native NP and AF cells cocultured with MSC, the goal being to induce the MSC differentiation to that of NP and AF cells.[21,22] Investigation into this method has begun, with some preliminary data suggesting the coculture with IVD cells can push MSC toward a phenotype more similar to either NP or AF cells.[21–23]

Simple coculture of NP cells with other cellular disc extracts (i.e., healthy disc tissue that has not had specific cells isolated) has been evaluated as well. It was shown that this system led to increased proliferation of the cells in preparation for injection into the degenerated rabbit IVD, although these cells alone were not able to reverse the degeneration.[24] More research is needed to elucidate the actual stimulating factors involved in this interaction so that it can be maximally exploited.

Notochordal Cells

Notochordal cells are commonly believed to be remnants of the notochord that was present during embryonic development of the spine. However, the exact source of these cells is not known. It is known that humans' IVD notochordal cells disappear ~10 years after birth. The function of these cells is currently very poorly understood, but it has been suggested these cells may have potential for biologic therapy for DDD.[25] Research has suggested the ability of notochordal cells to synthesize extracellular matrix,[26] as well as regulate the production of proteoglycans by other cells.[27] It has even been suggested that the success of certain cellular therapies in regenerating any disc tissue, either in vitro or in vivo, could actually be due to the action of notochordal cells instead of the NP or AF cells.[25] However, much research is needed to further characterize this poorly understood cell population, as well as to define whether or not these cells represent a stem cell population, before application to the biologic therapy of DDD.

Extracellular Scaffolds

One of the newest proposed biologic therapies for DDD involves the use of extracellular scaffolds. Synthetic scaffolds consisting of various specific materials are seeded with NP and AF cells and cultured with the hope of essentially growing a new IVD in its entirety. The resulting organ would then be transplanted to replace a degenerated one; thus resulting in biologic total disc arthroplasty. Investigation has begun into different scaffold materials as well as culture methods to optimize this process.

Alini et al[28] used a three-dimensional scaffold consisting of collagen and hyaluronate. They were able to successfully culture IVD cells within the matrix, but found difficulty in maintaining the synthesized proteoglycan within the scaffold. Using a different scaffold matrix consisting of calcium polyphosphate, Séguin et al[29] found that the resulting NP-like tissue had similar compressive mechanical properties

to a healthy bovine NP but still failed to achieve native levels of proteoglycan. Mizuno et al[30] cultured AF and NP cells in an extracellular scaffold of polyglycolic acid polymer and alginate/calcium sulfate, respectively. This construct was then cultured in the subcutaneous space of athymic mice. The resulting disc tissue generated consisted of extracellular matrix compositions similar to that of a native disc, but yet again was unable to maintain native levels of proteoglycan.

Summary

Cellular biologic therapy for the DDD includes a broad category of research topics. The advantage of this approach lies in restoration of native tissue without the use of viral vectors or gene overexpression. Cell viability is central to many of the therapies discussed, and thus optimization of viability is necessary. Concern over sources of donor cells also remains an issue. Autologous cell use virtually eliminates concern of tissue rejection, but the availability and necessary extraction procedures remain a major obstacle. Despite these issues, cellular therapy remains an active area of research with promising prospects.

■ Conclusion

Researchers around the world are actively investigating potential biologic therapies designed to repair, regenerate, or replace the degenerated IVD. Many strategies, ranging from the injection of growth factors, to either in vivo or ex vivo gene therapy, to cellular transplantation are being explored to discover and develop safe, effective, and pragmatic techniques and treatments for DDD. Although great strides and discoveries have been made, much work remains before these proposed hypotheses become effective therapeutic realities.

Acknowledgments   The authors thank Mary Synnott for her assistance with the creation of the gene therapy figure (Fig. 20.2).

References

1. Thompson JP, Oegema TR Jr, Bradford DS. Stimulation of mature canine intervertebral disc by growth factors. Spine 1991;16(3):253–260
2. Kim DJ, Moon SH, Kim H, et al. Bone morphogenetic protein-2 facilitates expression of chondrogenic, not osteogenic, phenotype of human intervertebral disc cells. Spine 2003;28(24):2679–2684
3. Masuda K, Takegami K, An H, et al. Recombinant osteogenic protein-1 upregulates extracellular matrix metabolism by rabbit annulus fibrosus and nucleus pulposus cells cultured in alginate beads. J Orthop Res 2003;21(5):922–930

4. Chujo T, An HS, Akeda K, et al. Effects of growth differentiation factor-5 on the intervertebral disc–in vitro bovine study and in vivo rabbit disc degeneration model study. Spine 2006;31(25):2909–2917
5. An HS, Takegami K, Kamada H, et al. Intradiscal administration of osteogenic protein-1 increases intervertebral disc height and proteoglycan content in the nucleus pulposus in normal adolescent rabbits. Spine 2005;30(1):25–31
6. Masuda K, Imai Y, Okuma M, et al. Osteogenic protein-1 injection into a degenerated disc induces the restoration of disc height and

structural changes in the rabbit anular puncture model. Spine 2006;31(7):742–754

7. Li X, Leo BM, Beck G, Balian G, Anderson GD. Collagen and proteoglycan abnormalities in the GDF-5-deficient mice and molecular changes when treating disk cells with recombinant growth factor. Spine 2004;29(20):2229–2234

8. Sprugel KH, McPherson JM, Clowes AW, Ross R. Effects of growth factors in vivo. I. Cell ingrowth into porous subcutaneous chambers. Am J Pathol 1987;129(3):601–613

9. Biewenga JE, Destree OH, Schrama LH. Plasmid-mediated gene transfer in neurons using the biolistics technique. J Neurosci Methods 1997;71(1):67–75

10. Sobajima S, Kim JS, Gilbertson LG, Kang JD. Gene therapy for degenerative disc disease. Gene Ther 2004;11(4):390–401

11. Ziady AG, Kim J, Colla J, Davis PB. Defining strategies to extend duration of gene expression from targeted compacted DNA vectors. Gene Ther 2004;11(18):1378–1390

12. Shimer AL, Shimer AL, Sobajima S, Chadderdon RC. BMP-2 Gene transfer favorably alters course of disc degeneration in rabbit model. Paper presented at: 51st Annual Meeting of the Orthopaedic Research Society; February 20–23, 2005; Washington, DC

13. Nishida K, Kang JD, Gilbertson LG, et al. Modulation of the biologic activity of the rabbit intervertebral disc by gene therapy: an in vivo study of adenovirus-mediated transfer of the human transforming growth factor beta 1 encoding gene. Spine 1999;24(23):2419–2425

14. Yoon ST, Park JS, Kim KS, et al. ISSLS prize winner: LMP-1 upregulates intervertebral disc cell production of proteoglycans and BMPs in vitro and in vivo. Spine 2004;29(23):2603–2611

15. Le Maitre CL, Freemont AJ, Hoyland JA. A preliminary in vitro study into the use of IL-1Ra gene therapy for the inhibition of intervertebral disc degeneration. Int J Exp Pathol 2006;87(1):17–28

16. Roberts S, Caterson B, Menage J, Evans EH, Jaffray DC, Eisenstein SM. Matrix metalloproteinases and aggrecanase: their role in disorders of the human intervertebral disc. Spine 2000;25(23):3005–3013

17. Zhang Y, Li Z, Thonar EJ, et al. Transduced bovine articular chondrocytes affect the metabolism of cocultured nucleus pulposus cells in vitro: implications for chondrocyte transplantation into the intervertebral disc. Spine 2005;30(23):2601–2607

18. Sakai D, Mochida J, Iwashina T, et al. Differentiation of mesenchymal stem cells transplanted to a rabbit degenerative disc model: potential and limitations for stem cell therapy in disc regeneration. Spine 2005;30(21):2379–2387

19. Steck E, Bertram H, Abel R, Chen B, Winter A, Richter W. Induction of intervertebral disc-like cells from adult mesenchymal stem cells. Stem Cells 2005;23(3):403–411

20. Risbud MV, Albert TJ, Guttapalli A, et al. Differentiation of mesenchymal stem cells towards a nucleus pulposus-like phenotype in vitro: implications for cell-based transplantation therapy. Spine 2004;29(23):2627–2632

21. Le Visage C, Kim SW, Tateno K, Sieber AN, Kostuik JP, Leong KW. Interaction of human mesenchymal stem cells with disc cells: changes in extracellular matrix biosynthesis. Spine 2006;31(18):2036–2042

22. Richardson SM, Walker RV, Parker S, et al. Intervertebral disc cell-mediated mesenchymal stem cell differentiation. Stem Cells 2006;24(3):707–716

23. Vadala GI, Studer R, Sowa G, Denaro V, Gilbertson L, Kang J. The interaction of mesenchymal stem cells and nucleus pulposus cells in a co-culture system: differentiation stimulatory effects, without fusion. Paper presented at 53rd Annual Meeting of the Orthopaedic Research Society; February 11–14, 2007; San Diego, CA

24. Okuma M, Mochida J, Nishimura K, Sakabe K, Seiki K. Reinsertion of stimulated nucleus pulposus cells retards intervertebral disc degeneration: an in vitro and in vivo experimental study. J Orthop Res 2000;18(6):988–997

25. Hunter CJ, Matyas JR, Duncan NA. The notochordal cell in the nucleus pulposus: a review in the context of tissue engineering. Tissue Eng 2003;9(4):667–677

26. Souter WA, Taylor TK. Sulphated acid mucopolysaccharide metabolism in the rabbit intervertebral disc. J Bone Joint Surg Br 1970;52(2):371–384

27. Aguiar DJ, Johnson SL, Oegema TR. Notochordal cells interact with nucleus pulposus cells: regulation of proteoglycan synthesis. Exp Cell Res 1999;246(1):129–137

28. Alini M, Li W, Markovic P, Aebi M, Spiro RC, Roughley PJ. The potential and limitations of a cell-seeded collagen/hyaluronan scaffold to engineer an intervertebral disc-like matrix. Spine 2003;28(5):446–454

29. Séguin CA, Grynpas MD, Pilliar RM, Waldman SD, Kandel RA. Tissue engineered nucleus pulposus tissue formed on a porous calcium polyphosphate substrate. Spine 2004;29(12):1299–1306

30. Mizuno H, Roy AK, Vacanti CA, Kojima K, Ueda M, Bonassar LJ. Tissue-engineered composites of anulus fibrosus and nucleus pulposus for intervertebral disc replacement. Spine 2004;29(12):1290–1297

21 Intradiscal Therapy

Steven Helper and Curtis W. Slipman

The term "internal disc disruption" syndrome (IDDS) was coined by Crock[1,2] to identify the syndrome of low back pain (LBP) and nonradicular referred pain in the setting of degenerative disc disease; and has evolved to encompass the entity marked by radial and circumferential tears in the anulus fibrosus (AF) associated with back greater than leg pain, radiation in a somatic referral pattern, and no focal neurologic deficit. Treatment has traditionally been limited to either conservative medical management or surgical fusion. Surgical treatment of these patients has yielded mixed results.[3-12] Given the prevalence of this problem and the limited treatment options, the development of alternative treatment methods is the logical advancement of care. The recognition of the obvious disparity within the existing treatment paradigm has led to the evolution of minimally invasive, fluoroscopically guided, intradiscal procedures as another step in the treatment algorithm for chronic discogenic pain. These intradiscal methods include intradiscal electrothermal therapy (IDET), radiofrequency (RF) posterior ablation, intradiscal radiofrequency, intradiscal steroid instillation, percutaneous laser disc decompression (PLDD), and nucleoplasty (coblation). Despite early promising results, no single approach has proven itself to be the definitive minimally invasive solution to internal disc disruption.

■ Intradiscal Heating Procedures

Recently, the use of heat therapy for controlled contraction, or shrinkage, of collagenous tissues has been evaluated. The prominent modes of thermal energy used in surgical applications are laser and RF.[13-21] The advantage of RF thermal energy is its ability to precisely target tissue, while simultaneously being accurately measured with temperature control technology.

Percutaneous Intradiscal Radiofrequency Thermocoagulation

Letcher and Goldring[22] demonstrated that RF current and heat preferentially block smaller C fibers before the larger A-group, raising the possibility of using heat to modify nerves that transmit pain. It has been demonstrated that temperatures in and above the range of 42° to 50°C are

cytotoxic to nerve fibers.[23-25] This preference for small unmyelinated pain fibers, in combination with the accurate control over the location of the lesion, theoretically makes RF precise for treating various painful spinal ailments.[26-31] The antinociceptive effect of percutaneous intradiscal radiofrequency thermocoagulation (PIRFT) is hypothesized to be due to a temperature increase and subsequent ablation of free nerve endings in the outer AF.

Procedure

Patient positioning is identical to that of provocative discography.[32] A 20-gauge C15 cannula with a 10-mm exposed tip is introduced under fluoroscopic guidance. With the tip of the cannula in the center of the disc, the stylet of the cannula is replaced by the RF probe (Integra Radionics, Burlington, MA). Electrical stimulation is then performed to ensure that the electrode is not positioned near nerve structures. Stimulation at 50 and 2 Hz is used to rule out sensory and motor activation, respectively. A 90-second 70°C lesion is then made. Typically, this lesion is painless and no local anesthetic is required. Temperature monitoring is maintained throughout the procedure.

Clinical Outcomes

In their 1996 pilot study, Van Kleef et al[33] reported a 70% success rate, but the follow-up evaluation interval was only 8 weeks. In a subsequent prospective double-blind randomized trial of 28 patients, Barendse et al[30] failed to demonstrate a clinical effect of PIRFT for reducing pain, functional disability, and physical impairment in patients with chronic discogenic LBP. In this trial, patients with a history of at least 1 year of chronic LBP were selected based on a diagnostic analgesic discography. Twenty-eight patients with a single painful disc were selected and randomly assigned to receive PIRFT or a sham procedure. At 8 weeks after treatment there was one success (1 of 13 patients) in the RF group and two (2 of 15 patients) in the control group. Ercelen et al[34] conducted a randomized trial of RF lesioning using two different time modalities. In their study, 60 patients with chronic LBP were selected for provocative discography after failing 2 years of conservative management. Thirty-nine patients (39 of 60 patients) with positive discography results were randomly selected and divided into two groups. In the first group, treatment was performed for

120 seconds, and in the second group for 360 seconds, both at 80°C. Although the immediate, 1-week, 2-week, and 1-month Visual Analog Scale (VAS) scores were decreased significantly in both groups, no statistical differences were found for pain relief and functional improvement between the two groups. At 6 months, the VAS scores returned to baseline values demonstrating the absence of a sustained beneficial effect.

Houpt et al[35] challenged the validity of thermocoagulation of annular nociceptors with PIRFT as a means of treating discogenic pain. They measured temperature changes within the human IVD during transient intranuclear heating demonstrating that temperature changes at distances further than 11 mm were insufficient to raise the tissue temperature to that needed for neuronal cell death. The authors appropriately concluded the possible clinical effects of RF heating of IVDs are not due to thermal denervation of the disc. Overall, there remains no evidence to support the use of PIRFT in the management of lumbar internal disc disruption syndrome.

Intradiscal Electrothermal Therapy

IDET is an intradiscal heating technique that is founded on the notion that the IVD itself is an avascular structure. If an external heating mechanism such as IDET is used to elevate temperatures within the disc there tends to be minimal fluctuation due to the absence of a circulatory system buffer. Heating external to the disc is quickly dissipated by the "heat sink" created by the vascular and cerebrospinal fluid circulation outside the disc, thereby protecting adjacent structures from injury.[36,37] IDET transfers heat by conduction from a thermal resistive coil to the adjacent tissue. Temperature sensors deliver feedback to the generator, which adjusts power levels as necessary to reach and maintain set target temperatures.

Procedure

Using a standard discographic approach, a 17-gauge introducer is placed into the center of the disc (**Fig. 21.1**). A navigable intradiscal catheter with a 6-cm active electrothermal tip (SpineCATH; Smith & Nephew Inc., Andover, MA) is then advanced through the trocar to pass completely across the nucleus pulposus until it contacts the inner aspect of the contralateral anterolateral anulus. With continued insertion, the electrode deflects circumferentially back, along the inner perimeter of the anulus, toward the insertion side. The catheter is then attached to the RF generator and the disc is gradually heated to a temperature of 90°C over 12.5 minutes. This peak temperature is maintained for 4 more minutes. Postprocedure, a lumbar support brace is worn for 6 weeks to deter movements that might elevate intradiscal pressure (i.e., forward flexion).

Mechanism of Action

IDET was developed to address the failure of PIRFT to reach therapeutic temperatures at the target tissues.[35-37] The proposed mechanism is a combination of annular collagen shrinkage, stabilizing annular fissures, and thermocoagulation of native nociceptors and ingrown unmyelinated nerve fibers.

Effect on Nerves

Initial data on IDET, in cadaveric specimens and live human subjects, showed an average maximum temperature at the outer anulus of 44.8°C and 47.5°C, respectively.[36,37] Similarly, Shah et al demonstrated outer annular temperatures ~55°C, seemingly adequate to provide neural blockade.[38] Freeman et al followed suit in their detailed in vivo study on sheep disc. Again, thermal mapping seemed to demonstrate adequate heating. However, postoperative histology failed to substantiate denervation of nerve fibers in the outer lamellae of the anulus. Kleinstueck et al[40] gave a plausible explanation of this paradox. By their calculations, with the use of the existing protocol for the IDET procedure,[13,17,44] destruction of neural tissue is limited to within 6 mm of the IDET heating probe. According to Kleinstueck et al's data, neurotoxic temperatures were found in the outer annular fibers only 55% of the time.[40] Bono et al[44a] then demonstrated comparable although slightly higher temperatures at varying distances from the heating coil. In fact, more than 45°C was achieved in 71% of specimens at distances of 9 to 14 mm outside the coil. It is evident from the data of either study that not all discs will achieve sufficient temperatures for nociceptive denervation in clinically relevant regions of the disc. Perhaps this is one explanation for the modest clinical efficacy demonstrated in published trials.[13,14,17-19,21,44-46]

Effect on Collagen

Several studies have examined the histologic effects of targeted thermal therapy on collagen.[47-61] Hecht et al[47] and Naseef et al[49] have studied the effects of RF effects on collagen tissue. Significant ultrastructural alterations in collagenous architecture occur during capsular heating. Thermal coagulation or coagulation necrosis will occur in collagen exposed to temperatures greater than ~60° to 65°C for a duration of minutes.[47,50,51,62,63]

In Shah et al's histologic study,[38] outer annular temperatures reached 55°C, which should not be sufficient to cause collagen shrinkage. Nevertheless, electron microscopy revealed shrinkage and clustering of collagen fibrils, annular disorganization, and cellular debris. Kleinstueck et al[40] also failed to demonstrate temperatures in excess of 60°C in the outer annular fibers. Paradoxically, despite posterior annular temperatures exceeding 60°C in 28 of

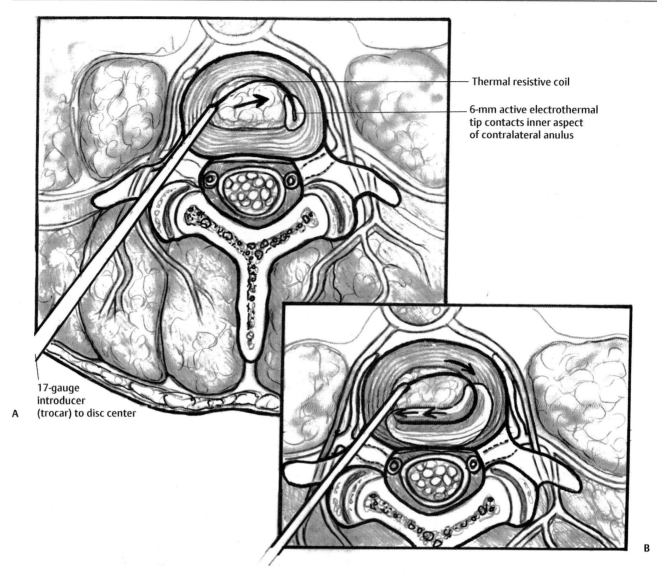

Thermal resistive coil

6-mm active electrothermal tip contacts inner aspect of contralateral anulus

17-gauge introducer
A (trocar) to disc center

B

Fig. 21.1 **(A)** Intradiscal electrothermal annuloplasty. Cross-sectional image of an intradiscal electrothermal annuloplasty catheter as it is coiled posteriorly along the inner annular fibers of the intervertebral disc. **(B)** Intradiscal electrothermal annuloplasty. Cross-sectional image of an intradiscal electrothermal annuloplasty catheter properly coiled within the lumbar disc.

40 levels (70%) on thermal mapping, Freeman et al[39] did not show a significant histologic effect on experimentally induced annular tears. Scientific inquiries to date suggest that the reported benefit from IDET appears to be related to factors other than annular collagen shrinkage or the stabilization of annular fissures. Even if the proposed theories of nociceptor ablation and collagen denaturation are valid, there remain variations of disc pathology and anatomy between patients and uncertainty regarding the exact pain source location.[64,65]

Alternate theories to explain the modest efficacy of IDET do exist. One possibility is that the procedure may denervate nerve endings in the adjacent endplate. Another relates to the prevention of leaching of chemical irritants through injured endplates or annular tears. Injured or herniated discs are known to produce chemical mediators such as phospholipase A2, nitric oxide, and metalloproteinase, which are associated with inflammation and repair. It is conceivable that IDET may reduce leakage of these chemical irritants through the annular tear so that periannular nociceptors are not stimulated.

Clinical Outcomes

In 1998, Saal and Saal[36] reported the preliminary results for 25 consecutive patients treated with IDET. Each patient underwent lumbar discography following failed conservative care for axial LBP. At a mean follow-up period of 7 months, 20 of 25 patients (80%) reported a 2-point reduction in their

VAS scores. A successful functional outcome as measured by the SF-36 Health Survey was achieved in 77% of the patients treated at a single level, 75% of the patients treated at two or more levels. In 2000, Saal and Saal[44] completed and published the first prospective case series on the success of IDET. Following a screening of 1116 consecutive patients, a cohort of 62 patients (0.6%) met the following inclusion criteria: at least 6 months of nonsurgical treatment; a normal neurologic exam; negative straight leg raise on exam; magnetic resonance imaging negative for neural compromise; and concordant pain on discography. Thirty underwent single-level IDET and 32 underwent multilevel treatment. The mean change between baseline and follow-up VAS score was 3.0 ($p < 0.001$), mean change in SF-36 physical functioning (SF-36-PF) score was 20 ($p < 0.001$), and mean change in SF-36 bodily pain (SF-36-BP) score was 17 ($p < 0.001$). Symptomatic improvement of SF-36-PF, SF-36-BP, and VAS was 71%, 74%, and 71%, respectively. Less favorable outcomes were observed in those patients with decreased disc height of at least 30%. The same authors later reported their 2-year outcomes on 58 of the original 62 patients.[13] The mean change between baseline and follow-up VAS score was 3.2, mean change in SF-36-PF was 31, and mean change in SF-36-BP was 22. Seventy-two percent of patients experienced at least a 2-point reduction on VAS, and 50% noted at least a 4-point reduction in pain. Symptomatic improvement of SF-36-PF, SF-36-BP, and VAS was 82%, 78%, and 72%, respectively. No significant statistical differences were noted between one-level and two-level IDET cases or between private pay patients and worker's compensation.

In 2000, Karasek and Bogduk published the first IDET prospective case-control outcome study.[14] Fifty-two patients with symptoms consistent with IDDS and positive provocation discograms, were studied. Thirty-five (35 of 52) of these patients were treated with IDET and were prospectively compared with 17 controls. This was not a randomized trial, as the control group was composed of patients who could not undergo IDET because their insurance company denied payment. Data were obtained before treatment and at 3, 6, and 12 months after treatment. At 1 year, 60% (95% CI ± 16%) of the IDET-treated group reported a satisfactory drop in their VAS pain scores. Only 23% (95% CI ± 14%) described complete pain relief. All but one patient (16 of 17 patients) within the control group continued to have persistent LBP. Interestingly, the lack of improvement seen in the control group seems to be worse than the rates of improvement by natural history alone.[15] Whether or not the natural history of IDDS is clearly known, the poor outcomes in the control group in Karasek and Bogduk's 2000 study[14] are subject to negative influence by patient expectations.[16] In 2002, the same authors[17] reported on their 2-year outcomes when compared with the 1-year data. Improvements observed at 1 year persisted in the IDET and were significantly different from the comparison group ($p < 0.001$).

Fifty-four percent of the IDET-treated group reported had continued pain relief of ≥50% (18 of 35 patients).

Derby et al[17,18] reported favorable outcomes in 62.5% of their IDET-treated cohort at 6 months. The mean VAS reduction was 1.84 (standard deviation [SD] 2.38), which may not be clinically significant. They also reported that 25% of IDET-treated patients did not appreciate any benefit at 12 months, and 12.5% of patients had a worsening of three out of four outcome scales.

In 2002, Gerszten et al[19] reported their results of a nonrandomized, prospective case series of 27 patients with 1-year follow-up. Seventy-five percent of patients noted improvement on the Roland-Morris Disability Questionnaire (RMDQ), yet only 47% improved on the SF-36 survey. As reported by Bogduk and Karasek,[14,17] no relationship was found between outcome and symptom duration ($p = 0.32$), number of levels treated ($p = 0.20$), and worker's compensation status ($p = 0.38$). In 2003, Lutz et al[63a] published the outcomes of their nonrandomized, prospective case series of 33 patients diagnosed with internal disc disruption by provocation discography. There was a mean follow-up of 15 months. A mean improvement of 3.9 points on the VAS ($p < 0.001$), a mean change in the lower limb VAS score of 3.7 ($p < 0.001$), and a mean change in the RMDQ of 7.3 ($p < 0.001$) was reported. Complete pain relief was achieved in only 24% of the patients and partial pain relief was noted in just 46% of the patients. No statistically significant difference was found between the demographics of responders versus nonresponders, single-level versus multilevel IDET outcomes, patients with low pressure (concordant pain at <15 psi above baseline opening pressure) versus high pressure (15 psi to 50 psi above baseline opening pressure) sensitive discs, and patients with workers' compensation versus no-fault cases.

In 2003, a bi-institutional, retrospective chart review study was published by Cohen et al[20] to determine complication rates and risk factors for IDET failure. Notwithstanding the title, the primary outcome measure for this study was pain relief. Over 50% reduction in pain 6 months postprocedure was defined as success and any other result was labeled as failure. Overall, 48% (38 of 79) of patients reported more than 50% pain relief persisting at their 6-month follow-up, with eight of these patients (10%) obtaining over 90% relief. To help explain their modest success rate, the authors draw attention to their liberal inclusion criteria.

The first double-blind, randomized, controlled trial for IDET was published in 2004. Pauza et al[21] identified 1360 potential subjects willing to submit to randomization and narrowed this number to 260 patients after clinical examination. Of these, only 64 proved discogram-positive and were randomized into the IDET treatment group ($n = 37$) or the matched sham control group ($n = 27$). Although both groups demonstrated mean improvements in pain, disability, and depression, the improvements were better in the IDET-treated group. In the IDET group, a mere 13.5% of treated patients had total pain relief, and only 40% had a partial response. That means 50% of the treated patients appreciated no significant benefit from IDET, which is in stark contrast to the 25% reported in the uncontrolled trial by Derby et al.[18] Thus, it seems that IDET may have a modest effect over placebo in only a limited percentage of well-selected individuals. Freeman et al[45] followed with their own randomized, double-blind, controlled trial.[45] Inclusion criteria included the presence of one- or two-level symptomatic disc degeneration with posterior or posterolateral annular tears as determined by provocative computed tomography discography. Fifty-seven patients were randomized with a 2:1 ratio: 38 to IDET and 19 to a sham procedure. Similar to Pauza et al,[21] the number of subjects included in each arm of the study was less than desired to achieve a power of 80%.[45] A comprehensive set of outcome measures was recorded at baseline and 6 months. There was no significant change in outcome measures in either group at 6 months. Freeman et al[45] concluded that IDET is no more effective than placebo for the treatment of chronic discogenic pain. The conclusions by Freeman et al[45] are quite different than those of Pauza et al.[21]

One study examined the use of IDET in a particular population.[66] Freedman et al[66] reported on the results of 36 active-duty soldiers (34 men, 2 women) who underwent IDET for chronic discogenic LBP unresponsive to conservative therapy. Data were collected through clinic chart review and follow-up questionnaires. Success was defined as a 50% decrease in pain from baseline. At 6 months, the success rate was 47% (17 of 36). These numbers deteriorated to 16% (5 of 31 patients)

at final follow-up (average 29.7 months). Almost 20% of patients felt worse at their most recent follow-up. Seven of 31 soldiers (23%), all men, went on to spinal surgery within 24 months of failed IDET. The authors concluded IDET was not an adequate alternative to spinal fusion for treatment of chronic discogenic LBP in active-duty soldiers.

One retrospective study that must be considered when attempting to determine the efficacy of IDET is the 1-year data by Davis et al.[46] They reported that 97% of post-IDET patients continued to have functionally limiting LBP, 29% reported having more LBP than before the IDET procedure, 29% required more narcotics than pre-IDET, and 53% of the patients were dissatisfied with their outcome. Interestingly, when queried as to whether they would undergo the procedure again, 53% said they would and 31% said they would not. The substantial percentage of patients willing to undergo a second IDET procedure, despite poor results as measured by the other outcome measures, may be related to the general preference of a patient to undergo a minimally invasive treatment before considering surgery.

Radiofrequency Posterior Annuloplasty

Procedure

Radiofrequency posterior annuloplasty (RFA) is also commonly known by the name of the device used to create the lesion, the DiscTRODE (Valleylab, Tyco HealthCare Group). Unlike the SpineCATH used with IDET, this flexible radiofrequency electrode can be directly placed in the posterior and posterolateral mid-anulus (**Fig. 21.2**). The electrode is inserted on the contralateral side to the annular tear and is

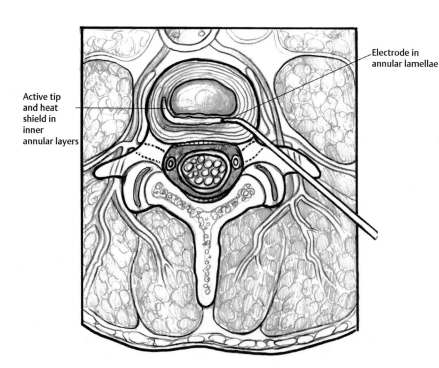

Active tip and heat shield in inner annular layers

Electrode in annular lamellae

Fig. 21.2 Radiofrequency posterior annuloplasty. Cross-sectional image of a DiscTrode catheter (Integra Radionics, Burlington, MA) properly situated within the inner annular fibers of the posterior lumbar disc.

navigated directly across the posterior anulus, between the annular lamellae. The depth of insertion is controlled by use of electrical impedance values and radiologic positioning. Once the electrode is placed, the anulus is heated so that the electrode registers incremental temperatures of 55° to 65°C over 14 minutes.

Clinical Outcomes

The first prospective trial, which found that RFA was more effective than conservative therapy, was published in 2005 by Finch et al.[67] Forty-six consecutive patients with a history of 6 months of chronic LBP, evidence of an annular tear on magnetic resonance imaging (MRI), and a subsequent single-level painful provocative discography at the same level, were offered RFA. Thirty-one patients underwent radiofrequency heating of their posterior annular tears. The remaining 15 patients, who mostly could not obtain funding for the procedure, continued with conservative management and acted as a control group. In the treatment group only, the VAS and Oswestry Disability Index (ODI) improved significantly at 12 months of follow-up. Using a control group that wished to proceed with the intended treatment, but was limited by financial barriers, has a tremendous negative impact on patient expectations; thus creating a control group destined to have a poorer outcome.

Kapural et al[31] followed with an RFA versus IDET head-to-head comparative study. All patients had been referred by spine surgeons with a request for lumbar discography; anticipating future fusion surgery or annuloplasty if indicated. The authors matched 42 patients (21 IDET and 21 RFA) for age, sex, weight, smoking history, manual labor, and number of IVDs treated. Ten patients in each group underwent annuloplasty at one level, while 11 patients were treated at two levels. From the 3rd to the 12th month after the procedure, the IDET group had significantly lower VAS pain scores than the RFA group. Despite the between group differences the VAS did show a statistically significant decrease from baseline to 1-year follow-up for both the RFA (6.6 ± 2.0 to 4.4 ± 2.4) and IDET (7.4 ± 1.9 to 1.4 ± 1.9) groups, individually. Pain disability index (PDI) scores in the IDET group had a statistically significant larger improvement than those for patients who received RFA.

Safety in Thermocoagulation

PIRFT, IDET, and RFA are relatively benign procedures, but do carry some inherent risk. Complications associated with discography or any percutaneous procedure directed into the IVD may also be associated with each of these three intradiscal thermal techniques. A recent meta-analysis by Appleby et al[68] places the overall complication rate of IDET at 0.8% (95% CI 0.2%, 1.4%).

In a multicenter study by Saal et al[69] the reported complication rate was 0.7% (12 of 1675). In contrast, Cohen et al[70] and Freedman et al[66] found complication rates as high as 10% (8 of 79 patients) and 16% (5 of 31 patients), respectively. The former, based on physician responses to questionnaires, identified disc herniations and nerve root injuries as the predominant complications.[69] In the latter two studies, based on patient self-report, transient non-dermatomal dysesthesias, radicular injury, increased low-back pain, disc herniation, and headache were the leading complications.[66,70]

Serious complications have been reported, including two reports of avascular necrosis of the vertebral body after IDET.[71,72] Although the risk of thermal endplate damage has not been supported in cadaver studies,[73] the above case reports confirm significant disc space narrowing and disc space collapse with biopsy evidence of heat injury of the endplates. There have been two reports of cauda equina syndrome when the IDET catheter was erroneously placed within the spinal canal.[74,75] Both cases were determined to be a result of technical error; it can be predetermined whether the catheter is outside the disc. Preprocedure preparation is necessary to ascertain if there is a focal protrusion of the disc one intends to treat. If the protrusion abuts a nerve root then the procedure should not be performed.

As with discography one of the major concerns is the potential for developing discitis. Only two cases have been reported to date.[46,76] Other problems, including the potential for bleeding, injury to the traversing nerve root, anulus, and dural puncture can all occur while introducing the needle and catheter into the disc.

Eckel et al[77] reported a catheter breakage rate of 1.1% (19 of 1675 patients) of cases.[46,77] Orr and Thomas[78] reported a case of a broken catheter tip migrating from the disc space into the thecal sac causing radicular pain.

■ Intradiscal Steroid Instillation

Feffer first reported the use of intradiscal steroid instillation (ISI) in 1956 to treat a patient with a disc herniation.[79] Several researchers and clinicians have theorized that ISI is a potential treatment for discogenic back pain based on the premise that the cause of symptoms is a consequence of an inflammatory process.[80–85] It is well established that inflammatory enzymes and mediators play a major role in the pathophysiology of degenerative disc disease.[40,56,86–100]

Clinical Outcomes

Simmons et al[101] performed the first prospective, randomized, double-blind study to test the therapeutic effect of intradiscal steroids in patients with LBP. Twenty-five patients with a concordant positive pain on provocative discography were randomized into two groups.[101] Group A (N = 14) received methylprednisolone [Depo-Medrol (Pfizer Pharmaceuticals, New York, NY) 80 mg/mL] and group B (N = 11) received bupivacaine [Marcaine (Abbott Laboratories, Abbott Park, IL) 0.5% 1.5 mL]. At 2 weeks, 21% (3 of 14) of group A patients showed subjective improvement and 79% no improvement, while none were clinically worse. In group B, 9% (1 of 11 patients) showing clinical improvement and 91% no improvement; none were clinically worse.

Khot et al[102] conducted a retrospective trial, which suggested positive results in 24.5% of patients at 6 weeks following injection. Subsequently, they performed a well-designed prospective randomized study.[102] One hundred twenty (120 of 274) patients with chronic LBP of discogenic origin met inclusion criteria, including a concordant pain response during awake sedated discography. At the time of discography, they were randomized to injection of normal saline or methylprednisolone (40 mg, 1 cc) into the disc space. The ODI and VAS scores were followed over the next 12 months. There was no significant difference between the two groups. The authors concluded that intradiscal steroid instillation is ineffective as a therapeutic option in discogenic pain.

More recently, researchers have investigated a subgroup of patients with discogenic LBP and associated inflammatory endplate changes on MRI.[103,104] Previous studies have shown a strong association between Modic I changes and LBP.[105–108] Modic changes appear to be a relatively specific but insensitive sign of a painful lumbar disc in patients with discogenic LBP.[109] Buttermann[104] prospectively studied 232 consecutive patients referred for treatment of DDD with and without inflammatory endplate changes on MRI. Potential candidates with at least one year of low-back pain were subject to the authors' therapeutic algorithm for discogenic LBP. Following a series of one to three epidural space steroid injections (transforaminal epidural steroid injection or interlaminar epidural steroid injection), patients who did not improve were offered repeat injections. If the injections were unsuccessful in significantly reducing pain, patients were then randomized to discography alone or in combination with intradiscal steroid instillation. Following ISI, those with persistent pain were offered lumbar fusion surgery. Pain and function were prospectively determined by a self-administered outcomes survey that included VAS, ODI, a pain diagram (PD), and opinion of success at 1 to 3, 4 to 6, and 7 to 12 months and at 1 to 2 years after the first injection. Ninety-three patients with inflammatory endplate changes and 139 patients without inflammatory endplate changes underwent ESI. Failures with inflammatory endplate changes (78 of 93 patients) or without inflammatory endplate changes (93 of 139 patients) underwent discography with or without intradiscal steroid in a nonspecified randomization process. Forty of 78 patients with inflammatory endplate changes and 46 of 93 without

endplate changes were randomized to discography with ISI. Within the group with inflammatory endplate changes, the rate of success was greatest at 1 to 3 months (27 of 40 patients; 68%) and diminished at 1 to 2 years (10 of 40 patients; 25%). In patients without inflammatory endplate changes the benefits were negligible at both short-term (8 of 46 patients; 17%) and long-term follow-up (5 of 46 patients; 11%). Fayad et al[110] further studied the relationship between symptomatic inflammatory endplate changes and the use of intradiscal steroid instillation. The purpose of this retrospective study was to analyze the association between the severity of Modic changes on MRI and the clinical response to intradiscal steroid instillation [1 cc (25 mg) of acetate of prednisolone] in chronic LBP. Seventy-four patients with LBP and inflammatory Modic changes, who showed no response to 3-month conservative treatment, received lumbar ISI. Patients were categorized by endplate changes on MRI as Modic type I (n = 37); those with a mixture of Modic type I and type II changes, but predominantly edema changes as Modic I-2 (n = 25) and those with predominantly fatty changes as Modic II-1 (n = 12). All patients underwent awake single-level discography prior to steroid instillation. Discography was used only at the suspected levels and pain provocation was not considered a primary goal. Discography was used solely to ensure an intranuclear location for steroid instillation. At 1 month, reduction in VAS pain score was significantly higher in the Modic I and Modic I-2 groups than in the Modic II-1 group (30.2 ± 26.6 and 29.4 ± 21.5 versus 5.3 ± 25.5; p = 0.009 and p = 0.017, respectively). At 3 and 6 months, ISI appeared to be more effective in the Modic I and Modic I-2 groups, but these findings were not statistically significant. No complications were reported.

To date, the use of intradiscal steroid instillation has been based mostly on conjecture. The findings from Buttermann[104] and Fayad et al[103] despite flaws in methodology, suggest that this minimally invasive spinal intervention for LBP due to degenerative disc disease may be reasonable in the properly selected patient. It is conceivable that ISI may prove to be a short-term efficient treatment for patients with chronic LBP and predominantly inflammatory endplate changes when conservative treatments have failed.

Safety

Complications specific to intradiscal instillation of corticosteroids include arachnoiditis,[65,111] escalated disc degeneration (destructive discopathy),[112–114] intradiscal calcification,[113] and epidural calcification.[115] Perhaps the most studied complication is destructive discopathy.[112–114] Aoki et al[113] demonstrated rapidly destructive changes in rabbits receiving intradiscal methylprednisolone acetate (Depo-Medrol). This was compared with discs receiving methylprednisolone (Sol-Medrol; Upjohn Company, Kalamazoo, MI) or saline alone. In the latter two groups, no accelerated gross or microscopic destructive changes were demonstrated. It appears the effects of Depo-Medrol on tissue degeneration originate from its vehicle, polyethylene glycol.[116-118] In a recent observational trial, Benyaha et al[114] showed a disc space collapse rate of 20% and 25% at 6 months and 12 months, respectively. Interestingly enough, they also demonstrated a clinical success rate (good or excellent results) of 71.8% at 1 month, 55.3% at 3 months, and 43.5% at 6 months.

The gravest risk to the patient receiving intradiscal steroid instillation is the development of discitis. The prevalence should be identical to that reported after lumbar discography utilizing a two-needle technique. A review of the available world literature on discography shows the prevalence of discitis ranges between 0.10 to 0.70% of patients and 0.07 to 0.14% of discs investigated.[119-123] In our experience at The Penn Spine Center (Philadelphia, PA), there has been only case of discitis in more than 5,000 procedures and more than 15,000 discs evaluated or treated.

■ Discussion

Only two randomized controlled clinical trials exist that describe a comparison of the efficacy of surgery to nonsurgical management of chronic low back pain due to degenerative disease of the lumbar spine.[5,10] The inconclusive results[5,10] demonstrate the lack of a clearly defined gap between surgical and nonsurgical outcomes for the treatment of lumbar degenerative disc disease. Given the prevalence of this problem and the limited treatment options, the development of minimally invasive alternative treatment methods is the logical advancement of care. Fluoroscopically guided intradiscal procedures have emerged as the possible missing link in the treatment algorithm for chronic discogenic pain. Currently, the literature is far too sparse to make any definitive conclusions as to the superiority or inferiority of any single intradiscal technique. More randomized clinical trials are necessary to determine the true efficacy of intradiscal therapies for low back pain caused by degenerative disc disease of the lumbar spine.

References

1. Crock HV. A reappraisal of intervertebral disc lesions. Med J Aust 1970;1:983–989
2. Crock HV. The presidential address: ISSLS, internal disc disruption: a challenge to disc prolapse fifty years on. Spine 1986;11: 650–653
3. Wetzel FT, LaRocca SH, Lowery GL, et al. The treatment of lumbar spinal pain syndromes diagnosed by discography: lumbar arthrodesis. Spine 1994;19:792–800
4. Zdeblick TA. A prospective, randomized study of lumbar fusions: preliminary results. Spine 1993;18:983–991
5. Brox JI, Sorensen R, Friis A, et al. Randomized clinical trial of lumbar instrumented fusion and cognitive intervention and exercises in patients with chronic low back pain and disc degeneration. Spine 2003;28:1913–1921
6. Bjarke-Christensen F, Hansen ES, Laursen M, et al. Long-term functional outcome of pedicle screw instrumentation as a support for posterolateral spinal fusion: randomized clinical study with a 5-year follow-up. Spine 2002;27:1269–1277
7. Christensen FB, Hansen ES, Eiskjaer SP, et al. Circumferential lumbar spinal fusion with Brantigan cage versus posterolateral fusion with titanium Cotrel-Dubousset instrumentation: a prospective, randomized clinical study of 146 patients. Spine 2002;27:2674–2683
8. Fairbank J, Frost H, Wilson-MacDonald J, et al. Randomised controlled trial to compare surgical stabilisation of the lumbar spine with an intensive rehabilitation program for patients with chronic low back pain: the MRC spine stabilisation trial. BMJ 2005;330:1233
9. France JC, Yaszemski MJ, Lauerman WC, et al. A randomized prospective study of posterolateral lumbar fusion: outcomes with and without pedicle screw instrumentation. Spine 1999;24: 553–560
10. Fritzell P, Hagg O, Wessberg P, et al. 2001 Volvo Award Winner in Clinical Studies. Lumbar fusion versus nonsurgical treatment for chronic low back pain: a multicenter randomized controlled trial from the Swedish Lumbar Spine Study Group. Spine 2001;26: 2521–2532
11. Thomsen K, Christensen FB, Eiskjaer SP, et al. 1997 Volvo Award Winner in Clinical Studies. The effect of pedicle screw instrumentation on functional outcome and fusion rates in posterolateral lumbar spinal fusion: a prospective, randomized clinical study. Spine 1997;22:2813–2822
12. Fritzell P, Hagg O, Wessberg P, et al. Chronic low back pain and fusion: a comparison of three surgical techniques. A prospective multicenter randomized study from the Swedish Lumbar Spine Study Group. Spine 2002;27:1131–1141
13. Hayashi K, Markel M. Thermal modification of joint capsule and ligamentous tissues. Op Tech Sports Med 1998;6:120–125
14. Naseef GS, Foster TE, Trauner K, et al. The thermal properties of bovine joint capsule: the basic science of laser and radiofrequency induced capsular shrinkage. Am J Sports Med 1997;25:670–674
15. Hecht P, Hayashi K, Cooley J, Lu Y, Fanton G, Thabit III G, Markel M. The thermal effect of monopolar radiofrequency energy on the properties of joint capsule: an in vivo histologic study using a sheep model. Am J Sports Med 1998;26(6)
16. Lopez M, Hayashi K, Fanton G, Thabit III G, Markel M. The effect of radiofrequency energy on the ultrastructure of joint capsular collagen. Arthroscopy 1998;14:495–501
17. Obrzut S, Hecht P, Hayashi K, Fanton G, Thabit III G, Markel M. The effect of radiofrequency energy on the length and temperature properties of the glenohumeral joint capsule. Arthroscopy 1998;14:395–400
18. Hayashi K, Thabit III G, Vailas AC, et al. The effect of nonablative laser energy on joint capsular properties: an in vitro histologic and biochemical study using a rabbit model. Am J Sports Med 1996;24(5)

19. Hayashi K, Nieckarz J, Thabit III G, et al. The effect of nonablative laser energy on the joint capsule: an in vivo rabbit study using a holmium:YAG laser. Lasers Surg Med 1997;20:164–171

20. Hayashi K, Thabit III G, Bogdanskc J, Mascio L, Markel M. The effect of nonablative laser energy on the ultrastructure of joint capsular collagen. Arthroscopy 1996;12:474–481

21. Hayashi K, Hecht P, Thabit G III, et al. The biologic response to laser thermal modification in an in vivo sheep model. Clin Orthop Relat Res 2000;373:265–276

22. Letcher FS, Goldring S. The effect of radiofrequency current and heat on peripheral nerve action potential in the cat. J Neurosurg 1968;29:42–47

23. Strohbehn JW. Temperature distributions from interstitial RF electrode hyperthermia systems: theoretical predictions. Int J Radiat Oncol Biol Phys 1983;9:1655–1667

24. Troussier B, Lebas JF, Chirossel JP, et al. Percutaneous intradiscal radio-frequency thermocoagulation: a cadaveric study. Spine 1995;20:1713–1718

25. Cosman ER, Nashold BS, Ovelman-Levitt J. Theoretical aspects of radiofrequency lesions in the dorsal root entry zone. Neurosurgery 1984;15:945–950

26. Mehta M, Sluijter M. The treatment of chronic back pain. Anaesthesia 1979;34:768–775

27. Sluijter ME. The use of radiofrequency lesions for pain relief in failed back patients. Int Disabil Stud 1988;10:37–43

28. Teixeira A, Sluijter ME. Intradiscal high-voltage, long-duration pulsed radiofrequency for discogenic pain: a preliminary report. Pain Med 2006;7(5):424–428

29. Oh WS, Shim JC. A randomized controlled trial of radiofrequency denervation of the ramus communicans nerve for chronic discogenic low back pain. Clin J Pain 2004;20:55–60

30. Barendse GA, van Den Berg SG, Kessels AH, Weber WE, van Kleef M. Randomized controlled trial of percutaneous intradiscal radiofrequency thermocoagulation for chronic discogenic back pain: lack of effect from a 90-second 70 C lesion. Spine 2001;26:287–292

31. Kapural L, Hayek S, Malak O, et al. Intradiscal thermal annuloplasty versus intradiscal radiofrequency ablation for the treatment of discogenic pain: a prospective matched control trial. Pain Med 2005;6:425–431

32. Slipman CW, Palmitier RA, DeDianous DK. Injection techniques. In: Grabois M., Hart H, Garrison J, Lehmhuhl D, eds. Physical Medicine and Rehabilitation: The Complete Approach. Blackwood, NJ: Blackwell Publishing; 1999:458–486

33. Van Kleef M, Barendse GAM, Wilmink JT, et al. Percutaneous intradiscal radiofrequency thermocoagulation in chronic non-specific low back pain. Pain Clin 1996;9:259–268

34. Ercelen O, Bulutcu E, Oktenoglu T, et al. Radiofrequency lesioning using two different time modalities for the treatment of lumbar discogenic pain: a randomized trial. Spine 2003;28:1922–1927

35. Houpt JC, Conner E, McFarland E. Experimental study of temperature distributions and thermal transport during radiofrequency current therapy of the intervertebral disc. Spine 1996;21(15):1808–1812

36. Saal JA, Saal JS. Thermal characteristics of lumbar disc: evaluation of a novel approach to targeted intradiscal thermal therapy. Paper presented at 13th Annual Meeting of the North American Spine Society; October 28–31, 1998; San Francisco, CA

37. Saal JA, Saal JS. Intradiscal electrothermal therapy for the treatment of chronic discogenic low back pain. Clin Sports Med 2002;21(1):167–187

38. Shah RV, Lutz GE, Lee J, et al. Intradiscal electrothermal therapy: a preliminary histologic study. Arch Phys Med Rehabil 2001;82:1230–1237

39. Freeman BJ, Walters RM, Moore RJ, Fraser RD. Does intradiscal electrothermal therapy denervate and repair experimentally induced posterolateral annular tears in an animal model? Spine 2003;28(23):2602–2608

40. Kleinstueck FS, Diederich CJ, Nau WH, et al. Temperature and thermal dose distributions during intradiscal electrothermal therapy in the cadaveric lumbar spine. Spine 2003;28:1700–1708

41. Damianou CA, Hynynen K, Fan X. Evaluation of accuracy of a theoretical model for predicting the necrosed tissue volume during focused ultrasound surgery. IEEE Trans Ultrason Ferroelectr Freq Control 1995;42:182–187

42. Graham SJ, Chen L, Leitch M, et al. Quantifying tissue damage due to focused ultrasound heating observed by MRI. Magn Reson Med 1999;41:321–328

43. Pearce J, Thomsen S. Rate process analysis of thermal damage. In: Welch AJ, Van Gemert MJC, eds. Optical-Thermal Response of Laser-Irradiated Tissue. London: Plenum; 1995:561–606

44. Saal JA, Saal JS. Intradiscal electrothermal treatment for chronic discogenic low back pain: a prospective outcome study with minimum 1-year follow-up. Spine 2000;25:2622–2627

44a. Bono CM, Iki K, Jalota A, et al. Temperatures within the lumbar disc and endplates during intradiscal electrothermal therapy: formulation of a predictive temperature map in relation to distance from the catheter. Spine 2004;29:1124–1129

45. Freeman BJ, Fraser RD, Cain CM, Hall DJ, Chapple DC. A randomized, double-blind, controlled trial: intradiscal electrothermal therapy versus placebo for the treatment of chronic discogenic low back pain. Spine 2005;30(21):2369–2377

46. Davis TT, Delamarter RB, Sra P, et al. The IDET procedure for chronic discogenic low back pain. Spine 2004;29:752–756

47. Hecht P, Hayashi K, Cooley AJ, et al. The thermal effect of monopolar radiofrequency energy on the properties of joint capsule: an in vivo histologic study using a sheep model. Am J Sports Med 1998;26:808–814

48. Hayashi K, Thabit G III, Vailas AC, et al. The effect of nonablative laser energy on joint capsular properties: an in vitro histologic and biochemical study using a rabbit model. Am J Sports Med 1996;24:640–646

49. Naseef GS III, Foster T, Trauner K, et al. The thermal properties of bovine joint capsule: the basic science of laser- and radiofrequency-induced capsular shrinkage. Am J Sports Med 1997;25:670–674

50. Wall MS, Deng XH, Torzilli P, Doty S, O'Brien S, Warren RF. Thermal modification of collagen. J Shoulder Elbow Surg 1999;8:339–344

51. Lu Y, Hayashi K, Edwards RB III, et al. The effect of monopolar radiofrequency treatment pattern on joint capsular healing: in vitro and in vivo studies using an ovine model. Am J Sports Med 2000;28(5):711–719

52. Osmond C, Hecht P, Hayashi K, et al. Comparative effects of laser and radiofrequency energy on joint capsule. Clin Orthop Relat Res 2000;375:286–294

53. Hayashi K, Hecht P, Thabit G III, et al. The biologic response to laser thermal modification in an in vivo sheep model. Clin Orthop Relat Res 2000;373:265–276

54. Hayashi K, Peters DM, Thabit G III, et al. The mechanism of joint capsule thermal modification in an in-vitro sheep model. Clin Orthop Relat Res 2000;370:236–249

55. Hayashi K, Massa KL, Thabit G III, et al. Histologic evaluation of the glenohumeral joint capsule after the laser-assisted capsular shift procedure for glenohumeral instability. Am J Sports Med 1999;27(2):162–167

56. Lopez MJ, Hayashi K, Fanton GS, et al. The effect of radiofrequency energy on the ultrastructure of joint capsular collagen. Arthroscopy 1998;14(5):495–501

57. Hayashi K, Thabit G III, Vailas AC, et al. The effect of nonablative laser energy on joint capsular properties: an in vitro histologic and biochemical study using a rabbit model. Am J Sports Med 1996;24(5):640–646

58. Hayashi K, Thabit G III, Massa KL, et al. The effect of thermal heating on the length and histologic properties of the glenohumeral joint capsule. Am J Sports Med 1997;25(1):107–112

59. Hayashi K, Markel MD, Thabit G III, et al. The effect of nonablative laser energy on joint capsular properties: an in vitro mechanical study using a rabbit model. Am J Sports Med 1995;23(4):482–487

60. Hayashi K, Thabit G III, Vailas AC, et al. The effect of nonablative laser energy on joint capsular properties: an in vitro histologic and biochemical study using a rabbit model. Am J Sports Med 1996;24(5):640–646

61. Obrzut SL, Hecht P, Hayashi K, et al. The effect of radiofrequency energy on the length and temperature properties of the glenohumeral joint capsule. Arthroscopy 1998;14:395–400

62. Chen SS, Humphrey JD. Heat-induced changes in the mechanics of a collagenous tissue: pseudoelastic behavior at 37 degrees C. J Biomech 1998;31:211–216

63. Lee JM, Pereira CA, Abdulla D, et al. A multi-sample denaturation temperaturetester for collagenous biomaterials. Med Eng Phys 1995;17:115–121

63a. Lutz C, Lutz GE, Cooke PM: Treatment of chronic lumbar diskogenic pain with intradiskal electrothermal therapy: a prospective outcome study. Arch Phys Med Rehabil 2003;84:23–28

64. Slipman CW, Patel RK, Zhang L, et al. Side of symptomatic annular tear and site of low back pain: is there a correlation? Spine 2001;26:E165–E169

65. Roche J. Steroid-induced arachnoiditis. Med J Aust 1984;140:281–284

66. Freedman BA, Cohen SP, Kuklo TR, et al. Intradiscal electrothermal therapy (IDET) for chronic low back pain in active-duty soldiers: 2-year follow-up. Spine J 2003;3:502–509

67. Finch PM, Price LM, Drummond PD. Radiofrequency heating of painful annular disruptions: one-year outcomes. J Spinal Disord Tech 2005;18:6–13

68. Appleby D, Andersson G, Totta M. Meta-analysis of the efficacy and safety of intradiscal electrothermal therapy (IDET). Pain Med 2006;7(4):308–316

69. Saal JA, Saal JS, Wetzel FT, et al. IDET related complications: a multi-center study of 1675 treated patients with a review of the FDA MDR data base. Paper presented at 16th Annual Meeting of the North American Spine Society; October 31 to November 3, 2001; Seattle, WA

70. Cohen SP, Larkin T, Abdi S, et al. Risk factors for failure and complications of intradiscal electrothermal therapy: a pilot study. Spine 2003;28(11):1142–1147

71. Scholl BM, Theiss SM, Lopez-Ben R, et al. Vertebral osteonecrosis related to intradiscal electrothermal therapy: a case report. Spine 2003;28:E161–E164

72. Djurasovic M, Glassman SD, Dimar JR Jr, et al. Vertebral osteonecrosis associated with the use of intradiscal electrothermal therapy: a case report. Spine 2002;27:E325–E328

73. Yetkinler DN, Nau WH, Brandt LL. Disc temperature measurements during nucleoplasty and IDET procedures. Paper presented at 6th International Congress on Spinal Surgery; September 4–7, 2002; Ankara, Turkey

74. Ackerman WE III. Cauda equina syndrome after intradiscal electrothermal therapy. Reg Anesth Pain Med 2002;27:622

75. Hsia AW, Isaac K, Katz JS. Cauda equina syndrome from intradiscal electrothermal therapy. Neurology 2000;55:320

76. Ercelen O, Bulutcu E, Oktenoglu T, et al. Radiofrequency lesioning using two different time modalities for the treatment of lumbar discogenic pain: a randomized trial. Spine 2003;28:1922–1927

77. Eckel TS, Ortiz AO. Intradiscal electrothermal therapy in the treatment of discogenic low back pain. Tech Vasc Interv Radiol 2002;5(4):217–222

78. Orr RD, Thomas S. Intradural migration of broken IDET catheter causing a radiculopathy. J Spinal Disord Tech 2005;18(2):185–187

79. Feffer HL. Treatment of low back pain and sciatic pain by the injection of hydrocortisone into degenerated intervertebral discs. J Bone Joint Surg Am 1956;38:585–592

80. Leao L. Intradiscal injection of hydrocortisone and prednisolone in the treatment of back pain. Rheumatism 1960;16:72–77

81. Feffer HL. Therapeutic intradiscal hydrocortisone: a long term study. Clin Orthop Relat Res 1969;67:100–104

82. Wilkinson HA, Schuman N. Intradiscal corticosteroids in the treatment of lumbar and cervical disc problems. Spine 1980;5:385–389

83. Graham CE. Chemonucleolysis: a preliminary report on a double blind study comparing chemonucleolysis and intradiscal administration of hydrocortisone in the treatment of back-ache and sciatica. Orthop Clin North Am 1975;6:259–263

84. Muro T. Treatment of lumbar disc herniation by intradiscal injection of corticosteroids: follow-up study. Paper presented at International Intradiscal Therapy Society Third Annual Meeting, March 7–11, 1990; Marbella, Spain

85. Nelson DA. Intraspinal therapy using methylprednisolone acetate: twenty-three years of clinical controversy. Spine 1993;18:278–286

86. Ozaktay AC, Kallakuri S, Cavanaugh JM. Phospholipase A2 sensitivity of the dorsal root and dorsal root ganglion. Spine 1998;23:1297–1306

87. Utzschneider D, Kocsis J, Devor M. Mutual excitation among dorsal root ganglion neurons in the rat. Neurosci Lett 1992;146:53–56

88. Palmgren T, Grönblad M, Virri J, Seitsalo S, Ruuskanen M, Karoharju E. Immunohistochemical demonstration of sensory and autonomic severe terminals in herniated lumbar disc tissue. Spine 1996;21:1301–1306

89. Peng B, Wu W, Hou S, et al. The pathogenesis of discogenic low back pain. J Bone Joint Surg Br 2005;87:62–67

90. Kang JD, Georgescu HI, McIntyre L, et al. Herniated lumbar intervertebral discs spontaneously produce matrix metalloproteinases, nitric oxide, interleukin-6, and prostaglandin E2. Spine 1996;21:271–277

91. Kawakami M, Tamaki T, Weinstein J, et al. Pathomechanism of pain related behavior produced by allografts of intervertebral disc in the rat. Spine 1996;21:2101–2107

92. Freemont AJ, Peacock TE, Goupille P, et al. Nerve ingrowth into diseased intervertebral disc in chronic back pain. Lancet 1997; 350:178–181

93. Palmgren T, Gronblad M, Virri J, et al. An immunohistochemical study of nerve structures in the annulus fibrosus of human normal lumbar intervertebral discs. Spine 1999;24:2075–2079

94. Ashton IK, Walsh DA, Polak JH, et al. Substance P in intervertebral discs, binding sites on vascular endothelium of the human annulus fibrosus. Acta Orthop Scand 1994;65:635–639

95. Weinstein J, Claverie W, Gibson S. The pain of discography. Spine 1988;13:1344–1348

96. Liesi P, Gronblad M, Korkala O, Karaharju E, Rusanen M. Substance P: a neuro-peptide involved in low back pain? Lancet 1983;1: 1328–1329

97. McCarthy PW, Petts P, Hamilton A. RT97- and calcitonin gene-related peptide-like immunoreactivity in lumbar intervertebral discs and adjacent tissue from the rat. J Anat 1992;180:15–24

98. Konttinen YT, Gronblad M, Antti-Poika I, et al. Neuroimmunohistochemical analysis of peridiscal nociceptive neural elements. Spine 1990;15:383–386

99. Ahmed M, Bjurholm A, Kreicbergs A, Schultzberg M. Neuropeptide Y, tyrosine hydroxylase and vasoactive intestinal polypeptide-immunoreactive nerve fibers in the vertebral bodies, discs, dura mater, and spinal ligaments of the rat lumbar spine. Spine 1993; 18:268–273

100. Burke JG, Watson RWG, McCormack D, et al. Intervertebral discs which cause low back pain secrete high levels of proinflammatory mediators. J Bone Joint Surg Br 2002;84(2):196–201

101. Simmons JW, McMillin JN, Emery SF, et al. Intradiscal steroids: a prospective double-blind clinical trial. Spine 1992;17(6, Suppl): S172–S175

102. Khot A, Bowditch M, Powell J, Sharp D. The use of intradiscal steroid therapy for lumbar spinal discogenic pain: a randomized controlled trial. Spine 2004;29(8):833–836 discussion 837

103. Fayad F, Lefevre-Colau MM, Rannou F, et al. Relation of inflammatory Modic changes to intradiscal steroid injection outcome in chronic low back pain. Eur Spine J 2007;16(7):925–931

104. Buttermann GR. The effect of spinal steroid injections for degenerative disc disease. Spine J 2004;4(5):495–505

105. Kjaer P, Leboeuf-Yde C, Korsholm L, et al. Magnetic resonance imaging and low back pain in adults: a diagnostic imaging study of 40-year-old men and women. Spine 2005;30(10):1173–1180

106. Toyone T, Takahashi K, Kitahara H, et al. Vertebral bone-marrow changes in degenerative lumbar disc disease: an MRI study of 74 patients with low back pain. J Bone Joint Surg Br 1994;76(5): 757–764

107. Weishaupt D, Zanetti M, Hodler J, et al. Painful lumbar disc derangement: relevance of endplate abnormalities at MR imaging. Radiology 2001;218(2):420–427

108. Sandhu HS, Sanchez-Caso LP, Parvataneni HK, et al. Association between findings of provocative discography and vertebral endplate changes as seen on MRI. J Spinal Disord 2000;13:438–443

109. Braithwaite I, White J, Saifuddin A, Renton P, Taylor BA. Vertebral end-plate (Modic) changes on lumbar spine MRI: correlation with pain reproduction at lumbar discography. Eur Spine J 1998;7(5): 363–368

110. Fayad F, Lefevre-Colau MM, Rannou F, et al. Relation of inflammatory Modic changes to intradiscal steroid injection outcome in chronic low back pain. Eur Spine J 2007;16(7):925–931

111. Johnson A, Ryan MD, Roche J. Depo-Medrol and myelographic arachnoiditis. Med J Aust 1991;155:18–20

112. Kato F, Mimatsu K, Kawakami N, et al. Changes in the intervertebral disc after discography with intradiscal injection of corticosteroids observed with magnetic resonance imaging (MRI). J Neurol Orthop Med Surg. 1993;14:210–216

113. Aoki M, Kato F, Mimatsu K, et al. Histologic changes in the intervertebral disc after intradiscal injections of methylprednisolone acetate in rabbits. Spine 1997;22:127–131 discussion 132

114. Benyahya R, Lefevre-Colau MM, Fayad F, et al. Intradiscal injection of acetate of prednisolone in severe low back pain: complications and patients' assessment of effectiveness. Ann Readapt Med Phys 2004;47(9):621–626 French.

115. Menkes CJ, Vallee C, Giraudet-Le-Quintrec JS. Calcification of epidural space after the injection of triaminolone hexacetonide. Presse Med 1989;18:1707

116. Chino N, Awad EA, Kottke FJ. Pathology of propylene glycol administered by perineural and intramuscular injection in rats. Arch Phys Med Rehabil 1974;55:33–38

117. Delaney TJ, Rowlingson JC, Carron H, Butler A. Epidural steroid effects on nerves and meninges. Anesth Analg 1980;58:610–614

118. Nelson AN. Intraspinal therapy using methylprednisolone acetate: twenty-three years of clinical controversy. Spine 1993;18: 278–286

119. Guyer RD, Collier R, Stith WJ, et al. Discitis after discography. Spine 1988;13:1352–1354

120. Guyer RD, Ohnmeiss DD. Lumbar discography: Position Statement from the North American Spine Society Diagnostic and Therapeutic Committee. Spine 1995;20:2048–2059

121. Collis JS Jr, Gardner WJ. Lumbar discography: an analysis of 1000 cases. J Neurosurg 1962;19:452–461

122. Wiley JJ, McNab I, Wortzman G. Lumbar discography and clinical applications. Can J Surg 1968;11:280–289

123. Aprill CN. Diagnostic lumbar injection. In: Frymoyer JW, ed. The Adult Spine. 2nd ed. Philadelphia: Lippincott–Raven Publishers; 1997:539–562

124. Eckel TS, Ortiz AO. Intradiscal electrothermal therapy in the treatment of discogenic low back pain. Tech Vasc Interv Radiol 2002; 5(4):217–222

125. Bull T, Sharp D, Powell J. The efficacy of intradiscal steroid injection compared to Modic changes in degenerate lumbar discs. J Bone Joint Surg Br 1998;80:47

22 Nucleus Augmentation

Thomas J. Raley, Qi-Bin Bao, and Hansen A. Yuan

Low back pain (LBP) is a common condition that affects the majority of the population[1,2] and economically impacts our society.[3,4] In fact, LBP is second only to the common cold for lost time at work.[5] The probability of returning to work decreases dramatically with increased time off work (roughly 50% at 6 months).[6,7] The true cause of LBP is unknown, but most likely it is associated with the degeneration of the intervertebral disc (IVD) and age-related deterioration.[8,9] With aging, the incidence of LBP, stiffness, and IVD changes increases,[10] preceding other degenerative changes in the spine.[11-13]

■ Normal Intervertebral Disc Function

The normal mechanical function of the IVD can be summarized as follows:

- The nucleus pulposus (NP) acts predominantly as a fluid under static loading conditions and generates large hydrostatic pressures. The swelling pressure mechanism, due to a high concentration of negatively charged proteoglycans in the NP, maintains disk height and contributes to the pressure mechanism of load support and transfer.[14]

- The high hydraulic permeability of the cartilage endplates allows load transfer uniformly across the anulus fibrosus (AF) and NP.

- The outer anulus, with the highest tensile modulus, is well suited for minimizing IVD bulging and AF strains generated during loading of the spine in compression, bending, or torsional loading.

- In contrast, the lower modulus of the AF allows viscoelastic dissipation. This fluid-flow generated frictional dissipation mechanism in the AF, along with dissipation resulting from NP deformation, is likely to be the mechanisms for energy dissipation and shock absorption for the entire IVD.

■ Nucleus Replacement for Intervertebral Disc Degeneration

After failure of all conservative treatment, the patient is eligible for surgical intervention. However, the appropriate surgical procedure must address the proposed pain generator.

Many treatment options have resulted in poor long-term outcomes. This has led to newer alternative technologies, including NP replacement, IVD replacement, and interbody fusion techniques. In this chapter we will focus on nucleus replacement.

Nucleus replacement is a novel approach to replace the degenerated NP and stop the degenerative cascade. Nucleus replacement is meant to mimic the normal function of the functional spinal unit by preserving motion and preventing adjacent segment degeneration. Nucleus replacements may be useful for the treatment of patients with early symptomatic disc disruption. In the future, they may be performed at the time of discectomy to maintain normal biomechanics of the spine and prevent future degeneration.

History

The idea of nucleus replacements originates in the 1950s. Initial attempts at maintaining disc space height and motion involved injection of polymethyl-methacrylate[15] or silicone[16] into the disc space after nucleotomy. Poor clinical results led to the abandonment of these procedures in favor of inserting preformed devices.

Historically, the first human implanted nucleus prosthesis was the Fernstrom ball in 1966. This device was a spherical endoprosthesis made of stainless steel.[17] It was meant as a spacer that allowed movement between the adjacent vertebral bodies. It did not restore normal load distribution and was abandoned because of concerns of implant migration and subsidence. However, encouraging long-term results led to further efforts in designing other nucleus replacements.[18] Failures with metal ball bearings led to Urbaniak's study on nucleus replacement with a silicone-Dacron composite device in chimpanzees.[19] This work spawned the idea for a preformed or contained implant. In 1981, Edeland[20] suggested the implantation of a device that behaved biologically and biomechanically similar to the NP. The device behaved in a viscoelastic fashion and the properties changed to adapt to the loads applied. In 1988, Ray and Corbin[21] developed a device based on Edeland's principles. It consisted of an outer woven polyethylene capsule, with thixotropic gel injected into the collapsed bags after implantation. This device exhibited swelling pressures similar to the natural NP. In 1991 and 1993, Bao and Higham patented hydrogel for nucleus replacement.[21,22] The Aquarelle hydrogel nucleus is composed of polyvinyl alcohol (PVA), which has a water content of 70%

under physiologic loading conditions, much like the natural nucleus. Three of 25 implants extruded through the annulotomy and one through a preexisting tear.[23] In the mid-1990s, Ray modified his device to a hydrogel core encased with a polyethylene jacket. This prosthetic disc nucleus was implanted in pairs. The device was implanted in a dehydrated state to facilitate insertion.

Biomechanics of Nucleus Replacement Implants

Biologically, the NP functions as a fluid pump, facilitating body fluid diffusion, which carries the nutrients and removes the metabolites from the avascular disc. Biomechanically, the nucleus inflates the anulus and shares a significant portion of compressive load with the anulus. Therefore, the main objective of nucleus replacement implants is to reestablish normal disc function by restoring disc turgor, tension in the AF, and the disc's ability to uniformly transfer loads across the disc space.

In addition to biocompatibility and fatigue strength, several features should be taken into consideration with the design of the nucleus replacement. First, the nucleus replacement should restore the normal and uniform load distribution to avoid excessive endplate wear. Second, the prosthesis should have sufficient stability in the disc space to avoid implant migration. Third, it should restore the normal body fluid pumping function to enhance nutrient diffusion for the remaining nucleus and inner anulus. Lastly, the implant should be able to be easily implanted.[24]

The nucleus replacement implants must be biocompatible and be able to endure a considerable amount of loading before failure. Assuming the average individual takes ~2 million strides per year, the average implant would be expected to take the loads of 100 million cycles over 40 years.[25] In addition to biocompatibility and withstanding load, the device must also (1) exhibit low wear characteristics with minimal wear debris; (2) allow uniform stress distribution under various physiological loading conditions to avoid subsidence and extrusion of the device; (3) fill the disc space to prevent excessive movement that may lead to extrusion; and (4) enable minimally invasive surgical implantation limiting destruction of the tissues and enhancing the stability of the implant.[24] Conceptually and ideally, the nucleus replacement should have the same mechanical properties, such as stiffness and viscoelastic property, as the natural nucleus. The key is to assure a good uniform stress distribution.

Materials and Types of Nucleus Replacement Implants

Choosing the appropriate material is paramount in preventing potential failures. Higher modulus of elasticity devices used in the past are believed to be too stiff for nucleus

devices. Most current nucleus prosthesis designs use various elastomers or designs having viscoelastic properties. At this time, nucleus replacements are categorized into two groups: intradiscal implants and in situ curable polymers. The intradiscal devices are biomechanically more similar to the native nucleus and the in situ curable polymers harden after implantation and allow for a less-invasive approach for implantation.

The first attempt of in situ formed nucleus prostheses was by Nachemson in 1960.[26,27] The main advantage is that it can be injected through a small annular window to reduce the risk of extrusion. It also has the advantage of better implant conformity leading to better stress distribution and implant stability. However, there are several challenges including fatigue of the material, biocompatibility, and leakage of the injectate through the annular incision or another annular defect. Preformed nucleus implants have more consistent polymer properties and biocompatibility. The disadvantages include mismatch with size and shape of the cavity and the need for a larger annular incision for implantation and therefore a risk of device extrusion.[28] Another preformed design concept is a device whose shape can be reduced or altered during implantation and restored after implantation. This may be achieved by inflating a balloon with incompressible fluid or by implanting dehydrated hydrogel that rehydrates in the disc.

Current materials used for nucleus augmentation include elastomeric materials, including both hydrogels and nonhydrogels, mechanical devices, and tissue-engineered implants. For the nucleus replacement devices made of elastomeric materials, they can be further divided into preformed and in situ formed.

Preformed Elastomeric Devices

Hydrogel materials closely mimic the functions of a normal disc. It has been demonstrated that PVA (nonionic hydrogel) has a similar swelling pressure characteristic as the natural nucleus; three-dimensional expandable polymers with variable water content and biomechanical properties suitable for nucleus replacement. These polymers increase in size and fill the disc space by absorbing water. Their high water content potentially mimics the hydrostatic load bearing and load distribution properties of an intact nucleus. One of the most important characteristics is the ability to absorb and release water depending on the applied load, much like the native nucleus.[29] Examples include:

- *Aquarelle (Stryker, Kalamazoo, MI)*: Aquarelle is made of PVA. Extensive preclinical studies have been conducted, including biocompatibility studies, swelling pressure studies, biomechanical studies using human cadaver models, fatigue studies (to 23.5 million cycles), and animal studies.

- *Prosthetic disc nucleus (Raymedica, Bloomington, MN)*: The current design is a pellet-shaped hydrogel encased within a polyethylene jacket. It absorbs water up to 80% of its weight. Biomechanical endurance tests have shown that the device is able to maintain its properties up to 50 million cycles with loads ranging from 200 to 800 N. The device shows a 10% implant migration rate.[30] The U.S. Food and Drug Administration (FDA) investigational device exemption feasibility studies have not been completed for its newer version of prosthetic disc nucleus (Hydraflex).

- *NeuDisc (Replication Medical, Inc., Cranbury, NJ)*: NeuDisc has been designed to replace the NP and restore function to the disc. The unique feature of this material is that it responds biomechanically and biologically like a natural NP. It can take up to 90% of its weight in water and can dehydrate and increase its stiffness when subjected to increased loads much like the native nucleus. The device is implanted in the dehydrated state and rehydrates anisotropically in the vertical direction. A jacket is not required because the implant has a "stacked" configuration, which includes layers of medical-grade polyester fiber mesh within the hydrogel layers. These layers restrict radial deformability (bulging) so that the device will not creep through a defect in the anulus. This product is not commercially available in the United States, but is being implanted in Europe.

- *Newcleus (Zimmer, Warsaw, IN)*: Newcleus is a polycarbonate urethane elastomer curled into a preformed spiral. The unique feature is that it does not function on a fixed axis, thus resisting compressive forces while allowing motion even if the component is not placed in the most optimal position. Polycarbonate urethane has shown biodurability up to 50 million cycles with loads up to 1200 N.[31,32]

In situ Formed Elastomeric Devices

These products are injected in a liquid state and solidify within the disc space. Current substrates used include serum albumin polymers, silk-protein polymers, silicone, and polyurethanes. The perceived advantage is that the injection can be done through a minimally invasive approach that will reduce the risk of migration after curing. Examples include

- *DASCOR (Disc Dynamics, Inc., Eden Prairie, MN)*: The DASCOR device consists of a two-part curable polyurethane polymer and expandable balloon, inserted into the disc after the nucleus has been removed. The polymer is then delivered under controlled pressure and completely fills the void created by the balloon, thus decreasing the risk of migration. The implant conforms to the shape and size of the nucleus cavity while distracting the disc space and maintaining disc height. DASCOR has been in clinical use outside the United States since 2003 and is currently under an investigational device exemption feasibility study.

- *NuCore (Spine Wave, Inc., Shelton, CT)*: NuCore is an injectable protein-based nucleus replacement. The NuCore material cures rapidly in situ forming a durable, adhesive hydrogel. It has been shown to be very resistant to extrusion due to a mechanical barrier that is formed since the bolus of the cured injectate is larger than the entry site and the adhesive hydrogel properties resist extrusion. The binary liquid of the silk elastin polymer with the chemical cross-linking agent is injected through a syringe after the nucleus material is removed. NuCore is currently under an investigational device exemption feasibility study.

- *Sinux ANR (DePuy Spine, Raynham, MA)*: Sinux ANR is a liquid polymethylsiloxane (PMSO) polymer that is injected into the disc space after the nucleus is removed. The polymer cures into an elastic mass in approximately 15 minutes and then the anulus is sutured. It has been commercially available in Europe since 2004.

- *BioDisc System (Cryolife, Inc., Kennesaw, GA)*: The BioDisc system is comprised of a protein solution (serum albumin) and a cross-linking component (glutaraldehyde). After the nucleus is removed, the two solutions are injected into the disc space and solidify to form a spacer that provides disc space distraction while acting as a glue to bind the vertebral bodies. The BioDisc system is not commercially available but has enrolled 10 patients in a pilot study being conducted in the United Kingdom in 2006. In 2009, Cryolife is still awaiting CE marketing and study results are still pending.

- *Geliflex (Synthes, Inc., West Chester, PA)*: Polymer-based hydrogels remain liquid at room temperature and solidify at body temperature. These hydrogels are injectables through a minimally invasive technique. This product is undergoing preclinical testing and is not commercially available in the United States at this time.

- *PNR (percutaneous nucleus replacement; TranS1, Wilmington, NC)*: PNR is an in situ formed nucleus replacement. The approach is transsacral to the lumbar spine, preserving the anulus and ligaments. Then, silicone is injected through the screw to fill the cavity and help maintain motion.

Mechanical Nucleus Replacements

The favorable clinical outcomes in both short-term follow-ups of Fernstrom's device recently prompted several companies to revisit the mechanical nucleus replacement. These new developments have been focused on using less stiff materials and having designs to allow better stress distribution to minimize subsidence. Some of the materials used include polyetheretherketone (PEEK), metal alloys, pyrolytic carbon, and Zirconia ceramics. Examples include

- *Regain Disc (Biomet Corp., Warsaw, IN)*: The Regain Disc is a rigid one-piece device made of pyrolytic carbon with a Young's modulus similar to cortical bone. The geometry of the device was designed to conform to the bony anatomy of the vertebral endplates. The lumbar device has been implanted in eight baboons, and 1-year follow-up has revealed no operative complications, no device migration, and no subsidence. The device is not commercially available in the United States, but clinical trials have started in Europe.

- *NUBAC (Pioneer Surgical Technology, Marquette, MI)*: NUBAC is made from PEEK. It is the only intradiscal device that utilizes articulating PEEK on PEEK. Extensive preclinical studies have been conducted.[33] It is a load-sharing device that provides uniform stress distribution. This design is intended to minimize potential subsidence and extrusion while maintaining disc height. It is currently commercially available in Europe under the CE ("Conformite Europeenne") mark and is under investigational device exemption feasibility study in the United States.

Nucleus Regeneration

It has been shown that reinserting NP cells may preserve the disc by slowing down the degenerative process.[33] The seeded cells could be mesenchymal progenitor cells or IVD cells. This matrix would serve as a scaffold to produce adequate mechanical properties, but would not be able to restore disc height. These tissue-engineered scaffolds would be natural or synthetic. Such approaches are currently under study.

See **Fig. 22.1** for a summary of all nucleus implants.

Diagnosis and Surgical Indications

The relationship between degenerative disc disease (DDD) and LBP is very controversial. There has been a poor correlation between DDD on imaging studies and symptoms reported by the general population. A high percentage of asymptomatic individuals have abnormal imaging studies.[34,35] Because of this, the decision of surgical intervention is patient dependent and requires a meticulous presurgical

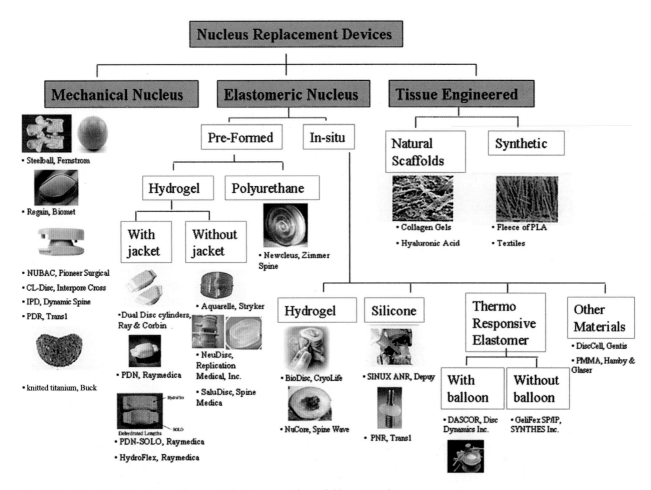

Fig. 22.1 Overview of nucleus replacement devices currently available or in trials.

workup that includes a thorough history relating to spinal complaints, a thorough physical examination looking for any abnormalities, and a diagnosis that correlates with the imaging studies.

The current relative indications for surgical intervention of lumbar discogenic back pain include chronic LBP of discogenic origin that has failed at least 6 months of conservative treatment, abnormal disc morphology on magnetic resonance imaging, positive concordant provocative discogram, and a normal psychological profile. For nucleus replacements, the indications should also include early degenerative changes with disc height more than 5 mm, competent anulus, spondylolisthesis less than grade I, and no Schmorl nodes.

Intradiscal nucleus replacement represents a possible alternative to spinal fusion procedures. The goal is to preserve the biomechanics of AF and cartilaginous endplates while replacing the NP. These implants should be designed to increase or maintain disc height, provide stable motion, restore turgor to the anulus, and stabilize spinal ligamentous structures.[27] To do so, the nucleus replacement has to maintain and re-create the functional characteristic of the disc.

Clinical Outcomes and Complications

To date, the only implant with significant experience is the prosthetic disc nucleus from Raymedica. The first human implantation was in 1996. In the first phase of 24 patients, an overall success rate of 83% was achieved. Following several shape and material changes, the success rate was reduced to 62% for the 17 patients in the phase II study. Further design changes were made in the phase III study of 26 patients with a success rate of 79%. In phase IV, the success rate was reported to be 91% for the 51 patients; however, there was still a 10% implant migration rate.[30] Four-year follow-up for the prosthetic disc nucleus implants showed a significant reduction in symptoms. Oswestry scores dropped from a presurgical mean of 52 to a mean of 10 after 2 years and further dropped to 8.3 after 4 years. Between the years of 1996 to 2002, prosthetic disc nucleus devices have been implanted in 423 patients. Of these, 10% have been explanted, with the main complication being endplate failure with subsidence and extrusion.

NUBAC has been implanted in over 100 patients since the end of 2004 in a prospective worldwide cohort study. The preliminary results were very encouraging. There have been no major intraoperative and postoperative vascular and neurologic complications in this series. The preliminary clinical data showed that there were significant decreases in both the Visual Analog Scale (VAS) and Oswestry Disability Index (ODI) after the NUBAC procedure. The average preoperative VAS was 76, which was decreased to 31, 31, 31, 27, and 11 at 6 weeks, 3, 6, 12, and 24 months postoperatively, respectively. The average ODI was decreased from 51 preoperatively to 31, 27, 24, 23, and 9 at 6 weeks, 3, 6, 12, and 24 months postoperatively, respectively.[36]

The DASCOR device from Disc Dynamics has enrolled 16 patients in its pivotal European trial, and 60 patients have been followed for up to 2 years. The device has demonstrated postoperative pain reduction, functional improvement, and a low complication rate.[37]

Newcleus's clinical results on five patients with an average follow-up of 23.6 months (range 6 to 64 months) have been reported. Results have been promising with improved Oswestry scores. There have been no extrusions or reoperations. All patients demonstrated vertebral body signal changes (Modic) on magnetic resonance imaging, a finding of unknown clinical significance.[38]

■ Conclusion

Nonfusion technologies have gained popularity. Nucleus replacement is an attractive technology due to its less invasiveness, and it may be a viable alternative to other more invasive nonfusion technologies, such as total disc replacement. Currently, there are several nucleus prosthesis designs that are at preclinical stage or just beginning feasibility studies. The ultimate success will be based on clinical outcome.

References

1. Weber H. Lumbar disc herniation: a controlled prospective study with ten years of observation. Spine 1983;8:131–140
2. Caillet R, ed. Low Back Pain Syndrome. Philadelphia: FA Davis; 1966
3. Cooper BS, Rice DP. The economic cost of illness revisted. Soc Secur Bull 1976;39(2):21–36
4. Bonica J. The nature of the problem. In: Caron H, Mc Laughlin R, eds. Management of Low Back Pain. Boston: John Wright PSG; 1982:1–15
5. National Health Interview Survey. Hyattsville, MD: National Center for Health Statistics; 1998
6. Andersson GB. The intensity of work recovery in low back pain. Spine 1983;8:880–884
7. McGill CM. Industrial back problem, a control program. J Occup Med 1968;10:174–178
8. Crock HV. Internal disc disruption: a challenge to disc prolapse fifty years on. Spine 1986;11:650–653
9. Aprill C, Bogudk N. High internsity zone: a diagnostic sign of painful lumbar disc on magnetic resonance imaging. Br J Radiol 1992;65:361–369

10. Praemer A, Furner S, Rice D, eds. Musculoskeletal conditions in the United States. Park Ridge, IL: American Academy of Orthopaedic Surgeons; 1992

11. Vernon-Roberts B, Pirie CJ. Degenerative changes in the intervertebral discs of the lumbar spine and their sequelae. Rheumatol Rehabil 1977;16:13–21

12. Mooney V, Robertson J. The facet syndrome. Clin Orthop Relat Res 1976; (115):149–156

13. Butler D, Trafimow JH, Anderson GB, et al. Discs degenerate before facets. Spine 1990;15:111–113

14. Ohshima H, Urban JP. The effect of lactate and PH on proteoglycans and protein synthesis rates in the intervertebral disc. Spine 1992;17:1079–1082

15. Hamby WB, Glaser HT. Replacement of spinal intervertebral discs with locally polymerizing methyl methacrylate. J Neurosurg 1959;16:311–313

16. Nachemson A. Some mechanical properties of the lumbar intervertebral disc. Bull Hosp Jt Dis 1962;23:130–132

17. Fernstrom U. Arthroplasty with intercorporal endoprosthesis in herniated disc and in painful disc. Acta Chir Scand Suppl 1966;355:154–159

18. McKenzie AH. Fernstrom intervertebral disc arthroplasty: a long-term evaluation. Orthop Int Ed 1995;3:313–324

19. Urbaniak JR, Bright DS, Hopkins JE. Replacement of intervertebral discs in chimpanzees by silicone-Dacron implants: a preliminary report. J Biomed Mater Res 1973;7(3):165–186

20. Edeland HG. Suggestions for a total elasto-dynamic intervertebral disc prosthesis. Biomater Med Devices Artif Organs 1981;9(1):65–72

21. Bao QB, Higham P. Hydrogel intervertebral disc nucleus. Patent 5,047,055;1991

22. Bao QB, Higham P. Hydrogel intervertebral disc nucleus. Patent 5,192,326;1993

23. Ordway NR, VanVanji V, Zhao J, Bao QB, Yuan HA, Mann KA. Failure properties of a hydrogel nucleus in the intervertebral disc. Paper presented at the North American Spine Society 14th Annual Meeting; October 20–23, 1999; Chicago

24. Bao QB, Yuan HA. New technologies in spine. Spine 2002;27:1245–1247

25. Kostuik JP. Intervertebral disc replacement: experimental study. Clin Orthop Relat Res 1997;337:27–41

26. Trout JJ, Buckwalter JA, Moore KC. Ultrastructure of the human intervertebral disc: II. Cells of the nucleus pulposus. Anat Rec 1982;204:307–314

27. Bao QB, McCullen GM, Higham PA, Dumbelton JH, Yuan HA. The artificial disc: theory, design, and materials. Biomaterials 1996;17:1157–1167

28. Hou TS, Tu KY, Xu YK, et al. Lumbar intervertebral disc prosthesis. Chin Med J (Engl) 1991;104:381–386

29. Thomas J, Lowman A, Marcolongo M. Novel associated hydrogels from nucleus pulposus replacement. J Biomed Mater Res A 2003;67:1329–1337

30. Klara PM, Ray CD. Artificial nucleus replacement: clinical experience. Spine 2002;27:1374–1377

31. Husson JL, Korge A, Polard JL, et al. A memory coiling spiral as nucleus pulposus prosthesis: concept, specifications, bench testing, and first clinical results. J Spinal Disord Tech 2003;16:405–411

32. Korge A, Nydegger T, Pollard JL, et al. A spiral implant as nucleus prosthesis in the lumbar spine. Eur Spine J 2002;11(suppl 2):S149–S153

33. Okuma M, Mochida J. Reinsertion of stimulated nucleus pulposus cells retards intervertebral disk degeneration: an in vitro and an in vivo experimental study. J Orthop Res 2000;18(6):988–997

34. Boden SD, Davis DO, Dina TS, et al. Abnormal magnetic resonance scans of the lumbar spine in asymptomatic subjects: a prospective investigation. J Bone Joint Surg Am 1990;72(3):403–408

35. Borenstein DG, O'Mara JW, Boden SD, et al. The value of magnetic resonance imaging of the lumbar spine to predict low back pain in asymptomatic subjects: a seven-year follow-up study. J Bone Joint Surg Am 2001;83-A(9):1306–1311

36. Bao QB, Songer M, Pimenta L, et al. NUBAC disc arthroplasty: pre-clinical studies and preliminary safety and efficacy evaluations. SAS Journal. 2007;1:36–45

37. Ahrens M, Donkersloot P, Maartens F, et al. Nucleus replacement with the DASCOR disc arthroplasty system: two year follow up results obtained from two prospective European multi-center clinical studies. Abstract presented at SAS 7th Annual Meeting; May 1–4, 2007; Berlin, Germany

38. Husson JL, Korge A, Polard JL, et al. A memory coiling spiral as nucleus pulposus prosthesis: concept, specifications, bench testing, and first clinical trials. J Spinal Disord Tech 2003;16(4):405–411

23 Interspinous Devices

Mario L. Pereira, Stephen H. Hochschuler, and Donna D. Ohnmeiss

The management of painful disc degeneration remains controversial, with traditional surgical treatment for painful degeneration being fusion. Ideally, interbody fusion could address the disc as the pain generator. Total disc replacements have been introduced as an optional alternative. These devices are designed to relieve pain and allow motion of the diseased segment. Given that narrowing of the foramen and mechanical loading of the facet joints play a role in degenerative back pain, devices that distract the foramen, unload the disc, and retain motion are appealing. In this chapter, we will review the various interspinous implants and the biomechanical and clinical findings to date, as well as issues related to their potential application in the treatment of painful disc degeneration.

■ Pathoanatomy of Biomechanical Load on the Intervertebral Disc

It has long been accepted that biomechanical load has a detrimental effect on the intervertebral disc. In animal studies, it has been described that following compression across the disc, distraction resulted in restoration of the disc.[1,2] Based on this finding and biomechanical studies suggesting that interspinous devices may unload the disc, there has been interest in using these devices to treat painful disc degeneration. However, there is very little information on this particular application. Below is an overview of the biomechanics of interspinous implants and the various types of interspinous devices available to date. Most of the investigation of these devices has dealt with their potential role in the treatment of spinal stenosis.

■ Biomechanics of Interspinous Decompression from Interspinous Implants

In an attempt to counter the detrimental effects of degenerative spinal conditions, primarily stenosis and disc degeneration, interspinous implants were developed. These devices are spacers between the spinous processes that limit extension at the symptomatic level, having little or no effect on rotation, side bending, or flexion of the lumbar spine. Implantation of an interspinous device is a minimally invasive procedure that may be implanted with MAC sedation and local anesthesia, resulting in a relatively quicker surgical recovery. A current limiting factor is that the design typically limits their use to levels above L5–S1.

The two primary therapeutic biomechanical changes associated with the use of interspinous devices are distraction of the neuroforamen and unloading of the intervertebral disc. These devices dissipate forces across the posterior spinal elements including the facet joints.[3–5] Biomechanical testing has found that interspinous devices do not affect the segments adjacent to the implant with respect to intradiscal pressure; motion;[5,6] neuroforaminal height, width, and area;[7,8] or facet loading.[4] Cadaveric studies suggest that a reduction in disc pressure at the posterior endplates does occur at the implanted segment.[5,6] Therefore, the effects of interspinous devices tend to be a local phenomenon, without any ill effects on the adjacent segments.[9] In a study using finite modeling, it was reported that implant forces were significantly impacted by the height of the implant, but not by stiffness of the device.[10] The size and stiffness of the device had only minimal effect on the disc pressure. However, the stresses in the vertebral arch were significantly increased. This relates to a potential concern with interspinous devices — by unloading the facet and possibly the disc, the load is transferred to the spinous processes. Little is known about the effect on bone integrity. Considering current indications for interspinous devices is stenosis, primarily seen in older patients, bone quality is a legitimate concern. Talwar et al[11] found that bone mineral density was significantly related to spinous process failure load. They also found that the insertion load was well below the failure load of the spinous processes. However, in patients with very low bone density, the fracture threshold may be reached; the authors encouraged caution be used when implanting the devices in patients with low bone mineral density.

■ Types of Interspinous Implants

Earliest Design

As described by Whitesides,[12] the earliest type of interspinous technology dates back to the 1950s when Dr. Fred Knowles inserted a steel plug that induced flexion to relieve symptoms while patients with stenosis improved with time. Some of the implants displaced and the device fell into disuse.

Wallis Interspinous Device

The Wallis interspinous device (Abbott Spine, Austin, TX) was initially designed as a titanium device by Sénégas in the 1980s. It was secured into place by two Dacron bands around the superior and inferior adjacent spinous processes. The indications for the Wallis implant have been reported to include postdiscectomy with significant loss of disc material, repeat discectomy after recurrence, discectomy for herniation of a transitional disc with a sacralized L5, disc degeneration adjacent to a fused segment, and patients with low back pain with isolated Modic I changes.[3] However, the implant has yet to be evaluated for all these conditions. In a nonrandomized study of patients with recurrent disc herniation, the original design of the implant combined with repeat discectomy was compared with discectomy alone.[3] The values for the group receiving the implant with discectomy appeared to be more favorable than in the discectomy only group, no statistical comparison was provided. Sénégas et al reported that the device decreased analgesic requirements and low back pain in patients undergoing repeat surgery for recurrent L4–L5 disc herniation.[13]

The potential role of the Wallis implant in preventing recurrent disc herniation was recently evaluated in a group of 37 patients undergoing discectomy augmented with a Wallis device implantation for the treatment of large herniations and in whom at least 50% of disc height was retained.[14] During follow-up (mean 16 months), the incidence of recurring leg pain was 13%, with two patients undergoing reoperation. The authors also had a rate of 13% recurrent symptoms following discectomy not supplemented with the Wallis implant. Therefore, they concluded that it did not provide any protective effect against recurrent disc herniation following discectomy.

Sénégas et al[15] reported a survival analysis of the first design of the Wallis implant in 142 patients with 14-year follow-up. Survival based on the failure endpoint of "any subsequent lumbar surgery" was 75.9% and for the endpoint of "implant removal" was 81.3%. The survivability of multiple-level procedures did not differ from single-level procedures. This long-term follow-up provided favorable support for the ability of these devices to perform as intended for more than a decade.

The Wallis device is now made of polyetheretherketone (PEEK) in an attempt to increase its elastic potential (**Fig. 23.1**). The new design of the Wallis device has been evaluated in biomechanical testing and computerized

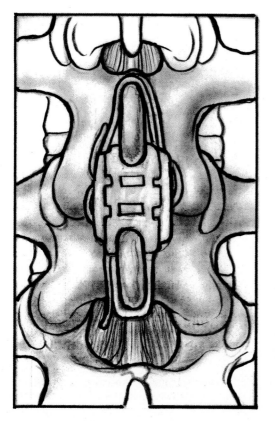
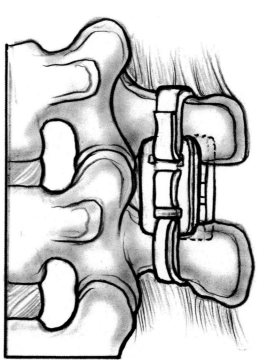

A   B

Fig. 23.1   Posterior (**A**) and side (**B**) views of an implanted Wallis device secured between the spinous processes.

modeling.[16] The implant resulted in reduced stresses in the disc at the implanted level and increased loads on the spinous processes. A prospective randomized trial is underway in the United States to evaluate the Wallis device in the treatment of mild to moderate symptomatic disc degeneration.

X-STOP

The X-STOP (Medtronic Sofamor Danek, Memphis, TN) is a titanium interspinous device designed for the treatment of symptomatic lumbar stenosis, specifically neurogenic claudication. This device has an oval shape with two wings, one of which is attached to the body of the implant for fixation between the spinous processes (**Fig. 23.2**). Initial studies found that the X-STOP increased the spinal canal dimensions and decreased pressure in the posterior annulus at the implanted level.[6] Changes in pressure were not seen at adjacent levels. In a cadaveric study the implant created 2 degrees of flexion resulting in a net decrease in motion at the implanted segment when moving from a position of lumbar flexion to extension.[17] Adjacent levels were not affected.

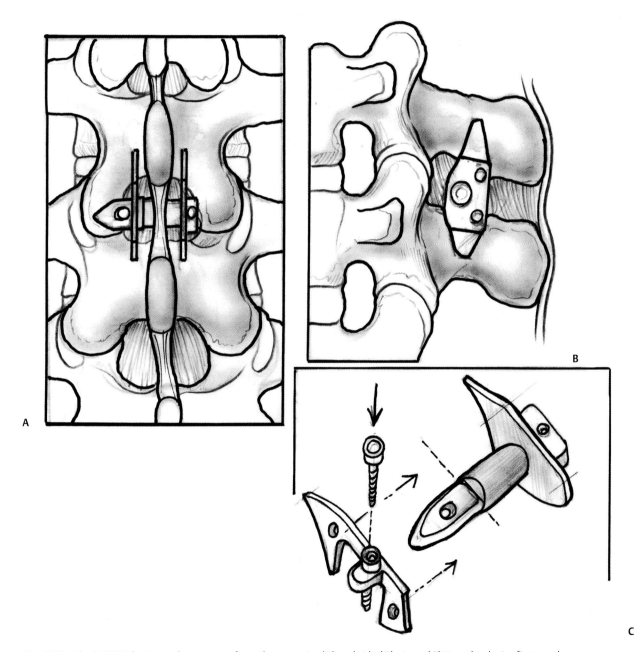

Fig. 23.2 The X-STOP device in place as seen from the posterior **(A)** and side **(B)** views. **(C)** How the device fits together.

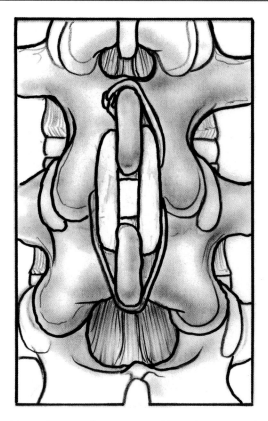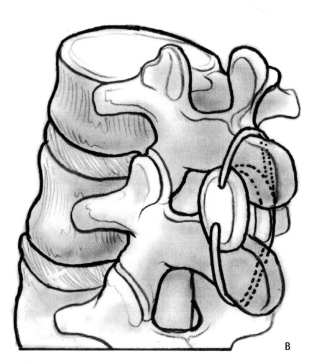

Fig. 23.3   The DIAM device as viewed from the posterior **(A)** and oblique lateral **(B)** views.

Perhaps the most comprehensive study to date for any of the interspinous devices has been the US Food and Drug Administration's (FDA's) investigational device exemption (IDE) trial evaluating X-STOP for the treatment of neurogenic claudication related to lumbar spinal stenosis.[18] The role of X-STOP in the treatment of degenerative disc disease (DDD) is unknown.

One concern that has arisen with the use of interspinous devices has been the potential for creating kyphosis at the implanted level. In a group of patients, magnetic resonance imaging (MRI) was performed before and after implantation of X-STOP.[19] Results revealed no evidence of malalignment of the spinal segments. Siddiqui et al[20] used upright MRI to analyze spinal kinematics following insertion of X-STOP at one or two levels. They found no change in endplate angles at the operated or adjacent segment. In single-level cases, there was no change in range of motion (ROM); however, in two-level cases, the ROM of the caudal level was significantly reduced with no changes in the adjacent segments. The authors found no significant changes in anterior or posterior disc height.

DIAM

The DIAM (Device for Intervertebral Assisted Motion; Medtronic Sofamor Danek, Memphis, TN) is a silicone interspinous device covered with polyethylene. A band around the spinous process above and below secures the device in place (**Fig. 23.3**). In one study, 22 patients had the device implanted for segmental degeneration. At 10-month follow-up, 16 patients had an excellent and 4 patients had a good outcome.[21] Favorable results were also reported in a study of 43 patients undergoing microsurgical nerve root decompression followed by implantation of a DIAM.[22] This device is currently in FDA IDE trials in the United States.

Coflex

Coflex (Paradigm Spine, New York, NY), a U-shaped titanium device (**Fig. 23.4**) originally called the Interspinous U, was developed in France. The design allows for adjacent segments to be instrumented. In a study performed in Korea, the authors compared Coflex to posterior lumbar interbody fusion (PLIF) for the treatment of stenosis with mild segmental instability.[23] At the 12-month follow-up, the clinical outcomes were very similar. Radiographically, the PLIF group had greater motion at the cephalad adjacent segment. The FDA IDE trial for this device is currently underway in the United States.

Minns Device

The Minns device is a silicone implant in the shape of a dumbbell of varying sizes, which limited extension at the

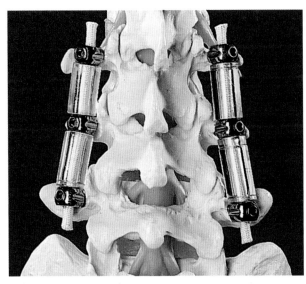

A

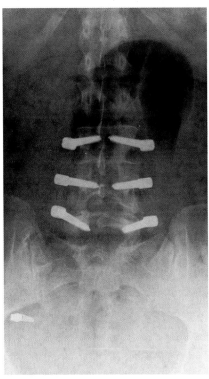

B

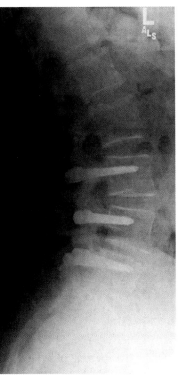

C

Fig. 24.1 **(A)** Dynesys implant. Postoperative anteroposterior **(B)** and lateral **(C)** radiographs of implanted Dynesys. (**A,** Courtesy of Zimmer Spine.)

segments.[11] Recently, a dynamic magnetic resonance imaging (MRI) study was performed of Dynesys in vivo. Beastall et al[12] noted a reduction of motion from the preoperative state at levels instrumented with Dynesys. They confirmed that no reduction occurred in posterior disc height, while a small decrement was noted in anterior disc height. They also noted no significant differences in adjacent segment motion when comparing adjacent levels to the preoperative state.

Stoll et al[13] reported very good results in 83 patients undergoing Dynesys in a multicenter trial. The indications were spinal stenosis, DDD, disc herniations, revision surgery, and others. They noted no screw breakage. The authors postulated that this might be due to the elasticity of the spacers/cord combination, which may cause cyclic peak load on the implant to be lower than in rigid constructs. Theoretically, offloading of the disc may result in reduced disc degeneration. Putzier et al[2] compared the results of 49 patients undergoing microdiscectomy alone versus 35 undergoing microdiscectomy with the addition of Dynesys stabilization. They noted that patients with Dynesys stabilization had no further degenerative changes in disc height, configuration, or morphology. They hypothesized that this was due to neutralization of intradiscal pressures and offloading of facet joints. These findings were similar to an earlier series from the same group suggesting Dynesys to be effective in reducing disc degeneration. The series noted this to be true with early disc degeneration, whereas patients with marked degeneration or deformity were deemed inappropriate candidates for Dynesys implantation.[2]

Grob et al[14] reported the results of 31 patients who had undergone Dynesys implantation. They reported a 67% improvement rate. The mean Visual Analog Scale (VAS) score improved from 7.0 and 6.66 to 4.7 and 2.8 for leg and back pain, respectively. They questioned, however, the value of Dynesys implantation as their late reoperation rate was 19%. Nevertheless, Grob et al assessed Dynesys implantation for a variety of indications including lumbar stenosis, spondylosis, disc degeneration, failed back surgery, degenerative listhesis, and extradural tumor. Given the small series and the very heterogeneous group of indications it is difficult to draw any firm conclusions.

Bordes-Monmeneu et al[15] reported 2-year outcomes in 94 patients undergoing Dynesys implantation. Indications for surgery included disc herniation, DDD, and lumbar stenosis. They reported a decrease in ODI from a mean of 56.8 to 21.4 along with remission of sciatica and back pain in nearly all cases. In conclusion, they noted that Dynesys might be useful when there is a need for "incorporating the functionality concept as opposed to restricting movement. This system can be defined as a disc prosthesis fitted externally to the disc."

Though not implanted in this trial for DDD as an indication, Welch et al[16] reported preliminary results from the Food and Drug Administration's investigational device exemption (FDA IDE) clinical trial of Dynesys. The study included 101 patients undergoing surgery at six trial centers for indications including spondylolisthesis, retrolisthesis, and stenosis, among others. They noted significant improvements at one year in both patient leg and back pain (ODI scores improved from 80.3 to 25.5 and from 55.6 to 26.3, respectively). The authors noted that Dynesys "may be preferable to fusion for surgical treatment of degenerative spondylolisthesis and stenosis because it decreases back and leg pain while avoiding the relatively greater tissue destruction and the morbidity of donor site problems encountered in fusion." They noted that this may be related to Dynesys preserving the disc and unloading the facet joints, permitting more normal motion.

Sengupta[4] developed two pedicle screw-based nonfusion stabilization systems that never achieved significant clinical use. Nevertheless, these represent important theoretical considerations in the development of the technology. The FASS (fulcrum-assisted soft stabilization) system was developed to avoid the theoretical limitations of the

Graf ligament. The Graf ligament resulted in lateral recess narrowing and increased loading of the posterior anulus. In the FASS system a fulcrum is placed between pedicle screws in front of an elastic ligament. This, in turn, distracts and unloads the disc anteriorly, changing any posterior compressive force into anterior distractive force. The implant also creates lordosis independent of the patient's musculature and resists the segment going into kyphosis. The dynamic soft stabilization (DSS) system utilizes titanium springs to unload the disc at rest. With motion, depending on the location of the instantaneous axis of rotation, the system would theoretically unload the disc further or become load bearing.[4]

■ More Recent Systems

Highsmith et al[17] noted that with widespread use of rigid pedicle screw-based instrumentation for spinal fusions, the incidents of adjacent-level disease appears to be increasing. It has been reported to be as high as 35% to 45%. They reviewed a new generation of spinal implants made of the semicrystalline thermoplastic polymer polyetheretherketone (PEEK). This includes a pedicle screw system utilizing a PEEK rod. The rod is attached to a modified top-loading multiaxial metallic screw (CD Horizon Legacy; Medtronic Sofamor Danek, Memphis, TN). They suggest that the semirigid hybrid of titanium pedicle screws and PEEK rods may have several clinical indications. They state the first scenario is the de novo treatment of spinal instability in which a solid osseous fusion is desired, with less potential adjacent-level stress. They also state a second clinical indication is for patients who have already undergone an instrumented fusion, but in whom adjacent-level disease has developed. Stabilization adjacent to the previous fusion may be desirable when the adjacent level can be stabilized with reduction of the risk of subsequent reoperation in neighboring levels. Finally, they suggest that their potential use of a hybrid PEEK rod/titanium screw construct is to create a tension band (e.g., in a patient with mobile or fixed spondylolisthesis). In these cases, the patient may not need an osseous arthrodesis, but placement of the screw rod construct may limit the progression of any deformity.

Recently, several other pedicle screw-based dynamic systems have become available (**Fig. 24.2**). These include AccuFlex (Globus Medical, Inc., Audubon, PA), PEEK rod (Medtronic Sofamor Danek), Agile (Medtronic Sofamor Danek), and Isobar (Scient'X, Guyancourt, France). Today, there are limited clinical and biomechanical data regarding these devices.

Kim et al[18] reported clinical results for BioFlex (BioSpine Co., Ltd, Sungdang-gu, Seoul, Korea), a nitinol spring rod dynamic pedicle screw-based stabilization system. Good results were reported using this device to augment

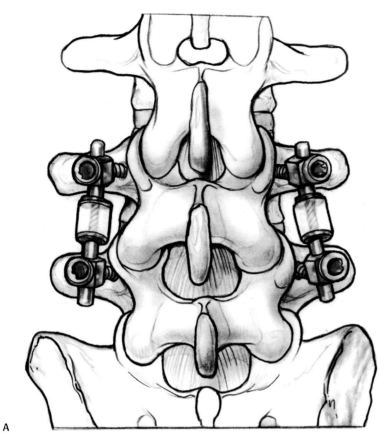

A

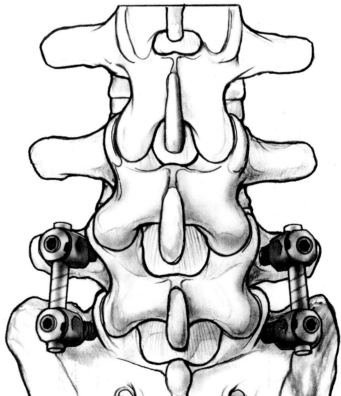

B

Fig. 24.2 Newer pedicle screw nonfusion stabilization systems including Agile (Medtronic Sofamor Danek, Memphis, TN, **A**); AccuFlex (Globus Medical, Inc., Audubon, PA, **B**); and Stabilimax (Applied Spine Technologies, Inc, New Haven, CT, **C**).

(Continued on page 202)

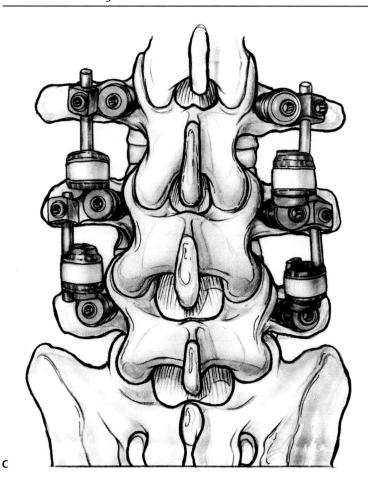

C

Fig. 24.2   *(Continued)*

posterior lumbar interbody fusion and also as an adjacent segment device in levels primarily treated with a posterior lumbar interbody fusion.

Mandigo et al[19] reported limited results with the Accu-Flex rod system. The AccuFlex like other posterior dynamic stabilization systems has been approved as a fusion device. Recently, Palmer et al[20] reported biomechanical and radiographic analysis of a novel pedicle screw-based device that limits extension. This device has been developed by Triage Medical (Irvine, CA) and is implanted into the pedicles at a single spinal level. Bumpers prevent the superior and inferior articular facets from coming in contact and thus limit extension. Additionally, the instrumented spine had 62% less motion during flexion and 49% less motion during extension compared with the intact spine when the device was inserted at L3–L4. Imaging analysis demonstrated 84% less compression of the posterior disc of the instrumented spine during extension and no difference during flexion when compared with the intact spine. Given the reduced motion seen with placement of this device, it may be considered a form of pedicle screw-based dynamic stabilization.

Another device in clinical trials is the Stabilimax NZ device (Applied Spine Technologies, Inc, New Haven, CT). This device is designed to reduce the neutral zone. Cadaveric studies have demonstrated reduced bending moments when compared with rigid screws and the Dynesys system. Additionally, the hypothesis of Panjabi has been that the increase in the neutral zone seen in the injured spine creates increasing stresses on the surrounding soft tissue and musculature and this, in turn, increases inflammation responsible for pain generation. Thus, devices that restore the neutral zone (that limit movement to more normal movement) theoretically are associated with reduction in pain.[21]

■ Indications

Khoueir and colleagues[22] suggested various indications for posterior dynamic stabilization. They discussed the need for controlled motion in the iatrogenically destabilized spine. Hypothetically, laminectomy may result in substantial facet joint removal. In some instances, iatrogenic destabilization may occur. One possible role of the posterior dynamic stabilization would be to reduce motion after destabilizing laminectomy, thus avoiding arthrodesis. They also noted that posterior dynamic stabilization devices might be theoretically useful for increased anterior load sharing to augment interbody fusion. They also reviewed the above-mentioned indication of protection and restoration of degenerated disc and possibly facet joints and noted that treatment of discogenic pain is perhaps the least understood area where posterior dynamic stabilization may have a role. Adaptation of nonfusion stabilization techniques for the aging spine is mentioned as a possibility, as current rigid fusion devices provide a high degree of rigidity, which may not be optimal in case of osteopenia. The application of "softer stabilization" techniques may possibly be more desirable in these settings. Lastly, they mention that posterior nonfusion stabilization might be useful to minimize the risk of fusion-related sequelae such as adjacent segment degeneration, iatrogenic flatback deformities, and pseudarthrosis.

Scott-Young[23] described several possibilities for using posterior dynamic stabilization as a strategy for revision of lumbar disc arthroplasty. His suggestions included patients with facet arthropathy contributing to pain, following disc arthroplasty, patients who experience facet arthropathy years after disc replacement, patients with an eccentrically or undersized disc replacement device resulting in functional spinal imbalance, and lastly as an augmentation in patients with multilevel total disc replacement to avoid coronal imbalance.

In the United States, the Dynesys FDA IDE trial was for patients with predominant leg pain with or without spinal stenosis and/or grade 1 spondylolisthesis. The authors have reported off-label use of Dynesys as a posterior nonfusion stabilization system for degenerative disc disease.[24]

The authors have also reported on the use of Dynesys as a posterior stabilizing device in a hybrid construct.[25] Posterior instrumentation is performed here at two or more levels with fusion being performed at the markedly degenerated or unstable level and nonfusion stabilization at the less-degenerated levels. Good short- to mid-term results have been observed in well-selected patients.

Our indications today are based on preserving the disc, while at the same time stabilizing the degenerated segment in patients with mechanical loading back pain. Our ideal patient would have mechanical loading back pain with no secondary gain factors limited to one or two levels with the following imaging findings:

1. Disc collapse less than 60% of the normal adjacent disk
2. Up to grade 1 degenerative spondylolisthesis
3. Not more than grade 1 or 2 facet degenerative changes
4. No lateral listhesis
5. No scoliotic tilt or segmental collapse
6. Bone density T score greater than −1.5

Stenosis of any degree at the involved level is not a contraindication and we would perform a microscopic laminoforaminotomy to achieve decompression, avoiding a laminectomy.

■ Dynesys System Experience

We recently reported on 88 patients who underwent posterior nonfusion stabilization of the lumbar spine at 118 levels using the Dynesys system.[26] The indications were spondylolisthesis in 48 patients, 12 retrolisthesis, 52 central/lateral recess stenosis, 6 dynamic foraminal stenosis, and 36 DDD, and 4 patients were instrumented adjacent to a previous fusion. This article discussed the benefits of a paraspinal muscle-sparing approach for posterior nonfusion stabilization as compared with the conventional midline approach. There were no significant complications from surgery. The surgical time and estimated blood loss were 150 minutes and 350 cc, respectively, for the midline approach and 120 minutes and 300 cc for the paraspinal approach.

All outcome measures in both groups showed significant improvement at last follow-up. Between the groups there was significant difference in the reduction of the treatment intensity score (TIS) when measured at 1 week and 6 weeks (**Table 24.1**).[26,27] The preoperative 1-week and 6-week values for the midline group were 66, 48, and 40, respectively, and 80, 32 ($P < 0.05$), and 28 ($P < 0.05$) for the paraspinal group

Table 24.1 Treatment Intensity Score

The Treatment Intensity Score is calculated by adding all components up and multiplying by 4. Each component is assigned a value 0 to 5.

Please answer the questions below, choosing the answer that most closely describes your situation at present. We understand that there may be one or more alternatives that may apply to you, please choose the one you feel is most descriptive of your problem.

What medication are you taking for your pain?
- ❏ None
- ❏ Tylenol, aspirin, Motrin, Alleve or other non-prescription pain medication
- ❏ Prescription anti-inflammatories (Relafen, Celebrex, Vioxx, etc.) or muscle relaxants (Soma, Flexeril)
- ❏ Vicodin, Codeine, Norco
- ❏ Medrol dose pack/steroids
- ❏ Morphine analogs (Oxycontin, MS Contin, Percocet, etc.)

How long is the pain relieved before you need medication again?
- ❏ 24 hours or more (rarely take them)
- ❏ 12 hours
- ❏ 8 hours
- ❏ 6 hours

(Continued on page 204)

Table 24.1 *(Continued)* **Treatment Intensity Score**

❏ 4 hours

❏ Less than 4 hours

How long have you taken these medications?

❏ Use them occasionally only (i.e., do not need them every day)

❏ 6 weeks

❏ 3 months

❏ 6 months

❏ 1 year

❏ 2 years or more

Have you needed to seek other treatment options specifically because of pain in your neck or back?

❏ None

❏ Physical therapy, massage therapy, shiatsu, yoga, chiropractor

❏ Acupuncture, acupressure, alternative medicine therapies

❏ Pain management consultation

❏ Injections such as nerve root blocks or epidural steroids

❏ Spinal cord stimulator, morphine pump

How often have you had to see a doctor or therapist, or go to the emergency room, specifically because of unbearable pain (disregard any routine follow-up visits)?

❏ Never

❏ Once in 6 months or less

❏ Once in 3 months

❏ Every 6 weeks

❏ Every week or 2 to 3 times a week

❏ Need admission to the hospital for severe pain/surgery

Source: Anand N, Hamilton JF, Perri B, Miraliakbar H, Goldstein T. Cantilever TLIF with structural allograft and RhBMP2 for correction and maintenance of segmental sagittal lordosis: long-term clinical, radiographic, and functional outcome. Spine 2006;31(20):E748–753; reprinted with permission.

(**Fig. 24.3**). This trend continued through 3 months to 6 months though not statistically significant. At 12 and 24 months there was no difference between the two groups. The VAS scores similarly showed a nonsignificant trend to lower values in the first month in the paraspinal group when compared with the midline group. The ODI and SF-36 Health Survey scores similarly showed improvement in both groups, but no significant difference between the groups (**Table 24.2**).

We have also reported on the results of 35 patients undergoing Dynesys stabilization for back pain from lumbar DDD, average age was 44 years with 21 females and 14 males.[24] All patients had a clear history of discogenic back pain with no leg pain further corroborated by MRI and/or discogram. Average follow-up was 18 months. In our series, VAS scores were reduced from a preoperative average of 9 to 2.5. Additionally, there were significant reductions in SF-36 and ODI scores.

◾ Surgical Technique

All patients are positioned prone on the Jackson table with care taken to maximize lordosis. Patients needing decompression are operated through a midline approach with microscopic laminotomy/foraminotomy with or without a discectomy followed by posterior nonfusion stabilization. The facet capsule and facet joint are carefully preserved. The midline structures are preserved in all the cases with care being taken to suture the lumbodorsal fascia back to the midline at the end of the procedure. None had a complete laminectomy. Patients not needing decompression are operated with bilateral paraspinal muscle-sparing approaches. In this manner tissue damage is minimized. Additionally, great care is taken not to violate the facet capsules or any of the muscle attachment.

We feel it is imperative to preserve the soft tissue when nonfusion stabilization is performed. Significant muscle damage has been described after midline, muscle stripping approaches to the spine.[28-34] Similarly, increased inflammatory mediators have been demonstrated in patients undergoing conventional microdiscectomy versus minimally invasive microdiscectomy.[35] Increased edema has been described on MRI in the paraspinal muscles of patients undergoing the midline muscle-stripping approach for open fusion versus those undergoing surgery with a minimally invasive approach.[36] Panjabi originated the concept of the neutral zone in the lumbar spine as a region of intervertebral motion surrounding the neutral posture where little resistance is offered by the passive spinal column.[37] He observed that the neutral zone might be a clinically important measure of spinal stability function. The neutral zone may increase with injury or degeneration of the spinal column or with weakness of the muscles. This may lead to spinal instability or low-back pain. With an increase in the neutral zone the stresses on the surrounding musculature increased in an effort to maintain the neutral zone, which theoretically may result in pain. Panjabi concluded that the spinal stabilizing system adjusts so that the neutral zone remains within certain physiologic thresholds to avoid clinical instability. It is thus possible that in nonfusion surgery maintaining the soft tissue and musculature surrounding the spinal segment may be significantly more important than in fusion surgery to achieve segmental balance and maintain the neutral zone within physiologic limits. Niosi et al[38] confirmed in a cadaveric model that Dynesys implantation reduced the neutral

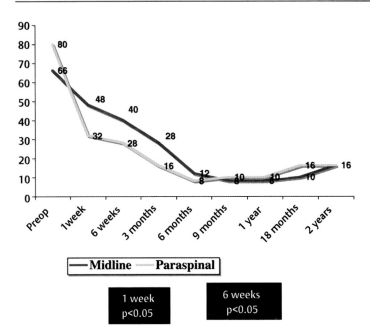

Fig. 24.3 Treatment intensity scores (TIS) following the midline versus paraspinal muscle-sparing approach for Dynesys implantation. There was a statistically significant difference seen up to 6 weeks postoperatively in TISs. (From Anand N, Baron EM, Bray RS. The benefit of paraspinal muscle-sparing approach compared to the conventional midline approach for posterior non-fusion stabilization: a comparative analysis of clinical and functional outcomes. SAS Journal 2007; reprinted with permission.)

zone to less than the intact spine; the injured spine typically had a significant increase in its neutral zone. We have seen improved functional results in early outcomes in patients undergoing the paraspinal approach for implantation of posterior nonfusion stabilization versus the midline approach.[39] We believe that posterior nonfusion stabilization is most likely of benefit to the patients with early evidence of disc degeneration. The patients who have severe disc degeneration or severe facet arthropathy are more likely to benefit from spinal fusion.

Considering the above, in terms of dissection for placement of pedicle screws, we prefer to use the term *modified muscle-sparing approach*, wherein a plane is teased apart by using a Langenbeck elevator, where the fibers of the multifidus are teased medially demonstrating a clear cleavage plane (**Fig. 24.4**). We use a narrow blade McCulloch retractor with a deep blade laterally and a shorter blade medially for retraction directly over the transverse process. This can be done very cleanly with minimal to no muscle bleeding being encountered if the proper plane is identified. Others have used the term *muscle-sparing* when discussing paraspinal approach using a tubular retractor.[40] We use the term, however, for this modified Wiltse approach in which muscle fibers are not grossly disrupted.

In terms of insertion of pedicle screws, when using posterior nonfusion stabilization, care must be taken not to

Table 24.2 VAS, ODI, and SF-36 Physical Component Scores in Patients Undergoing Posterior Nonfusion Stabilization

Time	VAS Scores			ODI			SF-36 Physical Component Score		
	Midline	Paraspinal	P Value	Midline	Paraspinal	P Value	Midline	Paraspinal	P Value
Preop	65	90		55	68		34	28.56	
6 weeks	35.62	30	0.64	50	50	0.50	30.38	30.38	0.50
3 months	30.63	20	0.82	29.1	25	0.62	36.78	36.78	0.42
6 months	30.81	25	0.93	25.6	25	0.62	36	36	0.39
12 months	24	20	0.98	20.2	20	0.61	38	35.4	0.21
18 months	22	25	0.95	22	22	0.60	38	34	0.09
2 years	24	22	1.00	20.4	22	0.52	36	34	0.05

Abbreviations: VAS, Visual Analog Scale; ODI, Oswestry Disability Index; SF-36, health survey.

Source: Anand N, Baron EM, Bray RS. The benefit of paraspinal muscle sparing approach compared with the conventional midline approach for posterior non-fusion stabilization: a comparative analysis of clinical and functional outcomes. SAS Journal 2007; reprinted with permission.

25 Lumbar Spine Arthroplasty

Charles W. Davis and Paul C. McAfee

Spinal fusion was traditionally the surgical solution to disabling arthritic conditions where stiffness and loss of function were acceptable trade-offs for relief of disabling pain. To date, most spine surgery consists of "salvage" procedures (e.g., correcting the effects of trauma, stabilizing and correcting deformity, fusing degenerate segments) and, similarly, does not address restoration of normal biomechanical function. In fact, although lumbar fusion is still the treatment of choice and the gold standard for many severe spinal disorders, it has been shown to restrict motion and increase stress on adjacent levels, which years later, could result in additional pain and surgery.[1,2]

Posterolateral lumbar fusion was described in the 1930s and was shortly thereafter followed by anterior lumbar interbody fusion (ALIF) in 1933, posterior lumbar interbody fusion in 1944, pedicles screw augmentation in the 1980s, and recombinant human bone morphogenetic protein (rhBMP-2) in 2003. Even with all these technical and scientific advancements, the average clinical success and fusion rates after fusion surgery still only reach 75% and 85%, respectively. This finding was presented in a recent review by Bono and Lee involving 4,454 patients from 78 reports over 20 years. The authors also reported that the length of time to fusion was 3 to 24 months. They hypothesized that fusion could cause adverse effects at adjacent levels and further discussed the complexity of surgical treatment for low back pain (LBP).[3,4] Despite these less-than-perfect clinical outcomes, however, Fritzell et al[5] prospectively demonstrated that compared with the nonoperative care, lumbar spinal fusion significantly improved outcomes in patients with chronic LBP.

Unlike fusion, lumbar total disc replacement (TDR) is intended to maintain motion at the spinal segment, restore proper disc height, and maintain segmental lordosis. Compared with arthrodesis, disc replacement presents two key theoretical advantages: (1) the risk for pseudarthrosis, a possible complication of fusion, is eliminated; and (2) by maintaining motion at the index level, adjacent segment disease may be minimized.

The effectiveness of arthroplasty devices to maintain motion was shown in both preclinical and clinical studies; several cadaveric studies demonstrated that artificial discs normalized disc motion.[1,6] Furthermore, clinical studies also confirmed restoration of radiographic motion.[7–9] Thus, although no long-term study has yet been published on the protective impact of arthroplasty on adjacent-level degeneration, early evidence has demonstrated some level of motion preservation at implanted levels.

The first disc replacement, developed by Hamby and Glaser in 1959, was an acrylic mass to be injected into an evacuated disc space after total discectomy. It showed no obvious clinical advantage and was soon replaced by an injectable silicone insert developed by Nachemson in 1962. This device, however, performed poorly in mechanical testing and did not proceed to clinical application. The first clinical series of disc replacements was performed by Dr. Fernstrom in the early 1960s; he evaluated a stainless steel ball bearing put in the disc space following discectomy.[10] After a short period of pain relief, the device predictably subsided into the vertebral body.

It took another 20 years for the next-generation device to enter the realm of clinical trials. The SB Charité I was first developed in 1984 by Drs. Schellnack and Büttner-Janz. It consisted of nonforged stainless steel and contained no special instrumentation.[11] This device was quickly followed by the Charité II in 1985 and then by the third generation in 1987, consisting of cast cobalt chrome endplates and an ultra- high-molecular-weight polyethylene (UHMWPE) sliding core. First released in 1987, discs were implanted worldwide and data on the clinical performance of the device became available soon thereafter.[12] The Charité artificial disc was then evaluated in the United States in a randomized controlled trial (RCT) against fusion with anteriorly placed stand-alone BAK cages and iliac crest autograft,[8,13] and obtained approval for market release in 2004.

In addition to the Charité artificial disc (DePuy Spine, Raynham, MA), other arthroplasty devices have recently been developed and are entering the market. Specifically, ProDisc-L (Synthes, Inc., West Chester, PA) was granted Food and Drug Administration (FDA) approval in 2006 and described in a recent peer-reviewed publication.[14] The Maverick artificial disc (Medtronic Sofamor Danek, Memphis, TN), Kineflex lumbar disc (SpinalMotion, Inc., Mountain View, CA), and FlexiCore lumbar discs (Stryker Spine, Kalamazoo, MI) completed their randomized enrollments and are currently in continued access nonrandomized modes. The Kineflex lumbar disc is the only lumbar disc, thus far, to be randomized against another disc (CHARITÉ) in FDA trials. All these ongoing and completed randomized clinical trials have generated a large body of evidence on the efficacy and safety of arthroplasty for lumbar spine.

Lumbar Spine Anatomy and Biomechanics

Understanding the biomechanics of healthy intervertebral discs (IVDs) is critical when evaluating new devices for spinal arthroplasty. A functional spine unit consists of two vertebral bodies and the intervening IVD. Included in this unit are also a pair of posterior facet joints and the associated complex of ligaments, tendons, and muscles. The IVD is avascular and consists of the anulus fibrosus, mostly made of type I collagen and the nucleus pulposus, made of type II collagen primarily. The nucleus consists of 88% water as well as proteoglycans (i.e., glycosaminoglycans). As for the anulus fibrosis, it presents a radial arrangement of type I collagen fibers that overlap in 90-degree biased layers. These layers resist distension and torsion forces. The IVD thus allows motion and absorbs compression forces. Uniform internal distribution of load and pressure can thus be found in a healthy disc.

Much like larger joints such as the knee, the motion in a healthy lumbar disc is characterized by a dynamic center of rotation (COR).[6,15] This moving core enables independent translation and rotation, which are key components of physiologic motion. With age, however, the disc tends to degenerate and respond with less elasticity and less uniform pressure distribution.

Two principal biomechanical designs are currently advocated by various device manufacturers: (1) to replicate this moving COR within the artificial disc, or (2) to replace the diseased disc with an artificial disc with a fixed COR. The theory behind the mobile core is that it attempts to maintain the motion of the operative spinal segment in a fashion similar to that of an intact nucleus. It has also been shown in biomechanical studies to decrease the load on the facets in flexion.[16] Replicating this moving COR has therefore been a key engineering focus for some of the lumbar arthroplasty devices, such as the Charité artificial disc. As for the fixed core design, it represents the "averaging" for instant access of rotation. This design is subject to less shear, which may protect the facets. It is, however, less forgiving to malpositioning as the COR of the device is fixed.

Indications and Contraindications

The biggest challenge with lumbar arthroplasty is not technical, but rather one of patient selection (**Fig. 25.1**). Arthroplasty is primarily used to treat discogenic pain. The cause of discogenic pain is not uniformly and conclusively known; however, recent studies indicate that production of proinflammatory mediators within the nucleus pulposus of degenerated discs may be causing the pain. Indeed, when comparing the levels of interleukin-6 (IL-6), interleukin-8 (IL-8), and prostaglandin E2 in explanted disc tissues from sciatica patients (i.e., no disc pain) versus fusion patients (i.e., high disc pain), a statistically significant difference in

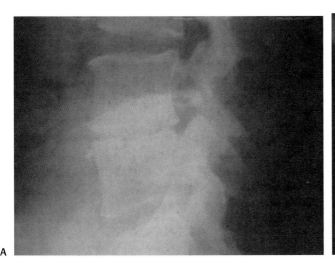

A

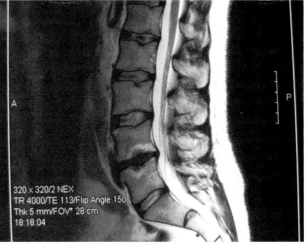

B

Fig. 25.1   Indications for lumbar arthroplasty: a typical case example. **(A)** A 47-year-old white male executive who has been disabled for 9 months due to lumbar spondylosis at L4–L5, mechanical back pain radiating down the posterolateral aspect of his right thigh with an Oswestry Disability Index of 55. **(B)** His sagittal MRI scan discloses single-level disc disease at L4–L5, Modic type II changes. His discogram

was also positive for concordant pain when his L4–L5 disc was stimulated, but not when L3–L4 or when L5-S1 were injected. He underwent in motion lumbar disc arthroplasty (the updated version of the Charité) with complete relief of his mechanical back pain, ODI = 5 postoperatively, and returned to work fulltime.

(Continued on page 210)

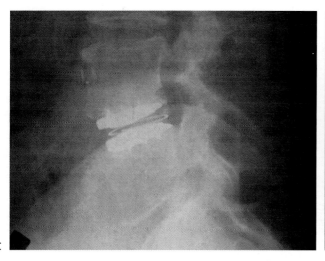
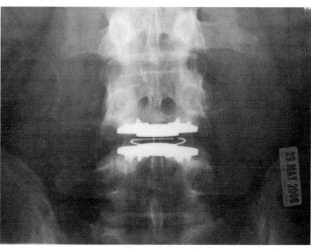

Fig. 25.1 *(Continued)*   **(C)** Postarthroplasty lateral radiograph, which demonstrates good restoration of disc space height, uniformly successful with many types of arthroplasty. **(D)** The anteroposterior radiograph with the in-motion Charité arthroplasty shows midline ideal position of this nonkeeled type of lumbar disc replacement.

the production of IL-6 and IL-8 was observed between the sciatica and fusion groups.[17]

The difference between a painful and an asymptomatic disc may therefore only be biochemical in nature and two radiographically identical "black discs" may elicit a completely different physiological response. In fact, up to 30% of all black discs are asymptomatic. This is why diagnosis of discogenic pain is challenging as imaging technologies such as magnetic resonance imaging (MRI) and computed tomography (CT) do not have the necessary specificity to precisely localize pain generators.[18]

In the early 1990s, analysis of the high-intensity zone (HIZ) on MRI was initially met with much enthusiasm as it reported sensitivity of 86% compared with discograms.[19] This enthusiasm, however, was soon mitigated by subsequent reports, devaluating the sensitivity of HIZ to much lower levels (27 to 31% and up to 52%) and further describing limitations of this technique, which also led to false-positives.[20,21] The key conclusion here is that surgeons must not fall prey to treating diagnostic results and must correlate the patients' clinical presentation with diagnostic studies to arrive at an outcome-oriented treatment plan. The best diagnostic approach to try and localize back pain, therefore, must include radiographic methodologies, such as CT and MRI, as well as pain-specific diagnostic tools, such as discograms or nerve block injections, to provide a clear connection between the radiographic dark disc and the actual source of pain.

Indications for use for the currently available lumbar arthroplasty devices (Charité artificial disc and ProDisc-L total disc replacement) are very similar. As an example, the Charité artificial disc is indicated for spinal arthroplasty in skeletally mature patients with degenerative disc disease (DDD) at one level from L4–SI, and ProDisc from L3–S1. These patients should have no more than 3 mm of spondylolisthesis at the involved level. Patients should have failed at least 6 months of conservative treatment prior to implantation of the prosthesis. Symptoms related to the degenerative segment can include chronic LBP with or without leg pain. Furthermore, foraminal stenosis secondary to disc space height loss may be relieved indirectly by disc height restoration. The contraindications are numerous and include active systemic infection or infection localized to the site of implantation, osteoporosis and osteopenia, bony lumbar stenosis, allergy or sensitivity to implant materials, pars defect, isolated radicular compression syndromes especially due to disc herniation, scoliosis with greater than 11 degrees of coronal deformity, instability (isthmic spondylolysis or retro or anterolisthesis >3 mm), central stenosis, tumor, advanced facet disease, and poor psychometric evaluation. Approach-related contraindications include anterior vascular calcification, previous major vessel surgery, a body mass index above 40, and previous retroperitoneal procedures.[8,13,22]

■ Surgical Techniques

As recently described, the surgical approach for TDR is similar to that for an ALIF.[23] The patient is supine on a radiolucent table. Arms should be positioned to not interfere with the lateral x-ray. An anterior retroperitoneal approach is preferred with a longitudinal incision lateral to the linea alba. Once the disc and posterior longitudinal ligament are excised and endplates are prepared, there are several key issues that the surgeon needs to understand to promote a successful outcome. First, the importance of sizing cannot be overemphasized. The implant must maximize coverage of the vertebral endplate. The endplate center and anterior perimeters are weaker than the posterolateral and periphery areas. Proper sizing therefore reduces the potential for subsidence. Care must be taken to avoid pushing any disc material into the spinal canal during placement of the prosthesis. Midline placement has also been shown to correlate with improved clinical outcomes. Most manufacturers have modular components, which allow for the surgeon to use lordotic endplates and minimize shear. The most lordotic endplate must then be placed inferiorly to make the joint plane more horizontal. This, in turn, neutralizes the forward displacement tendency and reduces any excessive shear load, unloading the facet joints.

■ Complications

Complications from spinal arthroplasty have been well documented, for both marketed products (such as the Charité artificial disc and the ProDisc-L) as well as devices in development (the Maverick total disc arthroplasty system).

Most complications requiring revision surgery were resolved by either fusion and/or disc replacement surgery. The revisability of spinal arthroplasty devices has been thoroughly described in the published literature.[24]

Beyond the general complication rates described in the main randomized controlled trials for Charité and the ProDisc-L publications, other investigators have reported various rates and causes of complications. Tropiano et al reported a 9% complication rate and a 6% revision rate in 53 patients treated with the ProDisc-L with an average follow up of 1.4 years.[25] Complications included vertebral body fracture, transient radicular pain, implant malposition, and transient retrograde ejaculation.

The issue of vertebral body fracture, a complication specific to devices with keels, was also recently described by Shim et al[26] in two cases that were not revised or treated surgically, but experienced prolonged back pain. An additional complication in the form of acquired spondylolysis was recently described by Schulte et al.[27]

Device failure and polyethylene wear debris, complications specific to devices containing UHMWPE cores, were presented by Punt et al and Van Ooij et al, both describing the same patient population.[28,29] It is worth noting that earlier devices were susceptible to this type of wear because of suboptimal sterilization processes. Nowadays, devices are sterilized in conditions that protect their biomechanical integrity.[30]

Neurologic complications were also evaluated within the RCT patient population that made up the Charité investigational device exemption (IDE) study. From these data, Geisler et al[31] concluded that the rate of neurologic complication

was "exceedingly low" in both, the fusion and arthroplasty groups, with no statistically significant differences between groups.

Metallosis and metal ion release from metallic arthroplasty devices have also been investigated as potential complications. An early case of device removal describing severe metallosis was recently published.[32] Zeh et al[33] further discussed release of cobalt and chromium ions from the artificial disc into the bloodstream. Authors described the concentrations of Cr/Co measured in the arthroplasty patients as "similar in terms of their level to the values measured in metal-on-metal THA [total hip replacement] combinations or exceed those values reported in the literature." Long-term clinical studies will thus be needed to further confirm the safety of these devices.

Despite all the above-mentioned possible complications, the most commonly reported failure is facet joint arthrosis. Facet degeneration is a contraindication for arthroplasty. In long-term studies, David and Lemaire et al described 5 cases (4.7%) and 11 cases (11%) of facet arthrosis at the latest time point (10-year postoperatively), respectively.[34,35] In other studies, facet degeneration was shown as high as 30% at 3-year follow-up. It is unclear, however, whether patients included in this 3-year study had completely healthy facet joints at time of surgery, or whether some level of degeneration had already occurred when the patients were admitted.[36]

Other complications, such as infection, malpositioning of the device, subsidence, and perivertebral heterotopic ossification, have low incidence with spinal arthroplasty, especially in the hands of experienced surgeons.[37,38]

■ Long-Term Clinical and Radiographic Outcomes

Two long-term studies were recently published describing the clinical and radiographic outcomes of patients more than 10 years postsurgery. The first account by Lemaire et al included 100 patients implanted with the Charité artificial disc, with a mean follow-up of 11.3 years. Authors reported overall 90% good or excellent results with a 92% rate of return to work. At the latest follow-up time point, the range of motion (ROM) at the index level was 10.3 degrees in flexion–extension and 5.4 degrees in lateral bending. Two percent patients presented with adjacent-level disease.[39]

The second long-term study was published by David. Although the latest results by David further confirmed Lemaire's excellent outcomes, he did address the fact that surgeon experience greatly impacts clinical outcome, a finding also presented by Regan et al.[38] The first clinical series by David—from surgeries performed in 1989, 1990, and 1991—had 69% excellent and good results,[40] whereas with more experience, as described recently, his success rate increased to 82.1%.[41] In addition, in his latest series, 89.6% patients returned to work. The mean ROM was 10.1 degrees in flexion–extension, and 4.4 degrees in lateral bending. Five "complete ossifications" around prosthesis were observed. Eight patients required revision via posterior instrumented fusion. There were five cases of postoperative facet arthrosis, three cases of subsidence, three cases of adjacent-level disease, and two cases of core subluxation.

In addition to these two 10-year studies, the 2-year follow-up randomized controlled IDE studies for both, the Charité and ProDisc-L were recently published, providing additional data on the safety and efficacy of the devices.

The Charité IDE trial was described in two recent publications, presenting clinical and radiographic findings.[8,13] This study evaluated the lumbar total disc replacement with the Charité artificial disc versus ALIF with BAK and iliac crest autograft. Investigators reported that Charité was a safe and effective alternative to fusion for the surgical treatment of symptomatic disc degeneration in properly selected patients. The Charité group demonstrated statistically significant

superiority in two major economic areas, a 1-day shorter hospitalization time, and a lower rate of reoperations (5.4% compared with 9.1%). At 24 months, the investigational group had a significantly higher rate of patient satisfaction (73.7%) than the control group (53.1%, $P = 0.0011$). This prospective randomized multicenter study also demonstrated an increase in postoperative return-to-work of 9.1% in the investigational group and 7.2% in the control group. Preoperative ROM in flexion/extension was restored and maintained in the Charité patients. In addition, arthroplasty resulted in significantly better restoration of disc space height and lower rate of subsidence than anterior interbody fusion with BAK cages. Clinical outcomes and flexion/extension ROM correlated with surgical technical accuracy of disc placement. A complete radiographic review confirmed that, despite participation of 15 sites and multiple coinvestigators, 83% cases presented with ideal disc placement.

At the request of the FDA, clinical and radiographic data from the Charité IDE study patients were further collected to 5 years postoperatively. The 5-year follow-up data were recently compiled and are pending publication.

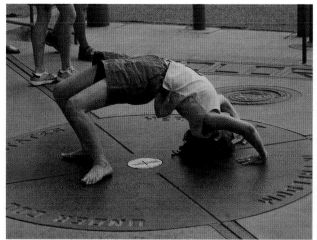
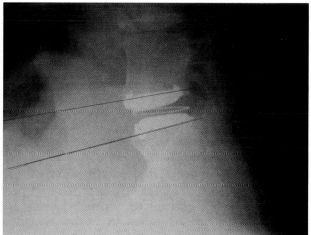
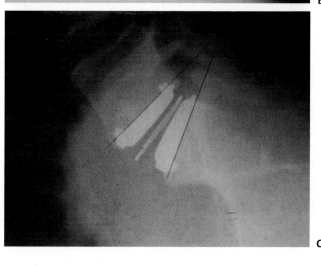

Fig. 25.2 The average postoperative segmental mobility is over 7-degree flexion–extension with lumbar arthroplasty. **(A)** This 52-year-old woman is 1 year after lumbar disc replacement and shows better global range of lumbar motion postoperatively than preoperatively due to resolution of pain and disability. She is performing a back bend with one extremity each in a different U.S. state ("The Four Corners" of Utah, Arizona, Colorado, and New Mexico). **(B)** The corresponding flexion lateral radiograph at 12 months postoperatively. **(C)** The accompanying lateral extension radiograph documents 18 degrees of flexion–extension range of motion.

The ProDisc IDE study similarly presented favorable clinical and radiographic outcomes. The control used for this study was a circumferential spinal fusion, and the indication included treatment of discogenic pain at one vertebral level from L3 and S1. At 24 months, 91.8% of ProDisc and 84.5% of fusion patients reported improvement in the Oswestry Disability Index from preoperative levels. Overall neurologic success in the investigational group was superior to that of the control group. Both groups showed statistically significant improvements in pain scores from preoperative to 2 years postoperative. Patient satisfaction was also statistically greater for arthroplasty patients as compared with control. Radiographic ROM averaged 7.7 degrees by latest follow-up.[14]

These two randomized controlled trials confirmed that arthroplasty is a safe and effective treatment for discogenic back pain (**Figs. 25.2 and 25.3**). Although overall superiority of arthroplasty over fusion was not proven in these "noninferiority" FDA trials, both the Charité and ProDisc-L trials confirmed that arthroplasty is a valuable treatment for discogenic back pain in carefully selected patients.

Herniated lumbar disc pathology was not included in the FDA studies for lumbar arthroplasty because this might have confounded the results with leg pain due to nerve root compression. There is no question, however, that the success rates of lumbar arthroplasty would have been improved if the FDA studies had included patients presenting with mechanical compression of neural elements and presenting with symptomatic radiculopathy. One should keep this fact in mind when interpreting "artificially pure" prospective FDA studies of lumbar arthroplasty.

■ Conclusion

Spinal arthroplasty was originally developed in an effort to restore motion at diseased levels and thereby minimize occurrence of adjacent-level degeneration, a long-term

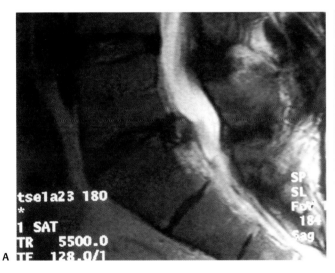
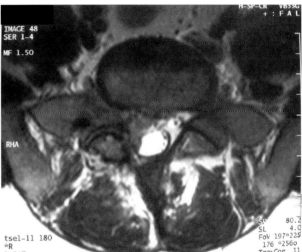
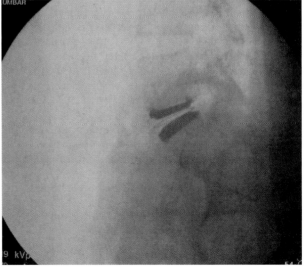

Fig. 25.3 Indications for anterior lumbar discectomy and arthroplasty with recurrent lumbar disc herniation. **(A)** This is a 27-year-old manual laborer who has a right-sided recurrent lumbar herniated disc at L5–S1. He had already failed two lumbar posterior laminectomies. The sagittal MRI scan documents a posterior free fragment herniation, severe right S1 nerve root compression, and posterior fibrosis. **(B)** The axial MRI image confirms the severity of the lumbar disc herniation at L5–S1. **(C)** This is a postoperative lateral radiograph following anterior retroperitoneal discectomy, removal of the herniated free fragment, and insertion of a lumbar disc replacement.

26 Spinal Fusion: Posterior Approaches

E. Andrew Stevens and Charles L. Branch Jr.

Damage and degeneration of the lumbar disc can be the result of aging, activity, and trauma. Biochemical degradation of the disc matrix and disc space narrowing can lead to segmental instability and pain.[1] Laboratory and clinical studies have identified the nucleus pulposus as a chemical irritant, able to incite an inflammatory response in surrounding tissues.[2] Intraoperative tissue stimulation has implicated the outer disc anulus as the primary generator of low back pain, with less of a contribution from facet joints and muscle.[3] Physiologic stress on an unstable joint sustains a cascade of inflammation, joint destruction, deformity, and scar formation with tethering and compression of neural elements. Lumbar fusion is used to try and halt this painful, progressive condition.

■ Biomechanical and Biologic Rationale for Treatment

Arthrodesis

The primary goal of fusion is to decrease movement and thereby decrease symptoms associated with pathologic movement. Fusion can alleviate pain that emanates from damaged or inflamed annular fibers as well as symptoms of neural compression related to positional instability, spondylolisthesis, and stenosis. A solid arthrodesis halts the progression of microinstability and associated tropism and stenosis.[4]

The posterior approaches to lumbar fusion are the most direct and familiar to most surgeons. Historically, posterolateral fusion (PLF), also known as transverse process fusion or dorsolateral fusion, has been the most commonly used method of lumbar arthrodesis. PLF generally involves the fusing of transverse processes and lateral facets through the onlay of autologous bone or allograft, with or without the addition of instrumentation or bracing. Paraspinous musculature permits vascular ingrowth, cellular migration, and delivery of growth factors necessary for fusion; however, muscular interposition may also prevent solid fusion.[5] PLF reduces motion in the posterior spinal column, but biomechanical studies have shown that some degree of motion is maintained through the disc space and may account for residual pain following solid PLF.[1] Circumferential fusion, through the addition of an interbody graft, is a more biomechanically rigid arthrodesis. Biomechanical advantages of interbody fusion include fusing the motion segment in the center of its axis of rotation, compressive forces on the graft, and an excellent local blood supply and bony surface for fusion in the vertebral body endplates.[4]

Deformity Correction and Prevention

Another biomechanical challenge faced by surgeons treating lumbar instability is the correction and prevention of spinal deformity. The idea of sagittal balance is becoming popular in the literature and is purported to influence the later effects of fusion on adjacent level degeneration.[6] Interbody fusion permits correction and maintenance of disc space height, foraminal patency, and restoration of lordosis. However, these advantages must be weighed against the additional adjacent-level stress created by these rigid constructs.

Neural Decompression

High-grade spondylolisthesis and gross instability can cause spinal stenosis, but microinstability can also cause stenosis through tissue inflammation and hypertrophy. The posterior approaches to lumbar fusion all allow for the examination and decompression of neural structures through laminotomy, foraminotomy, facetectomy, and discectomy as needed. Discectomy not only permits mechanical decompression of neural structures, it may also improve the local biochemical environment by removing a nidus of inflammation. Chemical irritation from disc material can cause a tethering of the thecal sac and nerve roots. A solid fusion can limit traction on tethered neural elements but should not replace attempts to decompress and release neural structures and remove inflammatory debris.

■ Indications

Recent literature supports the role of fusion surgery as part of a multidisciplinary approach to lumbar disc pathology.[7] Advantages of surgical over nonsurgical treatments have been demonstrated for chronic back pain,[8] lumbar stenosis,[9] and spondylolisthesis.[10] Exact criteria for lumbar fusion have not been established, but the broad indication for fusion is symptomatic or progressive instability of a spinal motion segment. Fusion has also been advocated in certain cases of recurrent disc herniation, massive midline or bilateral disc herniation, painful pseudarthrosis, traumatic or iatrogenic instability, and as an adjunct to anterior fusion.

Both PLF and posterior lumbar interbody fusion (PLIF) have been used successfully to treat any of the above diagnoses. However, because PLIF typically requires as least some retraction of the thecal sac and nerve roots, its use is relatively contraindicated above L3. PLIF is also commonly avoided in reoperations as a dorsal scar and neural tethering can increase the risk of dural and neural injury. Transforaminal lumbar interbody fusion (TLIF) was developed in an effort to avoid the neurologic complications associated with PLIF, while still permitting circumferential fusion through a single incision. TLIF may be used higher in the lumbar spine as the complete hemifacetectomy allows a more lateral trajectory to the disc space, avoiding retraction of the thecal sac. TLIF may also be advantageous in reoperations as the more lateral bone removal provides a fresh working channel to the disc space and avoids dorsal scar and retraction against tethered neural elements.[4]

■ Work-up

Before any patient is considered for lumbar fusion, it is mandatory that they have tried and failed an adequate nonoperative treatment attempt. Conservative management strategies vary, but should generally contain some combination of the following: nonsteroidal antiinflammatory medications, judicious use of oral corticosteroids or epidural injections, strengthening and stretching exercises, physical therapy, activity modification, low-velocity chiropractic or massage manipulation, and possibly bracing.[11] Furthermore, a thorough evaluation of any potential psychiatric, social, and medicolegal influence in a patient's life is strongly recommended as these factors have been shown to have a tremendous impact on outcome and disability.[12] The history, signs, symptoms, and exam findings suggesting lumbar instability or discogenic low back pain should be concordant with radiographic and/or provocative test results.

Imaging

Segmental instability is dynamic pathology by definition; therefore, it is essential that imaging studies include dynamic views. Flexion and extension as well as supine and standing x-rays in both AP and lateral planes should be routine.The absence of overt kyphotic or translational deformity on radiography does not completely rule out pathologic instability, however. Microinstability, characteristic of degenerative disease, manifests as disc narrowing, articular sclerosis, osteophytosis, synovial cyst formation, and other sequelae of inflammation. Magnetic resonance imaging (MRI) best demonstrates soft tissues including discs, ligaments, and synovium; it may also be helpful in identifying subtle fractures and potential neoplasia. Characteristic MRI findings in an unstable, degenerated motion segment may include dark narrowing of a desiccated disc and bright, hyperintense widening of the facet joint spaces on T2-weighted sequences (**Fig. 26.1**). Computed tomography (CT) scans best reveal bony architecture and bone quality, and they permit valuable measurements of pedicle diameter and vertebral body depth for instrumentation planning. It may also be helpful in preoperative planning to obtain complete spine x-rays to assess overall alignment and sagittal balance.

Discography

Although the above studies are sensitive in demonstrating disc degeneration and segmental instability, it is often difficult to determine which disc is symptomatic and most clinically relevant. Discography through the injection of an opaque medium into multiple lumbar discs may help to localize a symptomatic disc by eliciting the patient's symptoms. It is deemed most helpful if a patient has adjacent discs that do not elicit pain with injections that serve as controls. Information about adjacent levels may be helpful in predicting which patients will be likely to have persistent pain or accelerated degeneration at a transitional level after a fusion.[13] Although the accuracy of discography is debated, and currently there is no gold standard by which to test its validity, any information obtained while considering a patient for fusion should be considered potentially useful.

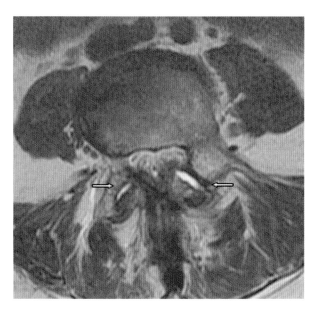

Fig. 26.1 T2-weighted bright MRI showing degenerated facet joints (*arrows*) in a hypermobile lumbar segment.

■ Surgical Technique

Patient Preparation and Positioning

Each of the posterior approaches to lumbar fusion discussed in this chapter are prepared and positioned similarly. Placement of a Foley catheter should be considered based on the anticipated surgical time and blood loss. Bilateral lower extremity sequential compression devices are used for deep venous thrombosis prophylaxis. A dose of prophylactic antibiotics is usually given during positioning. The patient is positioned prone on chest rolls to lower intraabdominal pressure and improve venous drainage. Typically, chest rolls are placed parallel to the operating table. However, occasionally for the morbidly obese we turn the rolls perpendicular to the table, placing one roll beneath the upper chest and shoulders and one roll beneath the anterior iliac crests, leaving the patient's breasts and abdominal pannus hanging between. Arms are placed on arm boards with abduction limited to 80 degrees as to prevent brachial plexus injury. Careful attention is paid to padding all appendages and pressure points. There should be no pressure on electrocardiogram leads, a pillow should be placed under the lower legs to protect the knees and toes, and padding should guard the spiral groove and ulnar nerve. Goggles and/or a ProneView (Dupaco, Oceanside, CA) or similar device should be used to protect the face, eyes, and endotracheal tube. A surgical "time-out" is executed prior to incision.

Transverse Process Fusion

A dorsal midline incision is made and subcutaneous tissues are dissected sharply or with monopolar coagulation until the deep fascia is encountered. The fascia is incised adjacent to the spinous processes bilaterally, preserving a midline ligamentous tension band. The paraspinous muscles are released from the laminae in a subperiosteal fashion, and the dissection is taken out to the facets bilaterally. Self-retaining retractors used for this exposure should be relaxed and repositioned intermittently to prevent inadvertent soft-tissue traction injury or ischemia. Lateral radiographs should be obtained to confirm the operative levels prior to arthrodesis.

Bleeding may be anticipated as the soft tissues around the facets are removed and the transverse processes are exposed. The terminal branches of the segmental lumbar vessels form a rich vascular network rostral, caudal, and lateral to the facet joints, overlying the pars interarticularis, and ventral to the transverse process (**Fig. 26.2**). Bipolar electrocautery is used for hemostasis to limit the transmission of thermal energy to surrounding tissues. To prevent injury to the nerve root or anterior transverse artery, the plane formed by the transverse process and intertransverse ligament should serve as the ventral boundary of the dissection.

Soft tissue and coagulation debris should be aggressively removed on and around the lamina, pars, facet joint, and dorsal transverse process, including the facet capsule and intrafacet synovium. Laminotomy and foraminotomy can

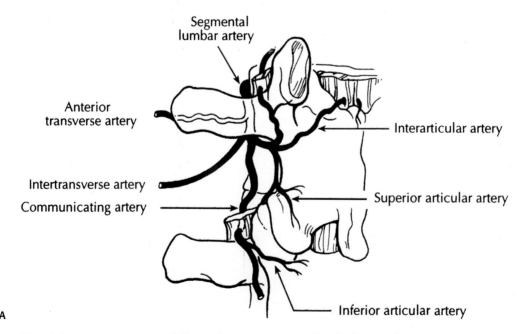

A

Fig. 26.2   **(A)** Anteroposterior view of the vascular anatomy surrounding the facets and transverse processes.

(Continued)

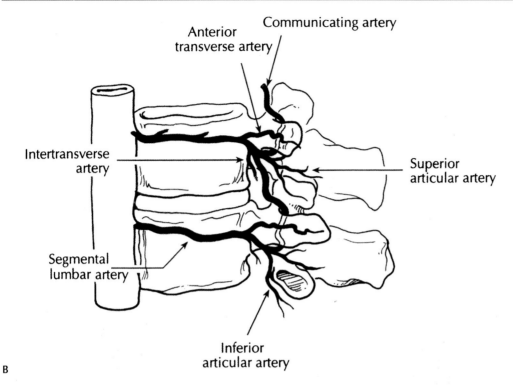

Communicating artery

Anterior
transverse artery

Intertransverse
artery

Superior
articular artery

Segmental
lumbar artery

Inferior
articular artery

B

Fig. 26.2 *(Continued)* **(B)** Lateral view of the vascular anatomy surrounding the facets and transverse processes. (From Wray SD, Jones DS, Branch CL. Transverse process fusion. In: Fessler RG, Sekhar L, eds. Atlas of Neurosurgical Techniques: Spine and Peripheral Nerves. New York: Thieme; 2006: 677; reprinted with permission.)

be performed as needed for neural decompression, and the facet and dorsal transverse process should be decorticated. All bone removed should be kept and further picked of any remaining soft tissue before being morselized. Pedicle screw and plate/rod fixation may be employed at this point as desired, and the fixation apparatus can help buttress the graft material in a dorsolateral position.

Hemostasis should be obtained and the wound copiously irrigated with antibiotic irrigation before the bone graft is placed; the use of bone wax is avoided. Autogenous bone, with or without the addition of any allograft or manufactured fusion enhancers, should be placed over the decorticated bony surfaces, beneath and around the instrumentation laterally (**Fig. 26.3**). The wound should be irrigated again, carefully as not to disrupt the onlay graft. The wound is closed in layers, and a subcutaneous drain is placed to prevent any hematoma formation.

Posterior Lumbar Interbody Fusion

A dorsal midline incision is made and the soft tissue dissection is performed as described above. Extent of neural decompression largely depends on the patient's symptoms and anatomy, but laminotomies and facetectomies are performed bilaterally in preparation of the interbody work. As

a rule, we place transpedicular instrumentation for all interbody fusions; therefore, liberal facetectomy is permitted and minimizes need for neural traction. In preparing the disc space for instrumentation, any epidural scarring is removed as to allow mobilization of the thecal sac and nerve roots without tether. Bleeding can be anticipated from epidural veins that must be breached as the disc space is entered. Care should be taken to protect neural structures with nerve root retractors. Aggressive discectomy and endplate preparation are performed using a combination of Kerrison and pituitary rongeurs, curettes, and interbody fusion instruments. Interbody rotating cutters are used to remove intradiscal material, and a combination of curettes and rasps are used to remove the cartilaginous endplates and ensure a richly vascular bed for the implants (**Fig. 26.4**). Trial spacers are inserted for distracting the disc space and gauging implant size. Morselized autogenous bone is packed anteriorly before the implants are placed. The implants are centered with the medial aspect of the pedicles bilaterally (**Fig. 26.5**). Pedicle screws and plates are placed and compressed to restore lordosis and promote fusion by graft compression. Exposed bony surfaces are decorticated and any remaining morselized bone is placed dorsolaterally. After hemostasis is ensured, the wound is irrigated and closed in layers, leaving a subcutaneous drain.

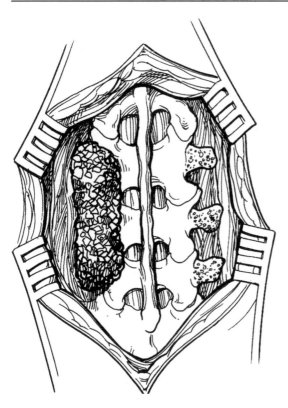

Fig. 26.3 Morselized bone graft over decorticated transverse processes. (From Wray SD, Jones DS, Branch CL. Transverse process fusion. In: Fessler RG, Sekhar L, eds. Atlas of Neurosurgical Techniques: Spine and Peripheral Nerves. New York: Thieme; 2006; 677; reprinted with permission.)

Transforaminal Lumbar Interbody Fusion

A dorsal midline incision is made and the soft tissue dissection is performed as described above. The extent of the necessary bony decompression is largely based on the patient's symptoms. Bone obtained from laminotomies and foraminotomies is saved and morselized. If the patient's symptoms lateralize, the interbody work is usually accomplished from that side. The facet joint of the level to be fused is removed with a Leksell rongeur or an osteotome. Bleeding is anticipated from the superior articular artery over the pars of the superior level and also from veins medial to the inferior pedicle. Hemostasis is important for visualization and can be attained with bipolar cautery and Gelfoam (Pfizer, Inc., New York, NY).

The superior and medial boundary of the pedicle of the lower level to be fused is an important orienting landmark that should be identified as soon as possible in the procedure. A large enough bony canal is created over the exposed foramen to allow safe passage of the interbody instruments and graft. The disc space is identified just rostral to the inferior pedicle and a square annulotomy is made at the lateral edge of the dura with a no. 15 blade scalpel. The dura can be

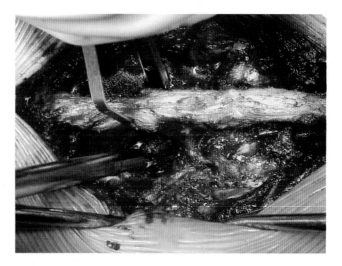

Fig. 26.4 Square rotating cutter used to remove disc material.

protected with a nerve root retractor, but the working channel should be prepared lateral enough such that retraction is not necessary. Bleeding is again anticipated from epidural veins during a radical discectomy. Disc material and endplate osteophytes are removed with a combination of instruments. Kerrison and pituitary rongeurs, straight and down-biting curettes, and interbody rotating cutters are used. Square rotating cutters should be inserted with their cutting edge parallel to the dura. Once inserted, they can be angled firmly against each endplate while rotated to remove additional disc material. The endplates are further scraped with round or oval curettes and rasps to ensure a richly vascular bed for the graft that is free of cartilage.

Trial spacers are used to distract open the disc space and gauge the implant size. Morselized autograft is packed anteriorly and contralaterally in the disc space. The interbody graft is inserted then impacted/rotated transversely into the coronal plane using a bone tamp and down-biting curette (**Fig. 26.6**). The ultimate position of the graft is as far anterior as possible under the anterior apophyseal ring, where a strong bone–implant interface reduces the risk of subsidence.[14] Morselized graft can then be packed around the implant. Pedicle screws and plates are placed and then compressed to restore lordosis and promote fusion by graft compression. Exposed bony surfaces can be decorticated and any remaining morselized bone can be placed dorsolaterally. After hemostasis is ensured, the wound is irrigated and closed in layers, leaving a subcutaneous drain.

■ Clinical Outcomes

Numerous studies have demonstrated the efficacy of fusion in treating lumbar disc disease and instability.[7–10] Each of the above techniques has been shown to achieve high

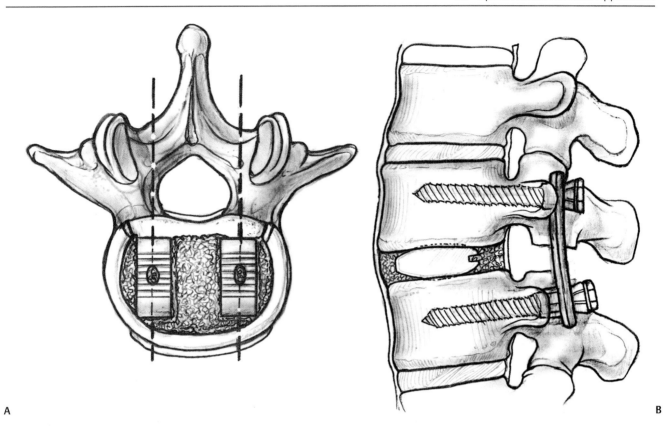

A   B

Fig. 26.5 **(A)** Axial view of posterior lumbar interbody fusion grafts seated in line with the medial border of the pedicles. **(B)** Sagittal view of anatomic lordosis wih interbody device, pedicle screws, and plates.

fusion rates and also clinical improvement in both short- and long-term follow up. In a review looking at all techniques employed in fusion for degenerative disc disease over the past two decades, Bono and Lee found an overall fusion rate of 87%. They reported fusion rates of 85%, 89%, and 91% for PLF, PLIF, and circumferential fusion, respectively.[15] Furthermore, they reported good and excellent clinical results in 75% to 79% of cases. Our review of the literature found fusion rates for PLF, PLIF, and TLIF to range from 40% to 100%, 80% to 100%, and 64% to 100%, respectively, with outcome and disability rankings generally improved, but equally varied.[16–24] Comparison of the different fusion methods is difficult due to a relative paucity in head-to-head studies and the wide variance in radiographic determination of fusion, inconsistent data reporting, and varied outcome measures.

Higher rates of fusion, lower rates of pseudarthrosis, and improved clinical outcomes have been shown with instrumented versus uninstrumented fusion.[25–27] Instrumentation also permits enhanced ability to correct deformity, allows earlier patient mobilization, and often obviates the need for bracing. The advantages of instrumentation must be weighed against technical challenges and risk. The incidence of pedicle screw malposition has

been quoted between 1% and 11%,[28] but Yuan et al found neural or vascular injury as a result in less than 1%.[25]

Choice of bone graft and the use of fusion extenders or osteoinductive proteins are widely debated topics. In Bono and Lee's review, no statistically significant difference in fusion rate was shown between the use of autograft and allograft.[15] Autogenous bone, whether local or harvested iliac crest, remains the most common source of graft material. However, graft harvest morbidity has led to studies demonstrating the safety and efficacy of potential bone substitutes.[29] Bone morphogenetic proteins show promise in their ability to promote fusion, but clear indications for their use do not yet exist. Current drawbacks include cost, potential for overexuberant bone growth, and coactivation of osteoclastic activity causing osteolysis and subsidence.[30]

Successful fusion surgery is not solely dependent on technique. Confounding variables include patient age, associated disease, number of levels fused, prior surgery, and smoking history. A report from the Swedish Lumbar Spine Study concluded that personality traits related to neuroticism predicted unfavorable surgical outcome, and a short sick leave prior to surgery predicted a better chance of returning to work.[31]

■ Complications and Complication Avoidance

Immediate or early complications associated with posterior approaches to lumbar fusion include nerve traction or compression injuries from malpositioning, deep venous thrombosis, excessive blood loss, dural tear, hardware malposition, vascular or neural injury, graft harvest morbidity, and hematomas. Excessive blood loss and associated sequelae can be avoided by a thorough knowledge of surgical anatomy, preoperative planning that includes possible use of technology such as CellSaver (Haemonetics Corp., Braintree, MA), and early communication with anesthesia when bleeding occurs. Hematomas may be prevented by careful attention to

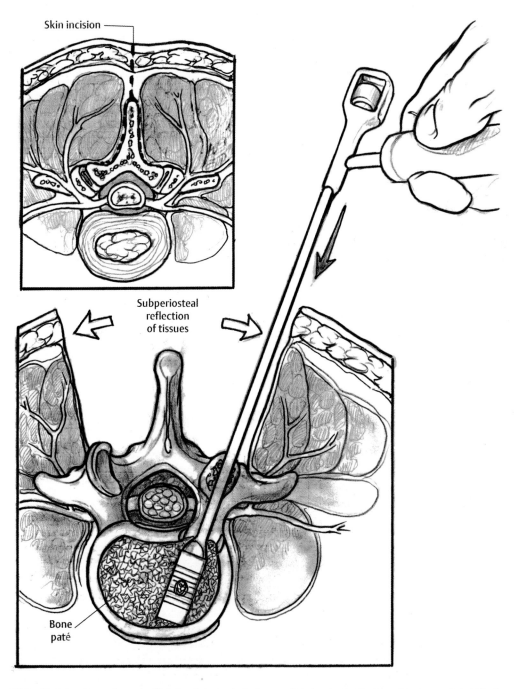

Fig. 26.6   Unilateral transforaminal lumbar interbody fusion graft is implanted in line with the pedicle **(A)**, then rotated transversely to sit beneath the anterior cortical apophyseal ring **(B).**

(Continued)

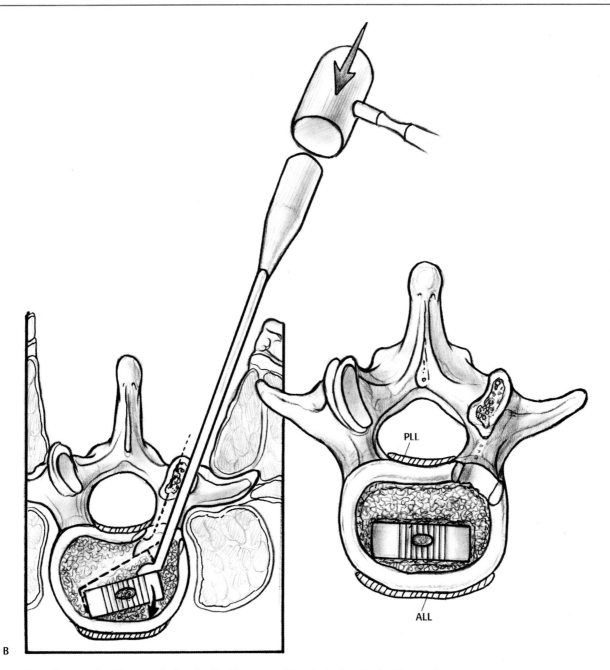

Fig. 26.6 *(Continued)*   PLL, posterior longitudinal ligament; ALL, anterior longitudinal ligament.

hemostasis and placement of a drain when prolonged tissue weeping may be likely, as in large exposures, interbody fusions, and bone graft harvests.

Greater technical difficulty and surgical risk are assumed with interbody fusion, especially PLIF. Dural tears are more common with PLIF as it requires displacement of the dura and the use of sharp instruments in the spinal canal bilaterally. Krishna et al[32] implicate inadequate decompression and nerve root swelling as the primary causes of neurologic complications following PLIF. Liberal facetectomy allows foraminal decompression and limits the need for traction on the traversing nerve root to access the disc space. The lateral approach afforded in TLIF is advocated to avoid the traction-related complications of PLIF.

Delayed complications include pseudarthrosis, hardware failure, graft dislodgement, graft subsidence, infection, and adjacent level degeneration. Hardware breakage and graft dislodgement are intimately linked to failure of fusion or pseudarthrosis. Prevention strategies are geared toward creating an environment most suitable for fusion: stabilization with instrumentation, aggressive bony decortication, adequate quantity and quality of bone graft material, graft compression, and circumferential fusion. Careful graft selection and placement under the cortical apophyseal ring can reduce the risk of implant subsidence by minimizing graft–host modulus mismatch.[14]

A higher percentage of superficial and deep wound infections are seen with interbody fusions compared with posterolateral fusion, likely secondary to increased operative time and tissue damage.[33] Infection rates for PLIF range from 0.2% to 7%.[4] Preoperative antibiotics, shorter operative times, and prevention of postoperative hematomas are recommended. The treatment of postoperative infections usually does not mandate hardware removal, but rather long-term antibiotics and tissue debridement as needed.[33]

Adjacent-level degeneration is a recognized complication of lumbar fusion that largely hinges on construct stiffness, sagittal alignment, and length of the fused segment.[34] Short-segment fusion and attention to restoring lordosis are thought to limit adjacent-level stress. However, the added ability to restore disc space height and sagittal alignment with interbody fusion must be weighed against the increased construct rigidity.

■ Conclusion and Future Directions

The surgical management of lumbar disc disease is a dynamic discipline. Minimally invasive techniques are limiting the operative morbidity associated with the current rubric of decompression and fusion for spinal disease. Motion-preserving instrumentation such as posterior dynamic stabilization devices seek to stabilize the spinal column without the increased adjacent level stress seen in fusion. Although the future of these devices as tools in our armamentarium appears promising, they fail to address significant pathology at the level of the disc.[35] Total disc arthroplasty is a proposed motion-sparing technique that more directly addresses disc disease; however, early clinical results have been mixed, and salvage procedures are difficult.[36,37] Nucleus pulposus replacement is an emerging technology that also seeks to restore motion, but with biomechanics more closely reflecting the native disc.[38] Currently experimental, this technology certainly follows a trend in past and future spinal innovation—trying to mimic nature's design.

References

1. Burkus JK. Interbody fusion devices: biomechanics and clinical outcomes. In: Vaccaro AR, ed. Principles and Practice of Spine Surgery. Philadelphia: Mosby; 2003:385–396
2. McCarron RF, Wimpee MW, Hudkins PG, Laros GS. The inflammatory effect of nucleus pulposus. Spine 1987;12:760–764
3. Kuslich SD, Ulstrom CL, Cami JM. The tissue origin of low back pain and sciatica: a report of pain response to tissue stimulation during operations on the lumbar spine using local anesthesia. Orthop Clin North Am 1991;22:181–187
4. Wiseman DB, Shaffrey CI, Lanzino G. Posterior lumbar interbody fusion. In: Benzel EC, ed. Spine Surgery: Techniques, Complication Avoidance, and Management. 2nd ed. Philadelphia: Elsevier; 2005:452–473
5. Bawa M, Schimizzi AL, Leek B, et al. Paraspinal muscle vasculature contributes to posterolateral spinal fusion. Spine 2006;31:891–896
6. Sears W. Posterior lumbar interbody fusion for degenerative spondylolisthesis: restoration of sagittal balance using insert-and-rotate interbody spacers. Spine J 2005;5:170–179
7. Mirza SK, Deyo RA. Systematic review of randomized trials comparing lumbar fusion surgery to nonoperative care for treatment of chronic back pain. Spine 2007;32:816–823
8. Fritzell P, Hagg O, Wessberg P, Nordwall A. 2001 Volvo Award Winner in Clinical Studies. Lumbar fusion versus nonsurgical treatment for chronic low back pain: a multicenter randomized controlled trial from the Swedish lumbar spine group. Spine 2001;26:2521–2532
9. Atlas SJ, Keller RB, Wu YA, Deyo RA, Singer DE. Long-term outcomes of surgical and nonsurgical management of lumbar spinal stenosis: 8–10 year results from the Maine lumbar spine study. Spine 2005;30:936–943
10. Weinstein JN, Lurie JD, Tosteson TD, et al. Surgical versus nonsurgical treatment for lumbar degenerative spondylolisthesis. N Engl J Med 2007;356:2257–2270
11. Bambakidis NC, Feiz-Erfan I, Klopfenstein JD, Sonntag VKH. Indications for surgical fusion of the cervical and lumbar motion segment. Spine 2005;30:S2–S6
12. Linton SJ. A review of psychological risk factors in back and neck pain. Spine 2000;25:1148–1156
13. Willems PC, Elmans L, Anderson PG, van der Schaaf DB, de Kleuver M. Provocative discography and lumbar fusion: is preoperative assessment of adjacent levels useful? Spine 2007;32:1094–1099
14. Tan JS, Bailey CS, Dvorak MF, Fisher CG, Oxland TR. Interbody shape and size are important to strengthen the vertebra–implant interface. Spine 2005;30:638–644
15. Bono CM, Lee CK. Critical analysis of trends in fusion for degenerative disc disease over the past 20 years. Spine 2004;29:455–463
16. Villavicencio AT, Burneikiene S, Nelson EL, Bulsara KR, Favors M, Thramann J. Safety of transforaminal lubar interbody fusion and intervertebral recombinant human BMP-2. J Neurosurg Spine 2005;3:436–443
17. Dimar JR, Glassman SD, Burkus KJ, Leah C. Clinical outcomes and fusion success at 2 years of single-level instrumented posterolateral fusions with recombinant human bone morphogenetic protein-2/compression resistant matrix versus iliac crest bone graft. Spine 2006;31:2534–2539
18. Lidar Z, Beaumont A, Lifshutz J, Maiman J. Clinical and radiological relationship between posterior lumbar interbody fusion and posterolateral lumbar fusion. Surg Neurol 2005;64:303–308
19. Ekman P, Moller H, Hedlund R. The long-term effects of posterolateral fusion in adult isthmic spondylolisthesis: a randomized controlled study. Spine J 2005;5:36–44
20. Lauber S, Schulte TL, Liljenqvist U, Halm H, Hackenberg L. Clinical and radiologic 2–4 year results of transforaminal lumbar interbody fusion in degenerative and isthmic spondylolisthesis grades 1 and 2. Spine 2006;31:1693–1698

21. Cutler AR, Siddiqui S, Mohan A, Hillard VH, Cerabona F, Das K. Comparison of polyetheretherketone cages with femoral cortical bone allograft as a single-piece interbody spacer in transforaminal interbody fusion. J Neurosurg Spine 2006;5:534–539

22. Sengupta DK, Truumees E, Patel CK, et al. Outcome of local bone versus autogenous iliac crest bone graft in the instrumented posterolateral fusion of the lumbar spine. Spine 2006;31:985–991

23. Fritzell P, Hagg O, Wessberg P, Nordwall A. Chronic low back pain and fusion: a comparison of three surgical techniques. Spine 2002; 27:1131–1141

24. Suk SI, Lee C, Kim W, Lee J, Cho K, Kim H. Adding posterior lumbar interbody fusion to pedicle screw fixation and posterolateral fusion after decompression in spondylolytic spondylolisthesis. Spine 1997;22:210–219

25. Yuan HA, Garfin SR, Dickman CA, Mardjetko SM. A historical cohort study of pedicle screw fixation in thoracic, lumbar, and sacral spinal fusions. Spine 1994;19:2279S–2293S

26. Fischgrund JS, Mackay M, Herkowitz HN, Brower R, Montgomery DM, Kurz L. 1997 Volvo Award Winner in Clinical Studies. Degenerative lumbar spondylolisthesis with spinal stenosis: a prospective, randomized study comparing decompressive laminaectomy and arthrodesis with and without spinal instrumentation. Spine 1997; 22:2807–2812

27. Fischgrund JS, Phillips FM. The argument for instrumented decompressive posterolateral fusion for patients with degenerative spondylolisthesis and spinal stenosis. Spine 2004;29:173–174

28. Okuda S, Akira M, Takenori O, Takamitsu H, Tomio Y, Motoki I. Surgical complications of posterior lumbar interbody fusion with total facetectomy in 251 patients. J Neurosurg Spine 2006;4:304–309

29. Vaccaro AR, Anderson DG, Patel T, et al. Comparison of op-1 putty (rhBMP-7) to iliac crest autograft for posterolateral lumbar arthrodesis: a minimum 2-year follow-up pilot study. Spine 2005; 30:2709–2716

30. Vaidya R, Weir R, Sethi A, Meisterling S, Hakeos W, Wybo CD. Interbody fusion with autograft and rhBMP-2 leads to consistent fusion but early subsidence. J Bone Joint Surg Br 2007;89:342–435

31. Hagg O, Fritzell P, Ekselius L, Nordwall A. Predictors of outcome in fusion for chronic low back pain: a report from the Swedish Lumbar Spine Study. Eur Spine J 2003;12:22–33

32. Krishna M, Pollock RD, Bhatia C. Incidence, etiology, classification, and management of neuralgia after posterior lumbar interbody fusion surgery in 226 patients. Spine J 2008;8(2):374–379

33. Mirovsky Y, Floman Y, Smorgick Y, et al. Management of deep wound infection after posterior lumbar interbody fusion with cages. J Spinal Disord Tech 2007;20:127–131

34. Sudo H, Oda I, Abumi K, Manabu I, Yoshihisa K, Akio M. Biomechanical study on the effect of five different lumbar reconstruction techniques on adjacent-level intradiscal pressure and lamina strain. J Neurosurg Spine 2006;5:150–155

35. Khoueir P, Kim AK, Wang MY. Classification of posterior dynamic stabilization devices. Neurosurg Focus 2007;22:E3

36. Ross R, Mirza AH, Norris HE, Khatri M. Survival and clinical outcome of SB Charite III disc replacement for back pain. J Bone Joint Surg Br 2007;86:785–789

37. Zigler J, Delamarter R, Spivak JM, et al. Results of the prospective, randomized, multicenter Food and Drug Administration investigational device exemption study of the ProDisc-L total disc replacement versus circumferential fusion for the treatment of 1-level degenerative disc disease. Spine 2007;32:1155–1162

38. Goins ML, Wimberly DW, Yuan PS, Fitzhenry LN, Vaccaro AR. Nucleus pulposus replacement and emerging technology. Spine J 2005;5: 317S–324S

27 Spinal Fusion: Anterior Approach

Selvon St. Clair and Isador H. Lieberman

The technique of spinal arthrodesis was first described by Albee[1] in 1911 for the treatment of Pott disease or spinal tuberculosis. The anterior lumbar interbody fusion operation (ALIF) was first described by Carpenter[2] and Burns[3] for the treatment of spondylolisthesis. The basic principles of the procedure were outlined starting with an anterior approach to the lumbar spine, complete anterior discectomy, subsequent segment reduction, and correction of spinal deformity and fusion with cadaveric tibial shaft rings supplemented with autologous bone graft. In an attempt to reduce the approach-related morbidity, there have been numerous modifications of the procedure to incorporate the minimally invasive philosophy. In addition to the classic open transperitoneal approach,[4] ALIF can now be effectively performed via the laparoscopic transperitoneal,[5] open retroperitoneal,[6] mini-open retroperitoneal,[7] and endoscopic retroperitoneal approaches.[8] Further, two new approaches for anterior lumbar fusion have recently been described and include the percutaneous transsacral[9] and the lateral transpsoas[10] approaches. Furthermore, the increased popularity of ALIF is attributed, in part, to the recent development of threaded metallic interbody cages and the available supply of allograft dowels and other osteogenic factors. Regardless of the specific approach, ALIF usually yields a consistently high fusion rate with good to excellent postoperative clinical outcomes, thereby representing a valuable option for anterior fusion of the lumbar spine.

■ Indications

Before the 1980s, the anterior interbody lumbar spinal fusion operation had only one widely accepted indication: the treatment of spondylolisthesis. Excellent clinical outcomes are expected when anterior interbody fusion is used to supplement posterior segmental instrumentation and fusion of spondylolytic spondylolisthesis.[11] This technique has been proven to be safe and effective for patients even with high-grade slippage.[12] Since its initial application, the indications for anterior lumbar interbody have expanded and are now effectively employed to treat a variety of disorders of the lumbar spine. At present, ALIF is used for the treatment of axial back pain from degenerative disc disease, recurrent disc herniation, failed posterior spine fusion, and postlaminectomy syndrome.[13,14] In addition, it is used for

the treatment of certain spinal infections and spinal tumors. Furthermore, in spinal deformity correction for both sagittal and coronal plane imbalances, anterior interbody fusion has the role of reestablishing a clinically acceptable degree of lumbar lordosis. Perhaps the most widely accepted role of ALIF is in providing the foundation for long spinal fusion and supplementation of posterior instrumentation and fusion. This is especially important for patients with poor bone stock and patients at risk for nonunions. Finally, anterior interbody fusion is also used for indirect foraminal decompression when posterior approaches are contraindicated.

■ Goals

The goals of interbody fusion are essential to keep in mind when planning to perform ALIF. There are three main goals of the procedure: the attainment of solid fusion; the restoration of lumbar spine anatomy; and finally, the reduction or minimization of approach-related complications (see Complication section). To ensure a solid arthrodesis, meticulous attention to the following techniques is paramount. First, a thorough discectomy and endplate preparation is done to ensure maximum bone to bone contact. This is accomplished by reaming or curettage. The goal is to establish clean endplates with sufficiently bleeding bone. Since the anterior longitudinal ligament is sacrificed, care must be taken to establish good soft tissue tension about the interspace to adequately secure the implants. Keep in mind, a carefully performed complete circumferential discectomy provides a large surface area for the interbody graft of choice to be implanted.

The availability and variety of graft materials has significantly increased for anterior interbody fusion. Coupled with the recent modifications of the anterior approaches to the lumbar spine, the availability of a new generation of interbody devices is directly related to the excellent outcome and popularity of ALIF. The graft materials include the gold standard: tricortical iliac bone. The utility of this graft is limited by the morbidity associated with anterior graft harvest, which can be as high as 30%.[14] In addition to the aforementioned limitation, the compressive strength of these grafts does not exceed physiologic axial loads during routine spine motion,[15–17] and have been shown to fatigue. These limitations can result in early failure as assessed by loss of disc space height, pathologic motion, and increased rate of pseudarthrosis.

The increased use of allograft bone for anterior interbody fusion is attributed to the morbidity associated with autologous graft harvest, its higher compressive strength relative to endplates and cancellous bone,[18,19] and the recent advances in allograft bone harvesting and preparation. Femoral allografts are now available in a precisely machined aseptic threaded bone dowel or femoral rings that can be implanted directly into the intervertebral space (**Fig. 27.1**). In addition, the center of the femoral allograft is usually filled with autologous bone, which has been demonstrated to yield a good fusion rate in several studies.[20–24] Further refinement of the femoral allograft by demineralization of its surface has been theorized to increase fusion rate, but evidence to support this claim is currently unavailable. The limitations of availability of allograft bone and the slight increased risk of disease transmission have somewhat curtailed the widespread use of this particular interbody graft material.

The development of metallic threaded interbody fusion devices (titanium and carbon fiber implants) is attributed, in part, to the inherent limitations of allograft bone materials. The devices are designed to be used as a composite graft with either osteoinductive or osteogenic materials. The metallic threaded interbody fusion devices facilitate fusion while concurrently providing immediate stability and maintenance of disc space height. Although first developed by Bagby to treat cervical stenosis (wobbler syndrome) in horses in the early 1980s, the concept was quickly adapted for the treatment of lumbar degenerative disc disease.[25–27] The first cage (BAK) was successfully implanted, in 1991, and was found to promote excellent interbody fusion (**Fig. 27.2A,B**). In biomechanical studies these devices have been shown to stabilize the spinal motion segments to reliably promote fusion.[19,28–32] Certain cylindrical cages are now designed with a tapered end, to more reliably restore lumbar lordosis (**Fig. 27.2C**).[31,33] Clinically, metallic threaded interbody fusion cages have been shown to stabilize the lumbar spine motion segment for fusion adequately without the requirement of supplemental fixation.[24,34,35] Finally, despite the lack of solid available clinical evidence to substantiate this claim,

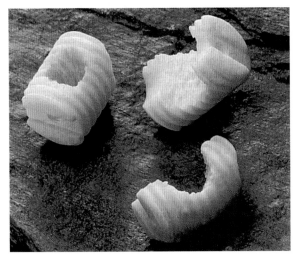
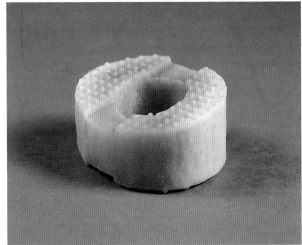

Fig. 27.1 Allograft graft materials. **(A)** Bone dowels. **(B,C)** Femoral ring allografts.

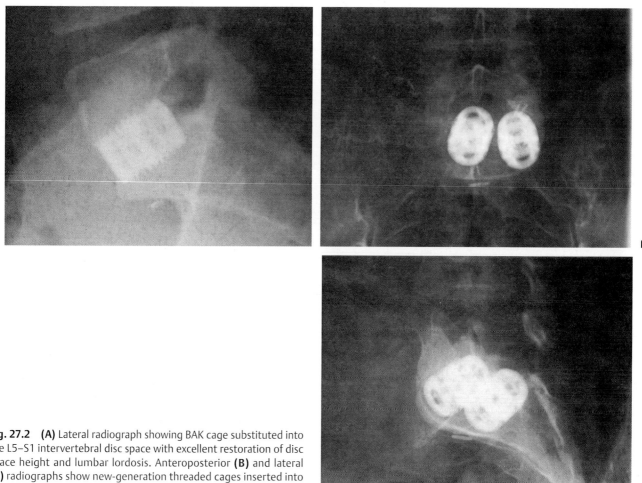

Fig. 27.2 **(A)** Lateral radiograph showing BAK cage substituted into the L5–S1 intervertebral disc space with excellent restoration of disc space height and lumbar lordosis. Anteroposterior **(B)** and lateral **(C)** radiographs show new-generation threaded cages inserted into the L5–S1 disc space.

carbon fiber composite implants are available and have been touted to improve fusion rates as a result of their modulus, which may allow for greater load sharing than the titanium implants.

Restoration of spinal anatomy is critical for successful anterior interbody fusion. Tensioning of the soft tissues and ligaments that surround the disc space restores the disc space height and enhances retention of the interbody graft. Furthermore soft tissue tensioning facilitates the use of larger interbody cages, which increases the surface area for fusion.[29–31,36,37] It is crucial to obtain or correct the proper spinal balance, in both the coronal and the sagittal planes, which is caused by intradiscal distraction and soft tissue conditioning. It has been demonstrated that perhaps more important than the use of tapered cages to restore adequate lordosis is the degree of intradiscal distraction and retensioning of the anulus. Another aspect in correction of spinal anatomy is indirect neuroforaminal decompression by restoration of foraminal dimensions that have been reduced as a result of disc space collapse. This is facilitated both indirectly by restoration of adequate disc space height and directly by anterior decompression of the radial bone spurs or disc material.[33]

■ Surgical Approaches

Surgical approaches to the anterior lumbar spine can be performed by either transperitoneal or retroperitoneal approaches. Recently, newer techniques have been described to gain access to the anterior lumbar spine. These are based on the minimally invasive principles and include the following approaches: the lateral transpsoas, the transsacral approach, the endoscopy- or laparoscopy-assisted approach, and the mini-open ALIF. The anterior lumbar approaches are performed by experienced orthopaedic and neurosurgery surgeons or by general or vascular surgeons. The techniques for these approaches will be discussed in detail below with emphasis placed on the more commonly employed approaches. Because surgical exposure of the different zones of the lumbar spine present unique challenges to the surgeon, the open approach to upper (T12–L2), middle

(L2–L5), and lower (L5–S1) lumbar zones will be described separately.

Patient Positioning

For approaches to the thoracolumbar junction patients are normally positioned in the lateral decubitus position. For the midlevel approach, they may be either lateral decubitus or supine; for lower lumbar regions, a combination of positioning may be appropriate but usually the patient is supine. The surgical team should ensure that bony prominences are well protected by padding and the patient is comfortably secured on the operating table. Pneumatic sequential compressive devices are applied to the patient's legs to reduce the risk of deep vein thrombosis. A Foley catheter is usually placed to assist with fluid management. The hips and knees are usually flexed to loosen any tension on the psoas muscle and lower extremity vasculature.

Open Approaches

Retroperitoneal

Thoracolumbar Zone (T12–L2)

The retroperitoneal approach to the lumbar spine was first described by Iwahara[38] and Harmon[39] in the early 1960s and later modified by Mayer,[40] who added the muscle-splitting component. For exposure to the thoracolumbar region, the senior author prefers an extrapleural or extracavitary approach to prevent potential complications associated the violation of the pleural cavity. An oblique thoracoabdominal incision is usually made over the 11th or 12th rib and is extended a few centimeters down onto the abdominal wall. Exposure to the rib of interest is then obtained by dividing the subcutaneous tissues and the serratus anterior and latissimus dorsi muscles. The intercostal muscles are then divided to expose the superior border of the rib, which is then partially resected after having been subperiosteally dissected free from surrounding tissues to protect the underlying neurovascular bundle. At this point, the external and internal oblique muscles are divided in line with their fibers. The underlying transversalis layer is split to gain access to the peritoneum, which is carefully dissected off the diaphragm and the psoas muscle for entry into the retroperitoneal space. At this time, proponents of an intracavitary approach will take the diaphragm down to gain access to the anterior thoracolumbar junction, but in our experience, this step can be bypassed.

To reduce extensive blood loss, careful vessel ligation is important. Overlying the vertebral bodies are the paired segmental vessels, which are dissected and divided as close to the aorta as possible to prevent disruption of the collateral circulation to the spinal cord. Preventing disruption of the collateral circulation to the spinal cord reduces the chance of catastrophic cord ischemia.[41,42] Access to the anterior disc space is then unhindered. Notably, careful attention should be paid to the artery of Adamkiewicz, which usually arises on the left between T8–T10, but may vary between T7 and L4. It provides blood flow to the anterior and posterior spinal arteries, in the thoracolumbar area, and its disruption can lead to paraplegia. At this anterior lumbar zone, injury to the retroperitoneal lymphatics is not uncommon but can be reliably managed by oversewing the lymphatic chain.

Midlumbar Zone (L2–L5)

The midlumbar spine zone is usually exposed via a retroperitoneal approach using a left anterior paramedian incision to avoid injury to the prominent sided vena cava and right common iliac vein. For exposure to the L3–L4 disc space, the skin incision should commence as close to the umbilicus as possible. The incision is then taken through the subcutaneous tissues down to the anterior abdominis rectus muscle and sheath, which is then divided in line with the skin incision, extending into the external oblique muscle. At the junction of the posterior rectus muscle and sheath is the arcuate line, an access corridor to the retroperitoneal space, which can be developed by bluntly separating the peritoneum off from lateral to medial direction to the posterior rectus sheath. The peritoneal sac is then dissected off of the psoas muscle and the left ureter, and the iliac artery and vein are then identified.

Self-retaining retractors are employed to maintain the exposure while the surgeon gains access to the disc spaces. A detailed understanding of the presacral neuroanatomy (**Fig. 27.3**) is paramount for careful dissection in this zone because one has to mobilize the left iliac artery and vein medially and the divided lumbar segmentals laterally. For exposure to the L2–L3, and L3–L4 levels, little or no segmental vessel ligation is needed. The exception is, on occasion, when the lumbar vessels along the anterior body of L4 must be divided for safe mobilization of the great vessels. Furthermore, the tethering of the iliac vein by the ileolumbar or ascending vein over the L5 is common and is usually sacrificed to gain adequate exposure to the L4/5 disc space. The ileolumbar vein can be quite large, between 3 to 5 mm at its entry to the left common iliac vein, and accidental injury can result in massive hemorrhage. To ligate this vessel, the sympathetic trunk is first identified along the anterior border of the psoas muscle. The groups of fibers that anchor this muscle to the superior and inferior vertebral margins are released to facilitate lateral retraction. The L5 nerve root is usually found in proximity to the ileolumbar vein and care must be taken to avoid its resection.

Lumbo–Sacral Zone (L5–S1)

Several incisions may be used for retroperitoneal access to the anterior lumbo–sacral junction. They include a paramedian incision, a transverse incision with either a muscle-cutting

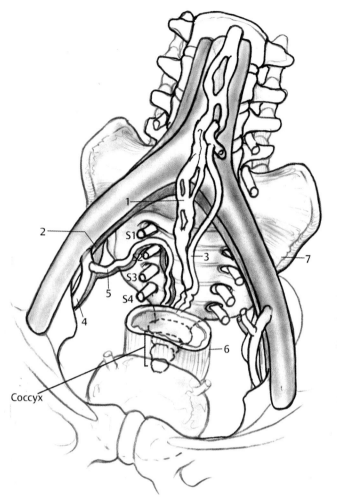

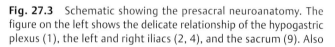

1 Inferior hypogastric plexus   6 Rectum

2 External iliac artery & vein   7 Sacrum

3 Middle sacral artery & vein

4 Internal iliac artery & vein

5 Superior gluteal artery & vein

Fig. 27.3 Schematic showing the presacral neuroanatomy. The figure on the left shows the delicate relationship of the hypogastric plexus (1), the left and right iliacs (2, 4), and the sacrum (9). Also depicted in the boxed figure on the right is the trajectory of the guide rod for the axial anterior lumbar interbody fusion.

or muscle-splitting approach,[39] an oblique incision extending from the iliac crest and ending a few centimeters proximal between the umbilicus and pubic symphysis, and a Pfannenstiel incision—low transverse incision. The incision is again carried through subcutaneous tissue down to rectus muscle, which is mobilized to the midline. The retroperitoneal space is then developed directly anteriorly by bluntly separating the peritoneal sac from lateral to medial because iliac arteries and veins cross the lateral aspect of the L5–S1 disc space. The ipsilateral ureter is normally identified and swept toward the midline along with the peritoneum. At this point, the sacral promontory and the L5–S1 disc are exposed by careful dissection between the iliac vessels. Division of the middle sacral vessels and resection of the thin anterior longitudinal ligament complete the approach. In the retroperitoneal approaches to the lumbosacral junction, fibers of the pelvic sympathetic plexus

may be damaged, resulting in retrograde ejaculation in a male patient. Although concerned patients have been advised to bank their sperm, retrograde ejaculation is a rare phenomenon and is ephemeral if it does occur.

Transperitoneal

The transperitoneal approach is less favored by most surgeons for access to the anterior lumbar compared with the retroperitoneal counterpart. However, there remain specific circumstances in which the transperitoneal approach is indicated. Such is the case for patients with previous surgery where excessive scar tissue makes the retroperitoneal approach very difficult and risky. In addition, the transperitoneal approach is used in very obese patients and in some cases for lumbosacral exposure, especially when the Ferguson angle is greater than 70 degrees.[43] The white line of Toldt is normally mobilized to expose the disc space after a standard paramedian or transverse incision is used to gain access to the abdominal cavity. The remainder of the dissection is similar to the retroperitoneal approach once the peritoneum overlying the anterior lumbar spine is split and retracted. Mobilization of the colon is unnecessary for access to the lower lumbar zone.

Minimally Invasive Approaches

Minimally invasive surgical approaches to the anterior lumbar spine have been developed to reduce the approach-related morbidity of standard open approaches. The theoretical advantages of less tissue damage, shortened hospital stay, less perioperative pain, and faster recovery are, in part, responsible for the increased popularity of these newer techniques. One caveat of the minimally invasive anterior interbody fusion is the protracted learning curve necessary to master the various techniques. In inexperienced hands, the surgical time can be excessive due to the inherent difficulty of positioning instrumentation and implants in a confined space and obtaining sharp and detailed intraoperative working images. Nevertheless, the most popular minimal-access anterior spinal procedures include mini-open ALIF, lateral transpsoas ALIF, axial ALIF via the transsacral approach, and laparoscopy- or endoscopy-assisted ALIF. The laparoscopic transperitoneal or balloon-assisted endoscopic retroperitoneal anterior lumbar procedures are less favored today because of their increased cost and the safety and effectiveness of the mini-open ALIF.

Mini-open ALIF

The application of laparoscopic techniques to access the anterior spine signaled a trend toward minimal invasive ALIF.

In 1996, Mayer redefined the mini-ALIF through his microscopic retroperitoneal anterior interbody fusion technique.[40] This technique is referred to as the mini-open approach because the skin incision may be as small as 4 cm. The approach is frequently performed with the patient positioned supine (**Fig. 27.4A**) on the operating room table. The patient is positioned in the Trendelenburg position to ensure that the abdominal contents are not encroaching on the operative side. After the disc space of interest is confirmed with fluoroscopy, an incision is made just below this level. The choice of incision, either vertical or horizontal, is surgeon dependent and is discussed with the patient in advance. For a typical L5–S1 exposure, a paramedian or 4-cm transverse skin incision is made 1 cm to the right of the midline that extends 3 cm to the left of the midline and two- to three-fingerbreadths above the pubic symphysis (**Fig. 27.4A**). The subcutaneous tissue is then sharply dissected through to the rectus abdominis fascia and muscle (**Fig. 27.4B**). The arcuate or semilunar line is then identified by bluntly separating the heads of the rectus to gain access into the retroperitoneal space (**Fig. 27.4C–E**). The retroperitoneal space is then developed from left to right and held in place with a retractor. The peritoneum is also dissected off the anterior lumbar column to the sacral promontory and along with the ureter, is retracted from left to right. At this point, to fully expose the L5–S1 disc space, the left common iliac vein and middle sacral vessels are mobilized (**Fig. 27.4F,G**). To avoid the rare risk of retrograde ejaculation, the presacral plexus is bluntly cleared from the midline. Often, the middle sacral artery and vein are attached to the anterior anulus and have to be sacrificed to limit excessive bleeding. Access to the disc level of interest is confirmed with fluoroscopy and prior to performing the discectomy. Adequate visualization of the working area is accomplished

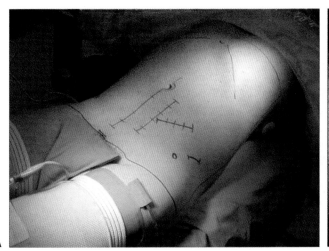
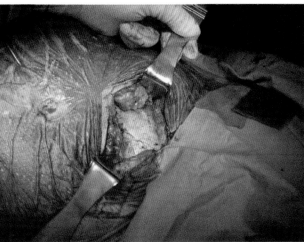

Fig. 27.4 Supine Trendelenburg open retroperitoneal approach to the midlumbar zone using a left anterior paramedian demonstrating the relevant anatomic structures encountered. **(A)** Patient position and surgical planning. **(B)** Anterior rectus sheath.

(Continued on page 232)

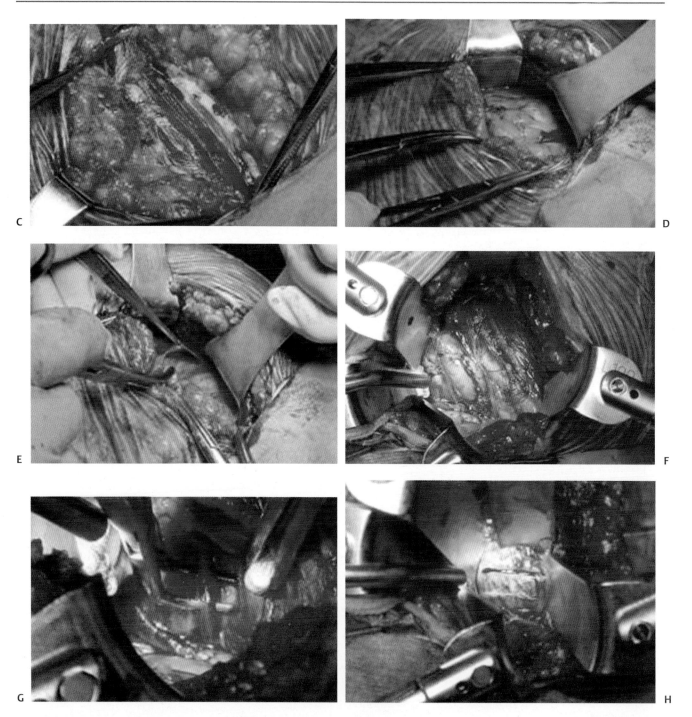

Fig. 27.4 *(Continued)* **(C)** Rectus abdominis. **(D)** Posterior rectus sheath. **(E)** Identification of the arcuate line. **(F)** Left common iliac artery and vein. **(G)** Midline sacral vessels. **(H)** L5–S1 anulus.

with either expandable tubular retractors, or a modified laparotomy table-based retractor system (**Fig. 27.4H**).

L4–L5 level can be exposed using the mini-open approach, but it is complicated by the bifurcation of the great

vessels. To circumvent this issue, exposure is obtained by retracting the major vessels to the right and creeping in posteriorly behind the vessels. As mentioned with the classic open approach, care must be taken to identify and ligate the iliolumbar vein if encountered to prevent significant and life-threatening hemorrhage.

Lateral Transpsoas Approach

Bergey et al described the endoscopic lateral transpsoas or extreme lateral interbody fusion (XLIF) technique.[9,44,45] The procedure is performed with the patient in the right lateral decubitus position. Following radiographic confirmation of the disc space of interest, two small incisions are made over that level at the lateral border of the paraspinous muscles (**Fig. 27.5A,B**). The retroperitoneal space is then bluntly developed and carried through to the psoas muscle. After entry into the psoas muscle, it is divided by sequential dilators to the level of the disc space under electromyographic monitoring of the psoas muscle. The genitofemoral nerve is at greatest risk during this exposure, and care must be exercised to avoid injury to this nerve. This can be done by staying in the anterior one third of the psoas muscle and by direct visualization of the nerve. The major advantage of the transpsoas technique over the mini-open anterior approach is that mobilization of the great vessels or sympathetic plexus is not necessary. Therefore, anterior exposure to the L1–L4 levels is effective and safely attainable.

Under limited circumstances, the lateral transpsoas technique can be performed to expose the L4–L5 or L5–S1 levels.[46] The first limitation is the presence of the great vessels, which require significant dissection and mobilization to expose distal to L4. The second drawback is the location of the iliac crest. Resection of the iliac crest may be necessary to gain access distal to the L3–L4 interspace.[47] As a result, the transpsoas approach to the ALIF is recommended for fusion only between the L1 and L5 levels.

Laparoscopic Approach (Transperitoneal) and Endoscopy-assisted Approach (Retroperitoneal)

In the 1990s, the incorporation of laparoscopy-assisted techniques in general and gynecologic surgery promoted the development of laparoscopy-assisted anterior interbody fusion. In 1991, Obenchain reported the first use of laparoscopy to the lumbar for discectomy.[48] Mathews et al in 1992 were among the first to report on a small series of stand-alone ALIF procedures using bone dowels in the interspace.[49] More

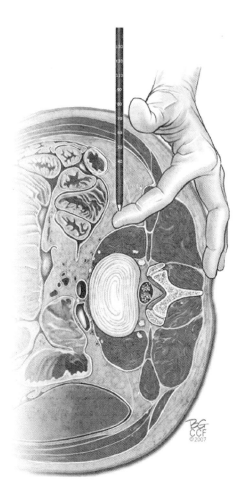

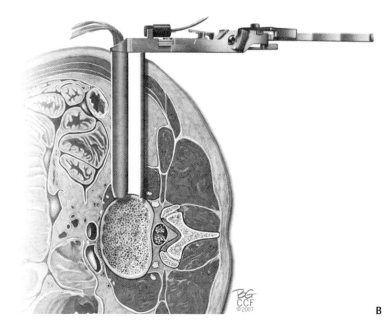

Fig. 27.5 Schematic showing surgical technique for the transpsoas approach. **(A)** Small incision over the psoas muscle and introduction of guide rod. **(B)** An expandable working canula is then inserted over the disc space after the psoas is divided to gain access to the retroperitoneal space. (Reprinted with permission of The Cleveland Clinic Center for Medical Art & Photography © 2007. All rights reserved.)

evidence for the utility of this technique was provided by Zucherman et al,[50] McAfee et al,[51] and Regan et al,[52] who successfully performed laparoscopy-assisted ALIF.

For this exposure, the patient is placed supine on the operating room table and lumbar lordosis accentuated with bolsters. The table is then positioned in the Trendelenburg position to ensure that the visceral contents are superiorly displaced out of the surgical field. Typically, four portals are established. Two paramedian incisions are made for a working portal and an instrumentation portal, respectively. The next two portals are positioned in the midline suprapubic region and the umbilicus for an instrumentation portal and a camera portal, respectively (**Fig. 27.6**). To safely expose the disc, both the middle sacral artery and vein are ligated and retracted out of the way. The iliac veins are then mobilized and retracted. At this point, a surgical disc is confirmed by fluoroscopy before discectomy is commenced.

Balloon-assisted endoscopic retroperitoneal gasless technique is another available option for exposure to the anterior lumbar spine.[53] This technique was first described by Gaur[54] and McDougall et al[55] for urologic procedures and later adopted for management of the lumbar spine pathology.

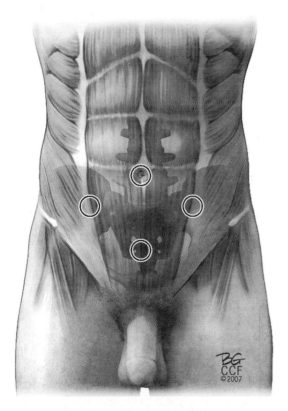

Fig. 27.6 Schematic showing the typical placement of laparoscopic portals. (Reprinted with permission of The Cleveland Clinic Center for Medical Art & Photography © 2007. All rights reserved.)

An inflatable balloon is used to expand the retroperitoneal space, which facilitates instrument and implant insertion, thereby avoiding the need for gas insufflation. The advantage of not needing gas insufflation or intraperitoneal entry is prevention of injury to the great vessels and to the hypogastric plexus. Although both the laparoscopy-assisted transperitoneal and the balloon-assisted endoscopic retroperitoneal gasless ALIF can be safely and reliably performed, they have fallen out of favor by most spine surgeons because of approach-related challenges and the associated long learning curve. Within the United States, excessive costs and the simpler and reproducible mini-open approach have significantly limited acceptability of the balloon-assisted endoscopic retroperitoneal gasless technique.

Transsacral Approach for Axial Lumbar Interbody Fusion at L5–S1

The transsacral access corridor to the lumbo-sacral junction was first explored by Cragg et al[10] for percutaneous lumbar interbody fusion at this level, and is called axial lumbar interbody fusion, AxiaLIF (TranS1, Wilmington, NC). For this technique, the patient is placed in the prone position and the presacral region is meticulously prepped and draped. A 2- to 4-mm incision is made on the right or left side adjacent to the paracoccygeal notch below the ischiolumbar ligament. Under fluoroscopic guidance, a trocar is then safely introduced along the anterior aspect of the sacrum and docked in the midline of the S1 body in both the anteroposterior and lateral views (**Fig. 27.7A–C**). Using specialized instruments, the disc is then completely evacuated and bone graft material substituted (**Fig. 27.7D,E**). A single translumbar axial rod is then inserted for rigid interbody fixation (**Fig. 27.7F–J**). Preliminary results suggest that this technique appears to be safe and may be effective for arthrodesis of the L5–S1 level.[10,56] Further study is required before this technique is routinely performed by surgeons.

■ Clinical Outcomes

A successful ALIF relies on both the rate of fusion and the clinical outcome, which can be measured by decreased pain and by functional restoration. Lane and Moore, in 1948, were the first to publish their outcomes following ALIF[57] to treat back pain and sciatica. Since that study, more data has become available in support of this technique as a bonafide alternative surgical option for the treatment of degenerative disc disease. For example, Harmon[58] reported a series of 244 patients with fusion rates of 98%, with 93% of the patients having a good to excellent clinical outcome. In this study the patients were treated with composite grafts of autogenous cortical and cancellous iliac dowels. Another study reported by Freebody et al[4] showed that, in a series of 243 patients, the fusion rate was 84%, with 92% good to excellent clinical outcomes. In addition, they found that patients with degenerative discs above the fusion level went on to failure as predicted.

High fusion rates and excellent clinical outcomes following ALIF are not always predictable. In fact, some studies have shown low fusion rates and poor clinical outcomes. Taylor's[59] review of 226 patients who had ALIF procedure

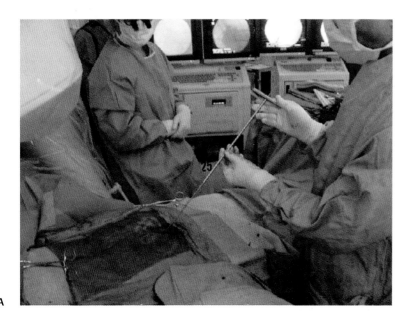

A

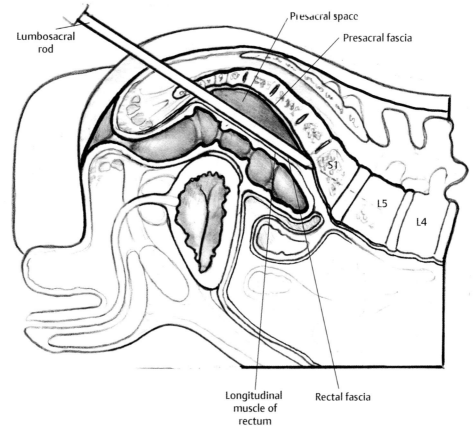

B

Fig. 27.7 The transsacral approach for anterior lumber interbody fusion at L5–S1. **(A)** Photograph showing position and setup of transsacral approach. **(B)** Trajectory of guide rod along the anterior sacrum, docking at the S1 vertebral body.

(Continued on page 236)

documented only a 44% fusion rate. Evaluation of the Mayo Clinic's experience by Stauffer and Coventry,[60] found a 56% fusion rate. Similarly, in Flynn and Houque's[61] review of 50 patients, a fusion rate of 56% was observed, with a 52% improvement in clinical outcomes. The apparent discrepancy in the fusion rates and the clinical outcomes reported in the 1960s and 1970s was, in part, due to poor patient selection, incomplete discectomy, poor endplate preparation, and limited choice of high-quality intervertebral graft materials.

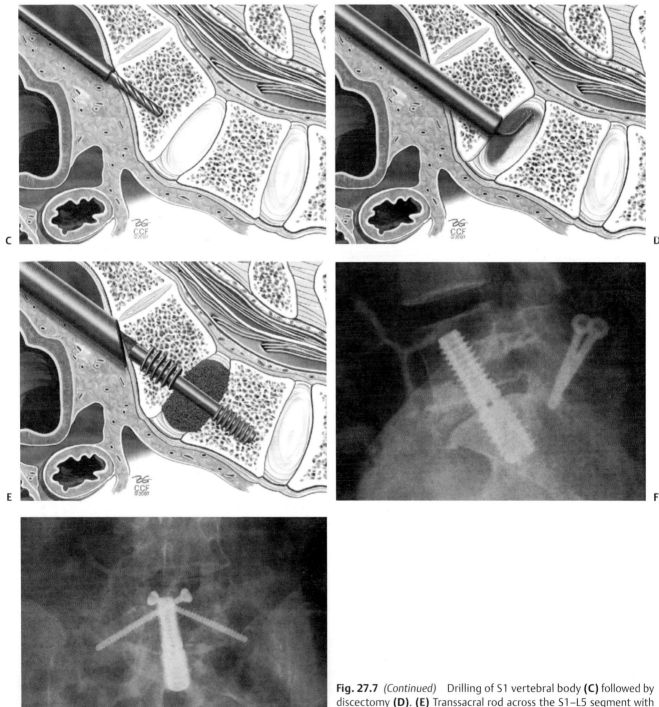

Fig. 27.7 *(Continued)*   Drilling of S1 vertebral body **(C)** followed by discectomy **(D)**. **(E)** Transsacral rod across the S1–L5 segment with bone graft material in the disc space. Anteroposterior **(F)** and lateral **(G)** radiographs of the axial anterior lumbar interbody fusion supplemented with translaminar screws.

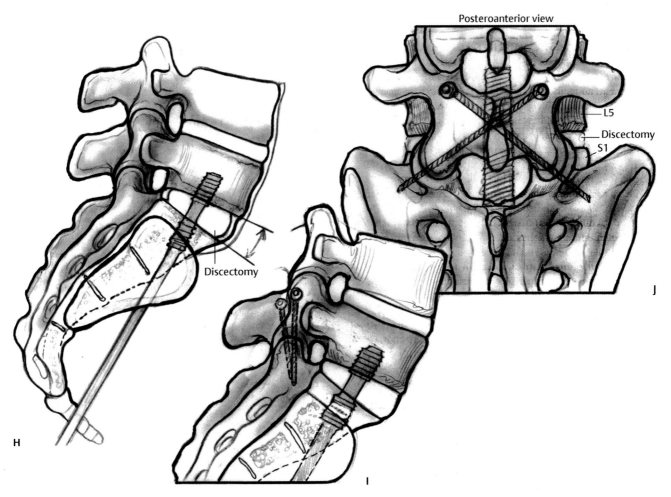

Fig. 27.7 *(Continued)* **(H–J)** Schematics of the axial anterior lumbar interbody fusion highlighting the desired positions of the transaxial rod both in the AP and L planes. (**C–E,** Reprinted with permission of The Cleveland Clinic Center for Medical Art & Photography © 2007. All rights reserved.)

In the 1980s and 1990s, in an attempt to improve the success of ALIF, advanced diagnostic techniques, to aid in proper patient selection, were incorporated in the preoperative planning phase.[62] This, along with embracing the theory of thorough endplate preparation, restoration of anatomic disc space height, the reduction of spinal deformities, and the use of combined structural allograft and cancellous autograph materials, led to reliably higher fusion rates with concomitant better clinical outcomes.[62–66] Furthermore, the recent development of threaded intervertebral fusion cages coupled with the availability of newer osteoinductive and osteogenic materials have resulted in improved fusion rates.[24,27,37]

The theoretical advantage of the minimally invasive ALIF is the reduction of approach-related morbidity, while at same time improving clinical outcomes. This remains to be fully substantiated with both long-term clinical observational studies and long-term prospective randomized controlled clinical trails. However, recent studies suggest that even though fusion rates are comparable to classic open procedures, clinical outcomes are overall slightly better following minimal invasive ALIF.[67] Finally, among the minimally invasive approaches there appears to be very little difference in clinical outcomes. Chung et al[7] found no significant difference in fusion rates and clinical outcomes between the laparoscopic approach and the mini-open approach for ALIF at 2-year follow-up.

■ Complications

Possible risks and complications following ALIF are due to injury to the anatomic structures encountered during the particular approaches. The potential complications are numerous and range from lymphoceles, ureteral injuries,[68–70] retroperitoneal fibrosis, rectus muscle hematoma, bowel obstruction, and pancreatitis. Vascular and neurologic injuries are not uncommon. For example, a significant potential risk of the extreme lateral or transpsoas approach is genitofemoral nerve palsy due to prolonged retraction of the psoas muscle.[9] Retrograde ejaculation and impotence have also been reported following anterior ALIF in the lower lumbar region due to damage to filaments of the presacral plexus. Furthermore, compression neuropathies involving the brachial plexus, femoral nerve, lateral cutaneous nerve of the thigh, and peroneal nerves have been reported following ALIF. In addition, sympathetic dysfunction manifested by increased warmth or uncomfortable sensations in one or both legs have been described.

It has been shown that there are higher rates of complications with the minimally invasive approaches, especially the laparoscopic ALIF. The risks include possible damage to the viscera, aorta, inferior vena cava, iliac vessels, and presacral plexus. Zdeblick and David found a 20% complication rate with the laparoscopic approach to L4–L5 compared with a 4% complication rate with the open technique.[71] Additionally, there appears to be a higher incidence of retrograde ejaculation with the laparoscopic technique compared with mini-open ALIF (45% versus 6%).[72] In the rare circumstances when the iliac artery and vein are injured and hemostasis cannot be controlled laparoscopically, conversion of the procedure to an open laparotomy becomes obligatory.[72]

Perhaps the most critical complication for both the patient and the surgeon is the potential risk of a painful pseudarthrosis. This can occur because of infection, lack of meticulous preparation of the endplates, or improper placement of the interbody graft material resulting in segmental spine imbalance, hardware fracture, implant subsidence or migration, and micromotion. A persistent painful nonunion usually mandates revision procedures. Finally, the rate of adjacent level degeneration or transitional syndrome is not insignificant and may have to be addressed at a later time by extending the fusion to incorporate the involved levels.

■ Conclusion

Although ALIF fusion has evolved since it was first described in the 1930s, to ensure a rigid fusion and an excellent clinical outcome adherent to the basic principles remains paramount. The steps are complete discectomy with removal of the cartilaginous endplates to expose bleeding bone, restoration of anatomic disc space height and reduction of spinal deformities, appropriate placement of intervertebral graft constructs, and the minimization of preventable complications. For degenerative disc disease, both high fusion rates and good clinical outcomes can be consistently achieved.

With the recent development of minimally invasive techniques, anterior interbody fusion can be safely performed with reduced morbidity and cost to the patient, thereby allowing a quicker return of function and improved postoperative outcomes. Nevertheless, further investigations, especially clinical outcome research, are mandatory to fully delineate the effectiveness of these newer minimally invasive techniques before their widespread acceptance as bona fide alternatives to the open and mini-open ALIFs can be achieved.

References

1. Albee RH. Transplantation of a portion of tibia into the spine for Pott's disease. JAMA 1911;57:885–887
2. Carpenter N. Spondylolisthesis. Br J Surg 1932;19:374–386
3. Burns BH. An operation for spondylolisthesis. Lancet 1933;1:1233–1239
4. Freebody D, Bendall R, Taylor RD. Anterior transperitoneal lumbar fusion. J Bone Joint Surg Br 1971;53:617–627
5. Zucherman JF, Zdeblick TA, Bailey SA, Mahvi D, Hsu KY, Kohrs D. Instrumented laparoscopic spinal fusion: preliminary results. Spine 1995;20:2029–2035
6. Burrington JD, Brown C, Wayne ER, Odom J. Anterior approach to the thoracolumbar spine: technical considerations. Arch Surg 1976;111:456–463
7. Chung SK, Lee SH, Lim SR, et al. Comparative study of laparoscopic L5–S1 fusion versus open mini-ALIF, with a minimum 2-year follow-up. Eur Spine J 2003;12:613–617
8. Zdeblick TA, David SM. A prospective comparison of surgical approach for anterior L4–L5 fusion: laparoscopic versus mini anterior lumbar interbody fusion. Spine 2000;25:2682–2687
9. Bergey DL, Villavicencio AT, Goldstein T, Regan JJ. Endoscopic lateral transpsoas approach to the lumbar spine. Spine 2004;29:1681–1688
10. Cragg A, Carl A, Casteneda F, Dickman C, Guterman L, Oliveira C. New percutaneous access method for minimally invasive anterior lumbosacral surgery. J Spinal Disord Tech 2004;17:21–28
11. Suk SI, Lee CK, Kim WJ, Lee JH, Cho KJ, Kim HG. Adding posterior lumbar interbody fusion to pedicle screw fixation and posterolateral fusion after decompression in spondylolytic spondylolisthesis. Spine 1997;22:210–219
12. Roca J, Ubierna MT, Caceres E, Iborra M. One-stage decompression and posterolateral and interbody fusion for severe spondylolisthesis: an analysis of 14 patients. Spine 1999;24:709–714
13. Stewart G, Sachs BL. Patient outcomes after reoperation on the lumbar spine. J Bone Joint Surg Am 1996;78:706–711
14. Tay BB, Berven S. Indications, techniques, and complications of lumbar interbody fusion. Semin Neurol 2002;22(2):221–230
15. Adams MA, Green TP, Dolan P. The strength in anterior bending of lumbar intervertebral discs. Spine 1994;19:2197–2203

16. Nachemson A, Morris JM. In vivo measurements of intradiscal pressure: discometry, a method for the determination of pressure in the lower lumbar discs. J Bone Joint Surg Am 1964;46:1077–1092
17. Burkus JK. Intervertebral fixation: clinical results with anterior cages. Orthop Clin North Am 2002;33:349–357
18. Dennis S, Watkins R, Landaker S, et al. Comparison of disc space heights after anterior lumbar interbody fusion. Spine 1989;14:876–878
19. Boyd LM, Estes BT, Liu M. Biomechanics of lumbar interbody constructs: effect of design and materials. In: Husson JL, LeHuec JC, editors. Chirurgie endoscopique et mini-invasive du rachis. Montpelier, France: Sauramps Medical; 1999:181–192
20. Kozak JA, Heilman AE, O'Brien JP. Anterior lumbar fusion options: technique and graft materials. Clin Orthop Relat Res 1994;300:45–51
21. Buttermann GR, Glazer PA, Hu SS, Bradford DS. Anterior and posterior allografts in symptomatic thoracolumbar deformity. J Spinal Disord 2001;14:54–66
22. Buttermann GR, Glazer PA, Bradford DS. Revision of failed lumbar fusions: a comparison of anterior autograft and allograft. Spine 1997;22:2748–2755
23. Buttermann GR, Glazer PA, Bradford DS. The use of bone allografts in the spine. Clin Orthop Relat Res 1996;324:75–85
24. Burkus JK, Dorchak JD, Sanders DL, et al. Single level anterior lumbar interbody fusion using threaded cortical bone allografts. Paper presented at the North American Spine Society Meeting of the Americas, May 15, 1999; Miami, FL
25. Bagby GW. Arthrodesis by distraction-compression method using a stainless steel implant. Orthopedics 1988;11:931–944
26. DeBowes RM, Grant BD, Bagby GW, et al. Cervical vertebral interbody fusion in the horse: a comparative study of bovine xenografts and autografts supported by stainless steel baskets. Am J Vet Res 1984;45:191–199
27. Bagby G. The Bagby and Kuslich (BAK) method of lumbar interbody fusion. Spine 1999;24:1857
28. Brodke DS, Dick JC, Kunz DN, et al. Posterior lumbar interbody fusion: a biomechanical comparison, including a new threaded cage. Spine 1997;22:26–31
29. Butts M, Kuslich S, Bechtold J. Biomechanical analysis of a new method for spinal interbody fixation. In: Erdman A, ed. 1987 Advances in Bioengineering. New York: The American Society of Mechanical Engineers; 1987:95–96
30. Hasegawa K, Ikeda M, Washio T, et al. An experimental study of porcine lumbar segmental stiffness by the distraction-compression principle using a threaded interbody cage. J Spinal Disord 2000;13:247–252
31. Tencer AF, Hampton D, Eddy S. Biomechanical properties of threaded inserts for lumbar interbody spinal fusion. Spine 1995;20:2408–2414
32. Zdeblick TA. Construct Stiffness Testing of the Threaded Interbody Fusion Device (TIBFD). Memphis, TN: Medtronic Sofamor Danek Group; 1994
33. Chen D, Fay LA, Lok J, Yuan P, Edwards WT, Yuan HA. Increasing neuroforaminal volume by anterior interbody distraction in degenerative lumbar spine. Spine 1995;20:74–79
34. Kuslich SD, Ulstrom CL, Griffith SL, et al. The Bagby and Kuslich method of lumbar interbody fusion: history, techniques, and 2-year follow-up results of a United States prospective, multicenter trial. Spine 1998;23:1267–1278
35. Hacker RJ. Comparison of interbody fusion approaches for disabling low back pain. Spine 1997;22:660–665
36. Lund T, Oxland TR, Jost B, et al. Interbody cage stabilization in the lumbar spine: biomechanical evaluation of cage design, posterior instrumentation and bone density. J Bone Joint Surg Br 1998;80:351–359
37. Oxland TR, Kohrs DW, Kuslich SD, et al. The BAK Interbody Fusion System: An Innovative Solution. Minneapolis, MN: Spine-Tech; 1994
38. Iwahara T, Ikeda K, Hirabayashi K. Results of anterior spine fusion by extraperitoneal approach for spondylolisthesis. Nippon Seikeigeka Gakkai Zasshi 1963;36:1049–1067
39. Harmon PH. Anterior excision and vertebral body fusion operation for intervertebral disk syndromes of the lower lumbar spine: three- to five year results in 244 cases. Clin Orthop Relat Res 1963;26:107–127
40. Mayer HM. A new microsurgical technique for minimally invasive anterior lumbar interbody fusion. Spine 1997;22:691–700
41. Anderson TM, Mansour KA, Miller JI Jr. Thoracic approaches to anterior spinal operations: anterior thoracic approaches. Ann Thorac Surg 1993;55:1447–1451
42. Gumbs AA, Bloom ND, Bitan FD, Hanan SH. Open anterior approaches for lumbar spine procedures. Am J Surg 2007;194:98–102
43. Ferguson AB. Roentgendiagnostic: Extremities and Spine. New York: Hoeber; 1949
44. Bradford DS, ed. Master Techniques in Orthopaedic Surgery: The Spine. New York: Lippincott Williams & Wilkins; 2004:321–334
45. Bradford DS. The Spine. New York: Lippincott Williams & Wilkins; 2004
46. Wright NM. XLIF: The United States Experience 2003–2004. Paper presented at the 12th International Meeting of Advanced Spine Techniques; July 7–9, 2005; Banff, Alberta, Canada
47. Ozgur BM, Aryan HE, Pimenta L, Taylor WR. Extreme lateral interbody fusion (XLIF): a novel surgical technique for anterior lumbar interbody fusion. Spine J 2006;6:435–443
48. Obenchain TG. Laparoscopic lumbar discectomy. J Laparoendosc Surg 1991;1:145–149
49. Mathews HH, Evans MT, Molligan HJ, Long BH. Laparoscopic discectomy with anterior lumbar interbody fusion: a preliminary review. Spine 1995;20:1797–1802
50. Zucherman JF, Zdeblick TA, Bailey SA, Mahvi D, Hsu KY, Kohrs D. Instrumented laparoscopic spinal fusion: preliminary results. Spine 1995;20:2029–2034
51. McAfee PC, Regan JJ, Fedder IL, Mack MJ, Geis WP. Anterior thoracic corpectomy for spinal cord decompression performed endoscopically. Surg Laparosc Endosc 1995;5:339–348
52. Regan JJ, McAfee PC, Guyer RD, Aronoff RJ. Laparoscopic fusion of the lumbar spine in a multicenter series of the first 34 consecutive patients. Surg Laparosc Endosc 1996;6:459–468
53. Vazquez RM, Gireesan GT. Balloon-assisted endoscopic retroperitoneal gasless (BERG) technique for anterior lumbar interbody fusion (ALIF). Surg Endosc 2003;17:268–272
54. Gaur DD. Laparoscopic operative retroperitoneoscopy: use of a new device. J Urol 1992;148:1137–1139
55. McDougall EM, Clayman RV, Fadden PT. Retroperitoneoscopy: the Washington University Medical School experience. Urology 1994;43:446–452
56. Marotta N, Cosar M, Pimenta L, Khoo LT. A novel minimally invasive presacral approach and instrumentation technique for anterior

L5–S1 intervertebral discectomy and fusion: technical description and case presentations. Neurosurg Focus 2006;20:E9

57. Lane JD, Moore ES. Transperitoneal approach to the intervertebral disc in the lumbar area. Ann Surg 1948;127:537–551

58. Harmon PH. Anterior excision and vertebral body fusion operation for intervertebral disc syndromes of the lower lumbar spine. Clin Orthop Relat Res 1963;26:107–127

59. Taylor TKF. Anterior interbody fusion in the management of disorders of the lumbar spine. J Bone Joint Surg Br 1970;52:784

60. Stauffer RN, Coventry MB. Anterior interbody lumbar spine fusion. J Bone Joint Surg Am 1972;54:756–768

61. Flynn JC, Houque MA. Anterior fusion of the lumbar spine. J Bone Joint Surg Am 1979;61:1143–1150

62. Crock HV. Anterior lumbar interbody fusion: indications for its use and notes on surgical technique. Clin Orthop Relat Res 1982;165:157–163

63. Blumenthal SL, Baker J, Dossett A, Selby DK. The role of anterior lumbar fusion for internal disc disruption. Spine 1988;13:566–569

64. Chen D, Fay LA, Lok J, et al. Increasing neuroforaminal volume by anterior interbody distraction in degenerative lumbar spine. Spine 1995;20:74–79

65. Leong JC, Chun SY, Grange WJ, et al. Long-term results of lumbar intervertebral disc prolapse. Spine 1983;8:793–799

66. Loguidice VA, Johnson RG, Guyer RD, et al. Anterior lumbar interbody fusion. Spine 1988;13:366–369

67. Lieberman IH. Minimally invasive spine surgery. In: Fardon DE. Garfin SR, eds. Orthopaedic Knowledge Update Spine 2. Rosemont, IL: American Academy of Orthopaedic Surgeons; 2002:469–476

68. Assimos DG, Patterson LC, Taylor CL. Changing incidence and etiology of iatrogenic ureteral injuries. J Urol 1994;152:2240–2246

69. Guingrich JA, McDermott JC. Ureteral injury during laparoscopy-assisted anterior lumbar fusion. Spine 2000;25:1586–1588

70. Oh BR, Kwon DD, Park KS, Ryu SB, Park YI, Presti JC Jr. Late presentation of ureteral injury after laparoscopic surgery. Obstet Gynecol 2000;95:337–339

71. Zdeblick TA, David SM. A prospective comparison of surgical approach for anterior L4–L5 fusion: laparoscopic versus mini anterior lumbar interbody fusion. Spine 2000;25:2682–2687

72. McAfee PC, Regan JR, Zdeblick TA, et al. The incidence of complications in endoscopic anterior thoracolumbar spinal reconstructive surgery: a prospective multicenter study comprising the first 100 consecutive cases. Spine 1995;20:1624–1632

28 Spinal Fusion: Combined Anteroposterior Approach

Richard D. Guyer and Thomas F. Roush

Despite recent biologic advancements such as improved osteoconductive and particularly osteoinductive materials and proteins, achieving a successful lumbar spinal fusion remains a difficult task. In many respects, the dorsal lumbar spine represents the worst of all anatomic regions for fusion due to the large dorsal tension forces on the lumbar spine, difficulty in immobilization, limited bony surface area available for biologic fusion, and poor avascular healing bed following surgical exposure via periosteal stripping. In contrast, the anterior interbody region is a favorable area for fusion, as witnessed by the roughly 80% share of spinal compressive load through the anterior and middle columns[1] in accordance with Wolff's law, 90% share of the spinal osseous surface area, and relatively strong and vascular bony endplates on which to obtain fixation strength. Additional proposed benefits are improved restoration of sagittal alignment and neuroforaminal height.[2] The surgical implementation of anterior lumbar interbody fusion (ALIF), however, destabilizes the spine in extension and axial rotation by the variable sectioning of anterior longitudinal ligament and outer anulus,[3] as well as possibly producing facet joint distraction. The sectioning of various stabilizing structures as is necessary during surgical procedures diminishes spinal stability in a complicated fashion not yet fully understood.[4] Furthermore, the original concept of "distraction compression"[5] due to the pretensioned anulus has been found to be short-lived due to the viscoelasticity of the ligamentous tissue.[6] Recognizing these drawbacks, combined anterior lumbar interbody/posterolateral lumbar fusion (ALIF/PLF) constructs have become increasingly popular in the treatment of recalcitrant lumbar disc degeneration.[7-13]

■ Biomechanical and Biologic Rationale

When considered independently, several biomechanical drawbacks exist for anterior and posterior fusions. ALIF has long been recognized to have limited control of extension and axial rotation.[14-18] Furthermore, these studies found that the addition of posterior fixation, either pedicle or facet screws, yielded significantly superior biomechanical stability. This improved stability was also noted during lateral bending and flexion. Posterolateral lumbar fusion (PLF) alone imparts even less stability to the lumbar spine and demonstrates deficiency in a multitude of loading conditions,[19-22] all of which are improved with the addition of interbody fusion. Intuitively, when the degenerated disc is implicated as the nociceptive generator, PLF as a treatment option makes little sense as the disc is not directly addressed. Even in the face of solid PLF, cantilever interbody motion remains,[23,24] thereby engendering motion about the disc. Bono et al[25] noted that this cantilever motion can yield sagittal range of motion of up to 6 degrees following solid PLF and, more interestingly, up to 3 degrees following solid ALIF. These residual motions have a clinical correlation in that further stabilization in the form of postoperative bracing following PLF leads to higher union rates.[26] Such findings indirectly support combined constructs such as anteroposterior (360 degrees or ALIF/PLF) lumbar fusion to yield more complete motion cessation. More direct evidence was offered by Oda et al,[10] who noted the importance of an ALIF/PLF construct to increase stiffness and decrease implant strain.

From a biologic standpoint, solid interbody fusion requires ample vascular surface area, which is difficult with a posterior interbody approach. Even in a controlled cadaveric setting, Manos et al[27] demonstrated ~50% to 60% disc material removal and adequate endplate preparation while performing a TLIF procedure. In addition to improved endplate preparation and fusion bed, ALIF affords improvements in sagittal balance,[28] particularly when coupled with PLF.[29] An additional concern of stand-alone ALIF constructs is subsidence,[30,31] which appears to be more problematic with recombinant human bone morphogenetic protein (rhBMP-2; INFUSE, Medtronic Sofamor Danek, Memphis, TN) use.[30,32] The combined ALIF/PLF approach possesses a sound biomechanical basis, but the concern as to the necessity of this more extensive procedure in the treatment of degenerative disc disease (DDD) remains despite improvements in technique that will be addressed in this chapter.

■ Indications and Work-up

Indications and work-up for ALIF/PLF are no different than the work-up for any other lumbar approach. We consider a patient a surgical candidate if they fail 6 months minimum of nonoperative treatment (medication, physical therapy, chiropractic manipulation, injections, etc.), and have radiographic evidence including plain x-rays, magnetic resonance imaging (MRI), computed tomography (CT), myelography-CT, and provocative testing in the form of discography (where deemed appropriate on a case-by-case basis) that corroborates the symptoms and isolates the degenerative level as the pathologic source, and that no contraindications to either procedure exist. Furthermore, the patient must be medically fit to undergo a 2- to 3-hour operation depending upon the levels involved. Nearly all patients considering surgery at our institution for back pain primarily undergo extensive psychological evaluation performed by a spine specialty psychologist, and must be deemed a surgical candidate following the evaluation. With the availability of various motion preservation strategies, we view more than two degenerative, nondeformed levels, as a relative contraindication to any lumbar fusion, though there are exceptions. Should a patient emerge with solid evidence that the pathologic disc is primarily responsible for symptoms, we proceed with providing them information on anterior and posterior surgery, and involve them in decision making concerning whether to have surgery and which approach to take.

■ Surgical Procedure

We begin all ALIF/PLF procedures with the anterior approach, which allows us to obtain improved restoration of disc height and lumbar lordosis. Following preoperative antibiotic infusion and application of mechanical deep vein thrombosis prophylaxis, patients are placed supine on a standard operating table configured to allow improved unencumbered fluoroscopic access under the table. It is imperative that the table be radiolucent, flexing and extending through the involved disc space. ALIF/PLF is particularly useful with advanced collapse of the degenerated disc to obtain better visualization and access to the entirety of the endplates. Endotracheal anesthesia is then commenced. The remainder of the surgery is based on the mini-anterior retroperitoneal approach as described by Brau.[33]

Each anterior surgical approach is performed by a general or vascular surgeon with expertise in such approaches. Transverse incisions are used whenever possible for cosmetic reasons. Hand-held retractors are used for efficiency and the perceived circulation improvement afforded by the transient relaxation of retraction pressure on the great

vessels. A single image intensifier is used to mark the appropriate level and center of the disc space via an anterior view, then the intensifier is converted to a lateral view for the remainder of the case to better assess posterior endplate preparation and implant sizing. The disc space is prepared as carefully as one would for a disc arthroplasty. That is, care is taken not to violate the endplates to prevent subsidence and clean the endplates down to bleeding subchondral bone with a variety of Cobb elevators, pituitary rongeurs, straight, angled, and ring curettes. After verifying by lateral C-arm images that the disc tissue has been evacuated to the posterior longitudinal ligament, a variety of implants can be placed including allograft bone, cylindrical tapered cages of metal or polyetheretherketone (PEEK), and PEEK grafts with or without incorporated screws and plates. Care should be taken not to overdistract the disc space greater than the next normal adjacent one. Implants can be used with autograft bone, demineralized bone matrix (DBM), or rhBMP-2. Our preference is allograft bone with rhBMP-2.

Following anterior wound closure and generous wound dressing to minimize removal during the transition to posterior procedure, a radiolucent Jackson table with either a Wilson or a four-post frame placed adjacent to the patient's operative table. The patient is transferred carefully, while intubated, to the prone position with ample padding of bony prominences and careful positioning of the upper extremities. The standard operating table is then removed from the room, and the Jackson table is then centered under the operative lighting. Prior to preparation and draping, two image intensifiers are positioned on either side of the table. The intensifier placed on the side of the surgical scrub technologist or nurse and operative instruments and implants is denoted the permanent lateral view, so as to minimize the bulkiness which is imparted when the intensifier is placed in an anteroposterior configuration. The image intensifier for the lateral view is then rotated whereby the bar connecting the x-ray source is rotated such that is moves in the cephalad direction until it reaches its limitation conferred by the underneath structure of the Jackson table. A second image intensifier then is introduced from the opposite side of the table and is designated as the anteroposterior image. Once a truly orthogonal view is obtained, which is centered on the image intensifier screen, sterile preparation and draping commence so that the image intensifiers are first covered in a sterile fashion, followed by sterile draping of the surgical site. We find that using biplanar fluoroscopy improves both the duration and accuracy of the posterior procedure. **Figure 28.1** shows the biplanar imaging configuration. Like all new techniques, however, experience must be rapidly gained by all involved; experienced fluoroscopists are vital to the success of such a technique.

Regardless of whether performing concomitant posterior fusion for DDD with or without spondylolysis or spondylolisthesis, we prefer to use the bilateral paramedian

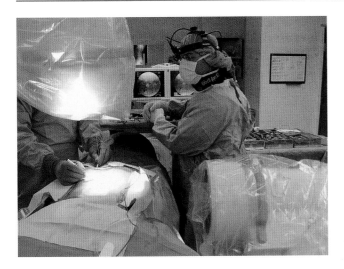

Fig. 28.1 The setup employed for biplanar fluoroscopy for the posterolateral fusion portion of the surgery.

Wiltse incisions due to improved biomechanical stability of bilateral over unilateral posterolateral fusion,[34] despite evidence[35–38] that unilateral PLF leads to similar clinical outcome. **Figure 28.2** shows the skin markings for the posterior approach. Care is taken to expose the relevant transverse processes/facet/pars complexes to prepare an adequate fusion bed. Following posterior instrumentation with pedicle screws taking care to avoid damaging the zygapophyseal articulation, a high-speed burr is used to decorticate the transverse processes, lateral aspect of the superior articular process, and pars interarticularis region. Following decortication, bone graft is placed over the surface and the pedicle screws and rods are placed. Bone grafting materials

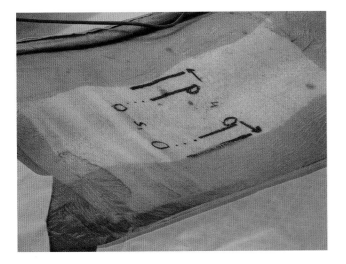

Fig. 28.2 Typical incision markings to guide the posterolateral fusion portion via an open Wiltse technique to ensure adequate decortication of bony elements and the promotion of bony fusion.

most commonly used include both osteoconductive and osteoinductive materials. A common combination is tricalcium phosphate for its osteoconductive properties and a DBM as a graft extender and osteoinductive source. Rarely, autograft from the posterior iliac crest is used. If a decompression is necessary, this can be performed from a separate midline approach and the local bone is admixed with DBM. Alternatively, if decompression is not needed, we favor the percutaneous pedicle screw technique using electrophysiologic pedicle screw monitoring that is demonstrated in the video. In these cases, we depend primarily on the anterior fusion, though the facet joints can be easily decorticated by the use of pituitaries and the guidance of the C-arm prior to rod placement.

Following placement of all graft materials and implants, final radiographs are obtained, and the wounds are closed in layered fashion with absorbable sutures. The patient is then turned to the supine position onto the standard hospital bed and extubated by the anesthesiologist.

Figure 28.3 shows the anteroposterior and lateral radiographic views of an ALIF/PLF procedure. Our patients typically are discharged from the hospital in 1 to 3 days. With the use of rhBMP-2 anteriorly, fusions may occur as early as 4 to 6 months. Pseudarthrosis is almost nonexistent and postoperative recovery is much faster compared with previous techniques.

■ Clinical Outcomes

The primary clinical advantages of ALIF/PLF pertain to fusion rates, restoration of sagittal alignment, and prevention of biomechanical failure of posterior implants. In many respects, this procedure represents a compilation of the virtues of stand-alone ALIF and PLF, while diminishing the untoward effects of each individual procedure. Spencer and DeWald[39] offered one of the earlier case series of a combined approach, albeit in the setting of complex spinal pathologies of the thoracic and lumbar spine. They described a simultaneous procedure of anterior application of iliac crest structural autograft and posterior application of Harrington instrumentation with two surgical teams accessing the patient placed in the lateral position. Walker[40] extrapolated this procedure to the treatment of primarily discogenic pain in a staged fashion. O'Brien et al[41] presented the earliest large series of ALIF/PLF for patients with disabling back pain secondary to spondylosis. In 150 patients, 60% were "suicidal" at the time of surgery due to chronic back pain. All of them were unemployed, and each had seen up to 34 physicians regarding their pain. Despite this highly morbid patient population, 86% were clinically improved following surgery, with 60% being significantly improved. Kozak and O'Brien[42] described 27 patients with disabling DDD with

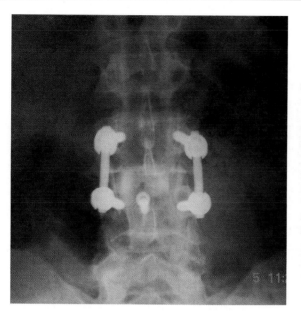
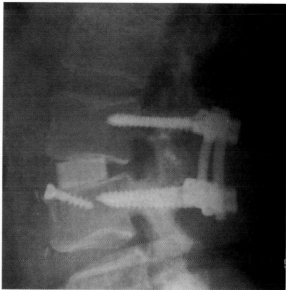

Fig. 28.3   Anteroposterior **(A)** and lateral **(B)** radiographs of our standard anteroposterior fusion construct.

no prior surgery whereby the authors employed a sequential anteroposterior approach under a single anesthetic and noted a fusion rate of 90% for one- and two-level procedures. The fusion rate decreased to 78% for three-level procedures. They noted acceptable clinical results in 82% (defined as minimum 26% improvement in back pain, return to work, mildly limited activities, and intermittent analgesic use) at minimum 1.6-year follow-up. Iliac crest structural autograft or femoral head allograft was used for the ALIF, and Knodt rods and iliac crest or allograft for the PLF. The complication rate was 23%, which included donor site pain.

By the mid-1990s, debate over the most effective treatment of DDD populated the literature, including an eloquent discussion by Nachemson, Zdeblick, and O'Brien.[43] Nachemson championed nonoperative care based on the heterogeneity in the diagnosis and the lack of quality evidence that surgical treatment is superior to natural history. Zdeblick supported instrumented PLF referencing his 86% or greater fusion rates translating to high clinical success. O'Brien cited the necessity to remove the nociceptive generator (intervertebral disc) and stabilize posteriorly with internal fixation as anterior fixation is "too hazardous because of the proximity of the vessels." He also cited the aforementioned studies of the 1980s,[40,41] which demonstrated superior radiographic and clinical results to the extant literature regarding anterior or posterior-only approaches.

Fraser compared the literature in the mid-1990s regarding interbody, posterior, and combined anterior/posterior fusion.[44] With respect to ALIF/PLF, he attributed the increasing popularity to the significant drop in fusion rate for multiple levels using a noncombined approach.

In 1997, the first study to directly compare combined anterior/posterior fusion surgery with an all posterior lumbar interbody fusion (PLIF)/PLF procedure for DDD was performed by Hacker.[45] Twenty-one patients underwent ALIF/PLF, and 54 subsequent patients underwent PLIF with threaded cages. Both groups received an uninstrumented PLF with iliac crest bone graft. When comparing clinical results, the PLIF/PLF group demonstrated significant improvements over the ALIF/PLF group in operative time, blood loss, hospital stay, and perioperative costs. Patient satisfaction was similar. Of note, there was a statistically higher percentage of workers' compensation patients in the ALIF/PLF group, and that group comprised the first patients of the retrospective study, which may signify the presence of the "learning curve." Furthermore, both surgeon and patient bias toward the PLIF/PLF procedure were likely as every patient given the option of ALIF/PLF versus PLIF/PLF chose the latter. Regardless, the findings of this study were in keeping with the trend toward greater morbidity with ALIF/PLF.

Not until the 21st century did a randomized, prospective study surface comparing surgical approaches to the lumbar spine for degenerative pathologies. Christensen et al[8] compared ALIF/PLF with isolated instrumented PLF for degenerative instability or isthmic spondylolisthesis. No cases of pure DDD were included. There were significant improvements in back pain, leg pain, sagittal lordosis restoration and maintenance, fusion rate, and reoperation rate in the combined fusion group. There was also a trend toward better overall outcome ($P < 0.08$) in this group. The authors concluded that combined fusion is the favored treatment over instrumented PLF in patients with complex lumbar pathology involving major instability, flatback, and previous disc surgery in younger patients.

The first prospective, randomized study comparing different surgical approaches for the treatment of recalcitrant primary DDD was published by the Swedish Lumbar Spine Study Group in 2002.[9] This study included 294 patients with a minimum 2-year history of chronic low back pain and radiologic evidence of disc degeneration at L4–5, L5–S1, or both. The radiologic evidence consisted of abnormalities on plain radiographs, CT scan, and/or MRI scan. Unfortunately, from a statistical standpoint, degenerative spondylolisthesis was not an exclusion factor, and the authors did not distinguish between patients with this condition from those with a stable spine and isolated symptomatic degenerative discs. Patients were randomized to three groups: uninstrumented PLF, PLF with pedicle screws connected by bendable plates, and circumferential fusion. The circumferential procedure included both ALIF/PLF and PLIF/PLF, though the authors did evaluate these groups separately. All groups had significant improvements in low back Visual Analog Scale, Oswestry Disability Index, Million score, and Zung Depression Scale scores. No differences in these values existed between groups. The only differences between groups occurred in hospital stay, operative time, and complication rate, all of which increased with the additional procedures. No differences were noted within the circumferential group when evaluating the subgroups undergoing ALIF or PLIF as the interbody component. Because the PLIF subgroup had only 19 patients, the authors surmised that the data in this group may have been subject to type II statistical error of inadequate power.

More recently, Videbaek et al[7] performed a prospective study of minimum 5-year results evaluating the same patient population reported at 2-year follow-up by Christensen et al.[8] Videbaek et al[7] demonstrated significantly improved outcomes in all validated questionnaires used in their study supporting combined fusion over instrumented PLF for their population of patients with degenerative instability or isthmic spondylolisthesis.

Clearly, additional clinical studies will be valuable as the surgical techniques and technology continue to evolve.

■ Complications and Complication Avoidance

Complication rates have long been the primary clinical concern of ALIF/PLF. Villavicencio et al[46] addressed this in a retrospective analysis of 124 patients who underwent TLIF as the interbody component compared with 43 patients

treated with ALIF in a combined anteroposterior procedure. They noted significantly less operative time, blood loss, hospital time, and complications in the TLIF group. However, their data regarding combined anteroposterior fusion are quite different from our experience. The authors noted a mean operative time for combined reconstruction of almost 8 hours, hospitalization of over a week, and a 76.7% complication rate, which is much less favorable than our experience with ALIF/PLF.

The recurring theme regarding the expected complications during ALIF/PLF relates to its complexity. As noted in the clinical studies cited above, operative time is critical. We cannot emphasize strongly enough the necessity of having a well-trained operative staff familiar with the procedure and a competent general or vascular surgeon to perform the surgical approach. We have noted a reduction in operative time of ~50% over the past 10 years that these procedures have been performed at our institution. We now schedule ~3 hours for a one- or two-level ALIF/PLF, which includes intraoperative repositioning. Such efficiency has greatly decreased our complication rates and hospital stay. Complications intrinsic to the anterior and posterior procedures, which have been discussed in the preceding chapters, remain. Regarding the anterior portion of the procedure, our incision size and dissection extent has greatly decreased, which has shortened the procedure while creating no notable shortcomings in visualization because the incisions tend to be precisely targeted.

By transitioning exclusively to the paramedian Wiltse approach for the posterior aspect of the procedure, we have noted clear improvements in postoperative pain and more rapid rehabilitation. Though we routinely perform simultaneous bilateral Wiltse approaches for instrumentation and fusion as two spine surgeons perform each case, the clinical data are currently such that unilateral Wiltse procedures may be performed with expectation of an identical clinical outcome to the bilateral technique.[35–37] Such a technique modification may further decrease the complication rate related to case duration if a single surgeon performs the posterior procedure.

■ Conclusion and Future Directions

As less-invasive techniques continue to develop, the morbidity of an ALIF/PLF will continue to decrease. We have already seen drastic improvements in patient satisfaction and clinical outcome with the obviation of iliac crest autograft harvest and shorted postoperative courses and return to work. The biomechanical data on ALIF/PLF remain unsurpassed, and we would anticipate that the improved restoration of disc height and sagittal balance via such a biomechanically stable construct will provide superior long-term clinical and radiographic results. The high

(97%) fusion rate for ALIF/PLF, as recently reported by Zigler et al,[13] also becomes significant in this era of cost-effective spine surgery, as none of the patients in their study received any commercially available osteoinductive graft materials (e.g., rhBMPs or DBMs), which have added a rapidly increasing cost to surgery. This study, which reflects our current experience, shows that no matter how future developments make the surgery less invasive and more expedient, the technical aspects of the surgical procedure remain paramount.

References

1. White AA, Panjabi MM. Clinical Biomechanics of the Spine. 2nd ed. Philadelphia: JB Lippincott; 1990
2. McAfee PC, DeVine JG, Chaput CD, et al. The indications for interbody fusion cages in the treatment of spondylolisthesis: analysis of 120 cases. Spine 2005;30(Suppl 1):S60–S65
3. Lund T, Oxland TR, Jost B, et al. Interbody cage stabilization in the lumbar spine: biomechanical evaluation of cage design, posterior instrumentation, and bone density. J Bone Joint Surg Br 1998;80:351–359
4. Lu WW, Luk KD, Holmes AD, Cheung KM, Leong JC. Pure shear properties of lumbar spinal joints and the effect of tissue sectioning on loadsharing. Spine 2005;30:E204–E209
5. Bagby GW. Arthrodesis by the distraction compression method using a stainless steel implant. Orthopedics 1988;11:931–934
6. Kettler A, Wilke HJ, Dietl R, et al. Stabilizing effect of posterior lumbar interbody fusion cages before and after cyclic loading. J Neurosurg 2000;92(Suppl 1):87–92
7. Videbaek TS, Christensen FB, Soegaard R, et al. Circumferential fusion improves outcome in comparison with instrumented posterolateral fusion: long-term results of a randomized clinical trial. Spine 2006;31:2875–2880
8. Christensen FB, Hansen ES, Eiskjaer SP, et al. Circumferential lumbar spinal fusion with Brantigan cage versus posterolateral fusion with titanium Cotrel-Dubousset instrumentation: a prospective, randomized clinical study of 146 patients. Spine 2002;27:2674–2683
9. Fritzell P, Hagg O, Wessberg P, et al. Chronic low back pain and fusion: a comparison of three surgical techniques: a prospective multicenter randomized study from the Swedish lumbar spine study group. Spine 2002;27:1131–1141
10. Oda I, Abumi K, Yu BS, Sudo H, Minami A. Types of spinal instability that require interbody support in posterior lumbar reconstruction: an in vitro biomechanical investigation. Spine 2003;28:1573–1580
11. Hinkley BS, Jaremko ME. Effects of 360 degree lumbar fusion in a workers' compensation population. Spine 1997;22:312–322
12. Moore KR, Pinto MR, Butler LM. Degenerative disc disease treated with combined anterior and posterior arthrodesis and posterior instrumentation. Spine 2002;27:1680–1686
13. Zigler J, Delamarter R, Spivak JM, et al. Results of the prospective, randomized, multicenter Food and Drug Administration investigational device exemption study of the ProDisc-L total disc replacement versus circumferential fusion for the treatment of 1-level degenerative disc disease. Spine 2007;32:1155–1162
14. Glazer PA, Colliou O, Klisch SM, Bradford DS, Bueff HU, Lotz JC. Biomechanical analysis of multilevel fixation methods in the lumbar spine. Spine 1997;22:171–182
15. Lund T, Oxland TR, Jost B, et al. Interbody cage stabilisation in the lumbar spine: a biomechanical evaluation of cage design, posterior instrumentation and bone density. J Bone Joint Surg Br 1998;80:351–359
16. Nibu K, Panjabi MM, Oxland T, Cholewicki J. Multidirectional stabilizing potential of BAK interbody spinal fusion system for anterior surgery. J Spinal Disord 1997;10:357–362
17. Oxland TR, Hoffer Z, Nydegger T, et al. A comparative biomechanical investigation of anterior lumbar interbody cages: central and bilateral approaches. J Bone Joint Surg Am 2000;82:383–393
18. Phillips FM, Cunningham B, Caradang G, et al. Effect of supplemental translaminar facet screw fixation on the stability of stand-alone ALIF cages under physiologic compressive loads. Spine 2004;29(16):1731–1736
19. Sudo H, Oda I, Abumi K, Ito M, Kotani Y, Minami A. Biomechanical study on the effect of five different lumbar reconstruction techniques on adjacent-level intradiscal pressure and lamina strain. J Neurosurg Spine 2006;5:150–155
20. Kanayama M, Hashimoto T, Shigenobu K, Oha F, Ishida T, Yamane S. Intraoperative biomechanical assessment of lumbar spinal instability: validation of radiographic parameters indicating anterior column support in lumbar spinal fusion. Spine 2003;28:2368–2372
21. Erulkar JS, Grauer JN, Patel TC, Panjabi MM. Flexibility analysis of posterolateral fusions in a New Zealand white rabbit model. Spine 2001;26:1125–1130
22. Totoribe K, Tajima N, Chosa E. A biomechanical study of posterolateral lumbar fusion using a three-dimensional nonlinear finite element method. J Orthop Sci 1999;4:115–126
23. Lee CK. Accelerated degradation of the segment adjacent to a lumbar fusion. Spine 1988;13:375–377
24. Ha KY, Kim YH. Bilateral pedicle stress fracture after instrumented posterolateral lumbar fusion: a case report. Spine 2003;28:E158–E160
25. Bono CM, Khandha A, Vadapalli S, Holekamp S, Goel VK, Garfin SR. Residual sagittal motion after lumbar fusion: a finite element analysis with implications on radiographic flexion–extension criteria. Spine 2007;32:417–422
26. Johnsson R, Stromqvist B, Axelsson P, et al. Influence of spinal immobilization on consolidation of posterolateral lumbosacral fusion: a roentgen stereophotogrammetric and radiographic analysis. Spine 1992;17:16–21
27. Manos R, Sukovich W, Weistroffer J. Transforaminal lumbar interbody fusion: minimally invasive versus open disc excision and endplate preparation. Paper presented at: International Meeting of Advanced Spine Techniques; July 7–9, 2005; Banff, Alberta, Canada
28. Goldstein JA, Macenski MJ, Griffith SL, McAfee PC. Lumbar sagittal alignment after fusion with a threaded interbody cage. Spine 2001;26:1137–1142
29. Pavlov PW, Meijers H, van Limbeek J, et al. Good outcome and restoration of lordosis after anterior lumbar interbody fusion with additional posterior fixation. Spine 2004;29:1893–1899

30. Vaidya R, Weir R, Sethi A, Meisterling S, Hakeos W, Wybo CD. Interbody fusion with allograft and rhBMP-2 leads to consistent fusion but early subsidence. J Bone Joint Surg Br 2007;89:342–345

31. Pradhan BB, Bae HW, Dawson EG, Patel VV, Delamarter RB. Graft resorption with the use of bone morphogenetic protein: lessons from anterior lumbar interbody fusion using femoral ring allografts and recombinant human bone morphogenetic protein-2. Spine 2006; 31:E277–E284

32. Choi JY, Sung KH. Subsidence after anterior lumbar interbody fusion using paired stand-alone rectangular cages. Eur Spine J 2006;15:16–22

33. Brau SA. Mini-open approach to the spine for anterior lumbar interbody fusion: description of the procedure, results and complications. Spine J 2002;2:216–223

34. Burton D, McIff T, Fox T, Lark R, Asher MA, Glattes RC. Biomechanical analysis of posterior fixation techniques in a 360 degrees arthrodesis model. Spine 2005;30:2765–2771

35. Fernandez-Fairen M, Sala P, Ramirez H, Gil J. A prospective randomized study of unilateral versus bilateral instrumented posterolateral lumbar fusion in degenerative spondylolisthesis. Spine 2007; 32:395–401

36. Suk KS, Lee HM, Kim NH, Ha JW. Unilateral versus bilateral pedicle screw fixation in lumbar spinal fusion. Spine 2000;25:1843–1847

37. Beringer WF, Mobasser JP. Unilateral pedicle screw instrumentation for minimally invasive transforaminal lumbar interbody fusion. Neurosurg Focus 2006;20:E4

38. Lowe TG, Tahernia AD, O'Brien MF, Smith DA. Unilateral transforaminal posterior lumbar interbody fusion (TLIF): indications, technique, and 2-year results. J Spinal Disord Tech 2002;15:31–38

39. Spencer DL, DeWald RL. Simultaneous anterior and posterior surgical approach to the thoracic and lumbar spine. Spine 1979;4:29–36

40. Walker E. 2-staged surgical procedure for more effective surgical relief of chronic disabling low back and sciatic pain. J Neurol Orthop Surg 1983;4:109

41. O'Brien JP, Dawson MHO, Heard CW, et al. Simultaneous combined anterior and posterior fusion: a surgical solution for failed spinal surgery with a brief review of the first 150 patients. Clin Orthop Relat Res 1986;203:191–195

42. Kozak JA, O'Brien JP. Simultaneous combined anterior and posterior fusion. An independent analysis of a treatment for the disabled low-back pain patient. Spine 1990;15:322–328

43. Nachemson A, Zdeblick TA, O'Brien JP. Lumbar disc disease with discogenic pain: what surgical treatment is most effective? Spine 1996;21:1835–1838

44. Fraser RD. Interbody, posterior, and combined lumbar fusions. Spine 1995;20(Suppl):S167–S177

45. Hacker RJ. Comparison of interbody fusion approaches for disabling low back pain. Spine 1997;22:660–665

46. Villavicencio AT, Burneikiene S, Bulsara KR, Thramann JJ. Perioperative complications in transforaminal lumbar interbody fusion versus anterior-posterior reconstruction for lumbar disc degeneration and instability. J Spinal Disord Tech 2006;19:92–97

29 Minimally Invasive Spinal Fusion Procedures

Mark P. Kuper, Mark C. Valente, William R. Taylor, and Choll W. Kim

Conventional open spinal approaches require extensive dissections to allow for the identification of anatomic landmarks for instrumentation and graft placement. Multiple studies have demonstrated that these approaches lead to paraspinal muscle atrophy and scarring with impaired spinal function.[1–6]

Open surgery requires prolonged tissue retraction that is associated with elevated contact pressures, tissue ischemia, decreased muscle density, and paraspinal electromyographic abnormalities.[1,5–8] Gejo and associates[3] studied 80 patients who underwent open lumbar surgery. They noted that prolonged retraction time resulted in a decrease in trunk muscle strength. The study also correlated prolonged retraction times to an increased incidence of low back pain. In addition, Datta et al[7] demonstrated that muscle retraction time was proportional to pain and disability scores.

Minimally invasive surgery (MIS) techniques have the potential to decrease the amount of muscle injury by using tubular retractors that produce less tissue ischemia.[9,10] In addition, these techniques eliminate muscle stripping that may denervate the paraspinal musculature. Several postoperative comparisons between open and MIS fusion techniques have supported this claim. Kim et al[10] compared open and MIS posterior fusion patients. The study demonstrated that there is a significant decrease in the multifidus muscle cross-sectional area and a clinically significant decrease in trunk extension strength seen only in the open posterior fusion patients.[10] In a similar study, Stevens et al[9] compared the magnetic resonance images (MRIs) taken from patients that underwent posterolateral lumbar fusion by either a standard open or a minimally invasive approach. They reported "striking visual differences in muscle edema" in the open posterolateral lumbar fusion group of patients compared with the minimally invasive patient group.[9] Hyun et al[11] retrospectively assessed a group of patients that underwent unilateral transforaminal lumbar interbody fusion (TLIF) with ipsilateral instrumented posterior spinal fusion via a standard open midline approach. An additional contralateral instrumented posterior spinal fusion was performed at the same level, employing a paramedian intermuscular approach. Postoperatively, there was a significant decrease in the cross-sectional area of the multifidus on the side of the midline approach. On the contralateral side

where the paramedian approach was used, no reduction in the multifidus cross-sectional area was measured.

The aforementioned muscle and soft tissue injury that result from open surgery have led to an intense focus to perform less tissue-disruptive spinal fusions. MIS fusions strive to follow several key concepts. First, the exposure should be limited to only the target surgical site, limiting the unnecessary resection of bone, tendons, and muscle. Through preoperative planning, the most direct surgical approach to the pathology is identified. When possible, the surgeon should utilize intermuscular, internervous, and/or intervascular planes to develop the surgical corridor. Second, elevated contact pressures that result from retraction must be avoided. Finally, surgeons should exploit the interbody space to achieve fusions. The interbody space not only provides for the best fusion environment but also constitutes an isolated tissue compartment. The ultimate goal of any MIS spine fusion is to limit surgical morbidity while achieving radiographic arthrodesis rates comparable to conventional open surgery.

■ Minimally Invasive Posterior Spinal Fusion

Posterolateral Fusion

Watkins[12] first described the posterolateral fusion (intertransverse process fusion) in 1953, which yielded superior to previous fusion techniques. This soon became the standard fusion procedure of choice for decades to come. Despite its popularity, it required an extensive soft tissue dissection to span the distance between the transverse processes, especially when a midline incision is used. MIS posterolateral lumbar fusions, on the other hand, can be done via a Wiltse approach using blunt dissection and gentle retraction. This approach therefore has the potential to limit muscle injury from denervation and retraction-induced ischemia.

Surgical Technique

In the posterior intermuscular (Wiltse) approach, the intraoperative C-arm is used to localize the midpoint between adjacent transverse processes to be fused ~4 cm off the

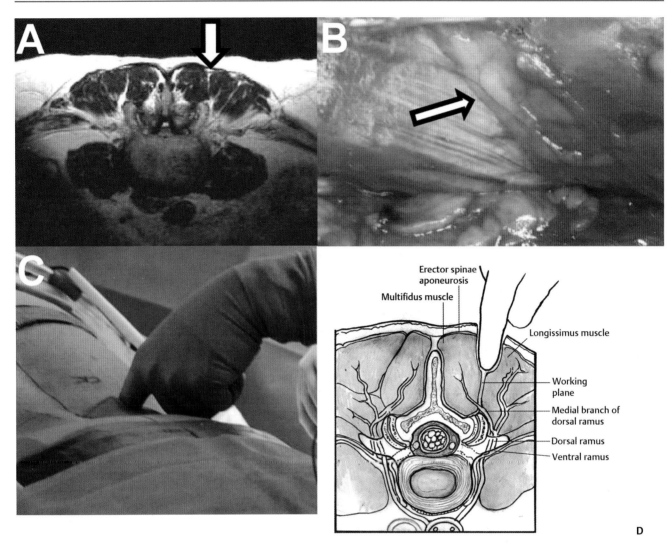

Fig. 29.1 **(A)** The cross-sectional anatomy as viewed on the axial MRI scan shows the intermuscular plane between the multifidus and longissimus muscles (*solid arrow*). **(B)** Once the incision is made, blunt finger dissection develops the plane between the multifidus and the longissimus muscles thereby preserving the neurovascular supply to the musculature (*arrow to nerve*). Intraoperative photo **(C)** and illustration **(D)** of finger dissection technique.

midline. A 2.5-cm longitudinal skin incision is then centered over this point. The dissection and decortication of the transverse processes can be achieved through expandable tubular retractors (**Fig. 29.1**).

Transforaminal Lumbar Interbody Fusion

By exploiting the interbody compartment, surgeons gain a large surface area to increase fusion rates. Interbody fusions also aid in deformity correction and better restore intervertebral height, which, in turn, can increase neuroforaminal and central canal volume. When considering a posterior approach for interbody fusions, two approaches are common: the TLIF and the posterior lumbar interbody fusion (PLIF). The TLIF has gained popularity in past years due to several advantages over PLIF. Because the TLIF approach is more lateral, less dural retraction is required to perform a discectomy and interbody fusion. This theoretically decreases the risk of iatrogenic neurologic injury and allows this technique to be safely used above L3. The PLIF technique, on the other hand, requires bilateral neural retraction. The 10% incidence of transient neurologic complications historically associated with the PLIF is likely due to excessive retraction and manipulation of the roots and thecal sac.[13]

Multiple authors have recently reported on the safe and effective use of MIS TLIF techniques for refractory mechanical low-back and radicular pain associated with spondylolisthesis, degenerative disc disease, and recurrent disc herniation.[14–17] Schwender et al[17] reported on 49 patients who underwent MIS TLIF through a paramedian, muscle-sparing approach using an expandable tubular retractor system. Of these patients, 26 patients had degenerative disc disease with herniated nucleus pulposus, 22 had spondylolisthesis, and 1 had a Chance-type fracture as the primary diagnosis. The minimum follow-up was 18 months with a mean follow-up of 22.6 months. Operative time averaged 240 minutes (110 to 310 minutes), average estimated blood loss was 140 mL (50 to 450 mL). No patients required a blood transfusion and there were no intraoperative complications. Length of hospital stay was 1.9 days on average (1 to 4 days). All 45 patients who had preoperative radicular symptoms had resolution of their symptoms. All patients with mechanical low back pain (LBP) had postoperative improvement of their pain. There were four complications noted postoperatively (two from malpositioned screws, one from graft dislodgement causing new radiculopathy, and the last from radiculopathy caused by contralateral neuroforaminal stenosis). Visual Analog Scale pain scores improved from 7.2 to 2.1, and Oswestry Disability Index scores improved from 46% to 14% at last follow-up.

Surgical Technique

The patient is placed prone. Intraoperative fluoroscopy is used to confirm the appropriate level and to position the patient in a true anteroposterior (AP) position relative to the floor. Longitudinal and transverse lines are drawn to delineate the landmarks to the spine. With the C-arm in the perfect lateral position, the initial dilator is positioned ~4 cm from the midline and directly in line with the disc space (**Fig. 29.2A**). A 2- to 3-cm longitudinal skin incision is centered over this entry point. The skin and dorsolumbar fascia are incised sharply with a scalpel followed by blunt digital dissection through the intermuscular plane between the multifidus and longissimus. This will place the tip of the finger at the lateral aspect of the superior articular process (SAP) as shown in **Fig. 29.1**.

The facet joint is palpated and a periosteal Cobb elevator is used to gently release the tendinous attachments of the facet joint and hemilamina of the cephalad level. Using the lateral fluoroscopic image, dilators are inserted to sequentially surround the facet joint. With gentle downward pressure, firm twisting motions of the dilators will help dilate and clear soft tissue away from the facet joint (**Fig. 29.2B**). Once the final dilator is placed, the retractor is inserted over the final dilator and placed in line with the disc space (**Fig. 29.2C**). A rigid articulating arm is attached to the retractor blade and fixed to the operative table.

The surgeon should always maintain constant downward pressure to prevent the retractor from backing out from the surgical site. A light source can then be attached to the retractor blades to illuminate the deep exposure. Final blade adjustments are then performed. Radiographically, the cephalad blade should expand to the inferior aspect of the superior pedicle. Likewise, the caudal retractor blade should expand for exposure to the superior aspect of the inferior pedicle. The surgical corridor will visualize the base of the spinous process, the cephalad inferior articular process and pars interarticularis, and the lateral edge of the caudal SAP (**Fig. 29.2D,E**).

A bayoneted electrocautery tip is used to gently expose these bony landmarks. A curette is used to sweep soft tissue out and under the retractor blades and a pituitary rongeur is used to remove any remaining soft tissue within the confines of the retractor.

A high speed matchstick drill, combined with fine curettes and Kerrison rongeurs, is used to remove the entire IAP and pars interarticularis. The ligamentum flavum is kept as a protective layer over the dural tube. Once a laminotomy window is identified, fine Kerrison rongeurs are used to complete the dorsal decompression. Removing bone at the base of the spinous process provides direct access to the opposite neuroforamen. A decompression of the contralateral nerve root is possible by undercutting the facet joint and thus achieving a full decompression of the canal (**Fig. 29.2E,F**).

The facetectomy is taken from the inferior margin of the cephalad pedicle and the superior margin of the caudal pedicle. This "pedicle-to-pedicle" exposure allows for a true transforaminal trajectory when performing the discectomy and placing the interbody spacer. The anulus is exposed medial and inferior to the exiting nerve root in the Kambin triangle (**Fig. 29.3A**). Abundant epidural veins are present and should be preemptively coagulated with a long, bayoneted bipolar electrocautery. Extreme care should be taken to avoid using the bipolar electrocautery near the dorsal root ganglion of the exiting nerve root (**Fig. 29.3A**). The discectomy is subsequently performed using a variety of specialized angled instruments. Even through this limited exposure, an aggressive discectomy and endplate preparation can be accomplished. The disc space is sized with a smooth trial (such as a rounded paddle distracter) and the spacer is diagonal across the interspace (**Fig. 29.3B–E**). A preferred technique is to use banana-shaped spacers that can be maneuvered into the anterior midline position. This places the spacer on the strong apophyseal ring and furthest away from the posterior tension band as well as creating additional space for bone graft. Autologous bone graft (usually from the facetectomy is combined) and/or bone morphogenetic protein are typically used to achieve the fusion.

Special consideration should be given to the insertion of the interbody spacer. In open TLIF techniques, the dorsolumbar fascia is incised. This allows the disc space to be adequately distracted using lamina spreaders between the lamina or spinous processes. In contrast to open TLIF techniques, the MIS TLIF techniques maintain the integrity of the dorsolumbar fascia. This makes distraction of the disc space extremely challenging. Without this distraction, the exiting and traversing nerve roots are at risk of injury during interbody spacer insertion. There are several techniques to overcome this obstacle. One reliable strategy is to use an insertion tool that acts as a shoe horn to open the disc space as the implant is inserted (**Fig. 29.3B–E**). Other techniques include the use of contralateral or ipsilateral

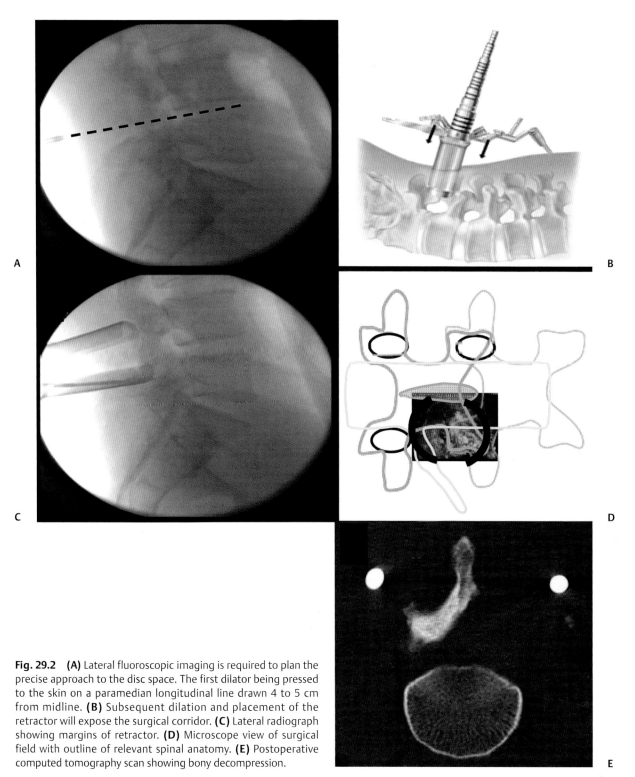

Fig. 29.2 **(A)** Lateral fluoroscopic imaging is required to plan the precise approach to the disc space. The first dilator being pressed to the skin on a paramedian longitudinal line drawn 4 to 5 cm from midline. **(B)** Subsequent dilation and placement of the retractor will expose the surgical corridor. **(C)** Lateral radiograph showing margins of retractor. **(D)** Microscope view of surgical field with outline of relevant spinal anatomy. **(E)** Postoperative computed tomography scan showing bony decompression.

(Continued on page 252)

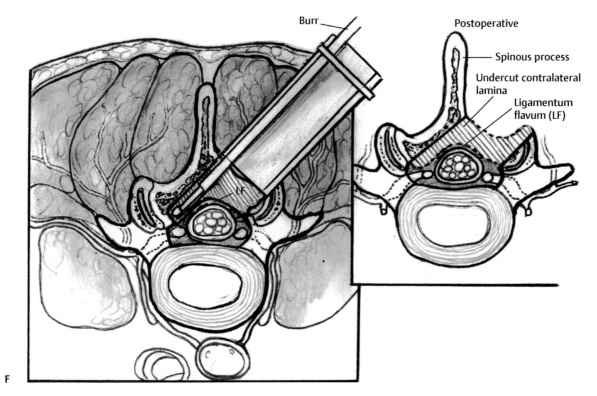

Fig. 29.2 *(Continued)* **(F)** The retractor is angled medially to undercut the base of the spinous process, thus allowing a contralateral decompression. LF, ligamentum flavum.

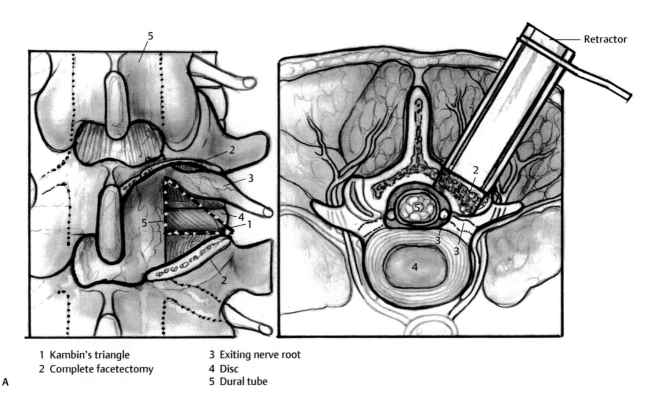

1 Kambin's triangle
2 Complete facetectomy
3 Exiting nerve root
4 Disc
5 Dural tube

Fig. 29.3 Once the surgical corridor is established, the facetectomy and decompression are performed. **(A)** Discectomy is performed in Kambin's triangle.

(Continued)

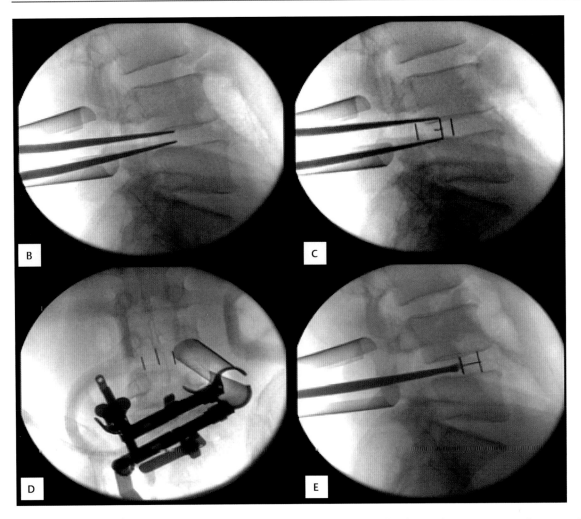

Fig. 29.3 *(Continued)* **(B–E)** After a complete discectomy, graft insertion is aided with special instrumentation that opens the disc space and protects the traversing and exiting nerve roots.

pedicle screws (placed at the beginning of the procedure) to maintain distraction. In some cases, adequate lumbar kyphosis using a Wilson frame may be sufficient to allow safe interbody implant insertion. Percutaneous pedicle screw instrumentation is used for stabilization (discussed below). A posterior fusion can be performed through a matching contralateral incision through which the surgeon can decorticate the contralateral facet and/or transverse processes. In most cases, the interbody arthrodesis alone will be sufficient to achieve a fusion.

■ Minimally Invasive Anterior Spinal Fusion

Anterior Lumbar Interbody Fusion

Anterior lumbar interbody fusion (ALIF) was first described in 1932 by Capener[18] and in 1933 by Burns.[19] Since that time, minimal access techniques have been developed and applied

to this technique. Today, ALIF may be achieved through transperitoneal laparoscopic, endoscopic retroperitoneal, and mini-open retroperitoneal approaches. In general, ALIF procedures avoid dural injury and the epidural scarring seen with posterior interbody fusion. Interbody grafts can also be placed with minimal risk to nerve roots. In general, larger grafts may be placed through the anterior approach, which corrects sagittal plane deformity through intervertebral height restoration. Disadvantages of the ALIF involve mobilization of the great vessels.

Laparoscopy-assisted transperitoneal or balloon-assisted retroperitoneal anterior lumbar fusion procedures have fallen out of favor in recent years in lieu of the less technically demanding mini-open techniques.[20,21] Laparoscopy-assisted ALIF typically requires three or four portals, each 1 to 2 cm in size. When the retroperitoneum is accessed, the fat must be bluntly dissected to avoid damage to the parasympathetic plexus. Most commonly, interbody fusion with this technique is performed at the L5–S1 interspace as the bifurcation of the great vessels is typically cephalad.

This approach is more difficult at L4–L5, as the aorta and vena cava often need to be mobilized. Additionally, the iliolumbar vein possesses some risk and should be ligated and divided if identified.

In 1995, two studies were published on laparoscopic ALIF.[22,23] One study found that laparoscopic anterior interbody fusion was associated with less blood loss and a shorter hospital stay than open anterolateral interbody fusion. However, it was associated with longer operative times and significantly higher complication rates (20% versus 4% for open surgeries).[24] When compared with mini-open anterolateral interbody fusion, the laparoscopic technique has also shown higher complication rates including retrograde ejaculation in males and vein laceration.[25,26] Other studies have shown complication rates from 10 to 20% including the need to convert to open procedures as a result of inadequate exposure and/or vascular injury.[27,28]

The paramedian, muscle splitting mini-open ALIF approach minimizes the incidence of exposure-related complications seen with the laparoscopic approach. Saraph and colleagues published a study comparing 33 patients who underwent conventional ALIF versus 23 patients who underwent mini-open ALIF.[29] Mean clinical follow-up was 5.5 years. They found no statistically significant difference in complications or fusion rates between the two groups. The mini-open approach did demonstrate significantly less intraoperative blood loss and operation time. In addition, the minimally invasive group showed significant improvement in postoperative back pain versus the conventional group. Today, the technique described by Mazer and modified by Brau et al remains the most popular minimally invasive technique.[30] The mini-open technique offers the benefits of minimally invasive surgery with less overall morbidity compared with laparoscopic or conventional open ALIF procedures.

Lateral Interbody Fusion

The lateral transpsoas approach is gaining popularity as an alternative minimally invasive technique for anterior interbody fusion. Gaur and McDougall et al were the first to describe a retroperitoneal approach for urologic procedures.[31,32] McAfee and associates published the first clinical series using a minimally invasive endoscopic lateral retroperitoneal approach for lumbar fusions.[33] The study demonstrated mean intraoperative blood loss of 205 mL, a mean hospital stay of 2.9 days, and no cases of implant migration or pseudarthrosis at a mean follow-up of 24.3 months. However, the technical difficulties of using the endoscope gave way to the direct lateral approach using expandable tubular retractors. Ozgur et al later reported on a series of 13 patients that underwent an extreme lateral interbody fusion (XLIF) procedure. The authors reported that there were no complications, transfusions, or intensive care admissions.[34]

Initial results suggest that XLIF is a safe and reproducible minimally invasive technique for anterior lumbar interbody fusion. This technique uses live, real-time neural monitoring while traversing the psoas muscle to access the lateral aspect of the disc. Rapid improvements in pain and function scores have been reported.[34] A key advantage of the lateral approach technique is the placement of the interbody spacer across the entire disc space (**Fig. 29.4**). This allows the implant to rest on the apophyseal ring, which remains the strongest portion of the endplate. The strength of the apophyseal ring, combined with the large size of the interbody spacer and the tethering effect of the anterior and posterior longitudinal ligament, allows for dramatic deformity correction. Sagittal balance can be maintained or improved by placing the implant anterior. Correction of coronal balance, as seen in degenerative scoliosis, can be achieved by placing the implant across the entire width of the interbody space.

The disadvantages to the lateral approach include iatrogenic injury to the psoas and the lumbosacral plexus. This is especially of concern when working at the L4–L5 interspace where the lumbar plexus rests farthest anteriorly, often at the midbody position where the discectomy is performed. The lumbar plexus resides more posteriorly in the L3–L4 levels and above. Furthermore, the iliac wing precludes access to the L5–S1 level. The lateral approach is therefore best suited for fusion of L2–L3, L3–L4, and L4–L5 using a retroperitoneal approach. The L1–L2 level is best accessed through a transthoracic approach with a small opening in the crus of the diaphragm. The transthoracic direct lateral approach also facilitates ready access to the thoracic spine up to T6. Similar to MIS TLIF, the XLIF may be coupled with percutaneous pedicle screw fixation. It is likely that anterior fixation systems will be developed to eliminate the need for adjunctive posterior fixation.

Surgical Technique

Meticulous positioning is a critical aspect of the procedure. The patient is placed in the lateral decubitus position. The patient should be positioned so that the bend in the table lies between the iliac crest and the greater trochanter. Once positioned, the patient must be secured to the operating table at the level of the greater trochanter and the shoulders. The operative table is now flexed to separate the iliac crest and the rib cage and to clear the iliac wing away from the L4–L5 level. A sterile C-arm is then brought under the table, where it is locked at 180 degrees. The surgical table is rotated to obtain a perfect anteroposterior (AP) image of the spine, thereby placing the patient in a true lateral position relative to the floor. By maintaining the trajectory of the instrumentation in a vertically straight position, the need for repetitive lateral C-arm imaging can be avoided.

With the C-arm in the upright position, the lateral image is used to mark the landmarks to the spine. The target disc is identified and a longitudinal 2.5-mm incision is marked and anesthetized with local anesthetic. From the lateral incision, blunt dissection is performed through the soft tissue until the retroperitoneal space is reached. Care should be taken not to perforate the peritoneum. The surgeon then bluntly sweeps the peritoneum anteriorly with the index finger. Some surgeons prefer using a small second posterior paraspinal incision through which a finger is introduced to clear the retroperitoneal space in an effort to ensure the safe placement of the laterally introduced dilators on the psoas muscle as described in the XLIF technique (**Fig. 29.4A**).

As the blunt finger dissection deepens, the surgeon will appreciate the psoas muscle, which is characteristically spongy and smooth to the touch. The transverse processes should also be palpated to confirm the exposure is in the anterior compartment. The first dilator is placed through the lateral incision, guided toward the psoas muscle with the surgeon's index finger. The blunt dilator initially rests on the anterior one third of the spongy psoas muscle. Lateral fluoroscopy aids the surgeon to position the dilator

directly over the disc space (**Fig. 29.4B**). A gentle back and forth "twirling" motion is used to spread the fibers of the psoas muscle as the first dilator is advanced to the disc space. With the initial dilator positioned directly over the midpoint of the disc, a guide wire is inserted into the disc. The C-arm is then brought under the table for an AP, image, and the subsequent dilators are advanced with a similar back and forth twirling motion with great care not to injure the lumbar plexus that lies in the posterior third of the psoas muscle. As the dilators are placed, an evoked electromyographic monitoring system allows detection of nerve roots within the surgical path. The nerve monitoring system emits an electrical signal that will search for the stimulus threshold of the lumbar nerves. When the nerve is triggered, it will be detected via the electromyographic monitoring on the distal extremities. It is preferable to use this nerve detection system during insertion of the retractor, particularly at L4–L5.

Once a thorough evaluation of the retractor's position is complete by visual inspection and fluoroscopy, the retractor is solidly fixed by the retractor arm and the guide wire is removed. Visualization through the tubular retractor is

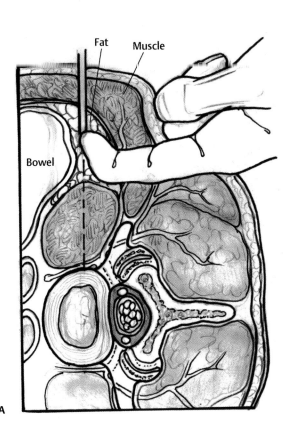 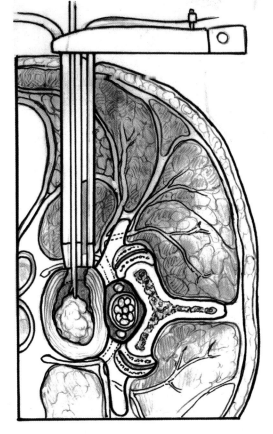

Fig. 29.4 The direct lateral approach relies on radiographic guidance for an accurate trajectory. **(A)** In addition to the working portal on the lateral flank, an additional posterior paramedian incision can be made to aid retroperitoneal dissection and safe passage of the initial dilator (*left*). The panel on the right shows the retractor placed through the psoas muscle and the grasping rongeur within the disk space.

(Continued on page 256)

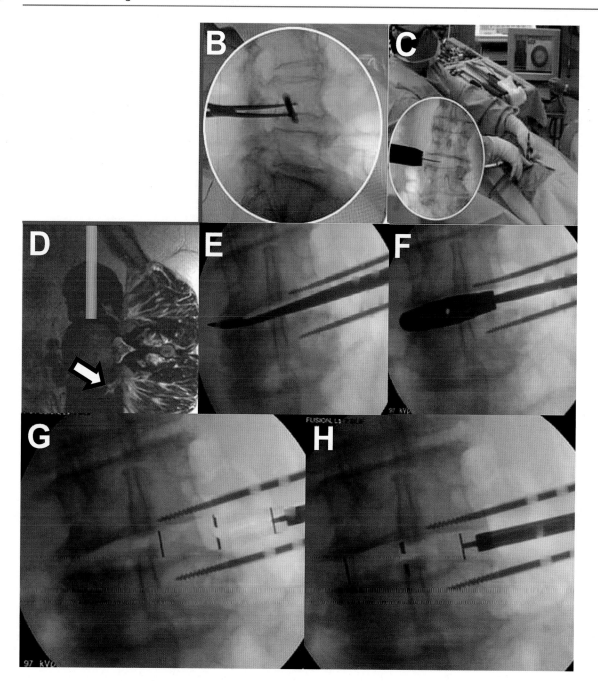

Fig. 29.4 *(Continued)*   **(B)** The initial dilator is docked on the disc at the midline. A guide wire is inserted through the dilator and into the disc. **(C)** The C-arm is then brought under the table for an anteroposterior image. Once the guide pin is placed, sequential dilation is performed followed by deployment of the retractor. **(D)** The surgical corridor is through the psoas muscle. Neuromonitoring is used to avoid the exiting nerve root, which can be near the midline at L4–L5 (*arrow* shows fat surrounding nerve root). **(E)** The Cobb elevator is used to release the contralateral anulus. **(F)** Smooth trials are used to dilate the disc space to restore disc height. **(G,H)** The large interbody spacer is inserted spanning the entire width of the vertebral body and resting on the apophyseal rings. Dramatic coronal and sagittal correction can be achieved with this technique.

enhanced by a fiberoptic light source. Further blunt dissection with bayoneted instrumentation is important to delineate the vertebral anatomy and expose the annulotomy site.

Long curettes, paddle shavers, and dilators are utilized for the discectomy. A Cobb elevator can be used to release the contralateral anulus (**Fig. 29.4C**). The release of the contralateral anulus is necessary if disc space restoration is desired. Extreme care should be used to pass the elevator in a perfectly lateral trajectory to avoid inadvertent injury to the great vessels anteriorly. Care must also be taken to avoid injury to the segmental vessels lying at the midvertebral body wall. The disc space is serially dilated with smooth trials of increasing size (**Fig. 29.4F**). The interbody implant is large, spanning the entire width of the vertebral body. This allows the implant to rest on the strong bony shelf of the apophyseal ring (**Fig. 29.4G,H**).

■ Minimally Invasive Spinal Pedicle Screw Placement

Pedicle screws provide stability during the fusion process. There are several minimally invasive techniques to place pedicle screws. The mini-open technique exposes the pedicle entry point for direct visualization. Unfortunately, this mini-open technique requires electrocautery dissection of the lateral aspect of the SAP where the multifidus tendons attach. The least invasive method utilizes a percutaneous technique as described below.

Surgical Technique

The patient is placed prone on a radiolucent table. Biplanar fluoroscopy can facilitate percutaneous screw placement. A perfect AP image is obtained by rotating the patient in relation to a fully upright C-arm. A Jamshidi needle is then placed through a small paramedian stab incision. If an MIS TLIF was performed, the same paramedian TLIF incision is used. Using fluoroscopy, the Jamshidi needle is docked on the lateral pedicle margin, midway between the superior and inferior aspects of the pedicle (**Fig. 29.5**). With subtle caudal and cephalad adjustments of the surgeon's hand, the needle can be adjusted. Each time the needle is advanced, fluoroscopic images should be obtained. To avoid excessive radiation to the surgeon's hand, hold the needle with a ringed towel clamp when obtaining fluoroscopic images. Gentle taps advance the tip into bone. Generally, we start with the bevel laterally (tip medially). By doing so, the needle advances from lateral to medial across the pedicle. The bevel is especially useful if the needle advances toward an undesired position. By simply rotating the tip, the needle can cut an improved trajectory across the pedicle.

The needle is advanced ~20 mm in the AP plane. If the correct trajectory has been taken, the needle should pass into the pedicle in a medial direction. By maintaining the tip lateral to the medial border of the pedicle wall, perforation into the canal is avoided. By doing so, the surgeon will not need to monitor the needle by lateral fluoroscopy. The goal is to advance the needle to the posterior vertebral body while not crossing the medial aspect of the pedicle on the AP view. The C-arm is then brought under the table for a lateral image. A guide wire is gently tapped 5 mm past the Jamshidi needle. The surgeon should carefully probe with the guide wire and be confident that bone is indeed engaged prior to tapping the guide wire. It is imperative that the guide wire is controlled at all times to avoid inadvertent advancement that could lead to catastrophic injury to the great vessels anteriorly. Sequential soft tissue dilators are used to create a path for the tap and screw. The outermost dilator can be used as a protective sleeve during pedicle tapping. As each level is tapped, hand position is monitored in relation to the guide wire to avoid advancement of the wire or cutting the guide wire by the sharp flutes of the tap. A cannulated pedicle screw is then placed over the guide wire. When the contralateral pedicle screw is placed, its position should be checked on AP, lateral, and oblique images in line with the pedicle. Segmental fixation is possible with various percutaneous rod insertion systems (**Fig. 29.6**).

■ Potential Pitfalls, Complications, and Drawbacks

The single-most important pitfall of MIS surgery is its difficult learning curve. MIS techniques deviate markedly from traditional spine training concepts. New paradigms must be appreciated during each step of the procedure. Seemingly straightforward tasks such as implant insertion, rod passage, endplate preparation, and decompression can be extremely difficult if specific methodologies are not strictly followed. For example, the intact dorsolumbar fascia prevents the use of a lamina spreader to distract the disc space during interbody cage insertion. If the retractor is not placed directly in line with the disc space, it may be impossible to perform an adequate discectomy. If curettes, rongeurs, and probes are not of the correct length, diameter, or angle, they may not fit down the MIS retractor. These drawbacks are mostly technical and thus amenable to correction through simple advancements in instrument design.

The limited exposure of MIS surgery can also lead to loss of anatomic orientation. If this is not appreciated, significant complications may be encountered, such as vessel laceration, nerve injury, and inadvertent durotomy. The repair of a durotomy is difficult through an MIS exposure. Various patch systems or fibrin sealants can be applied to the tear.

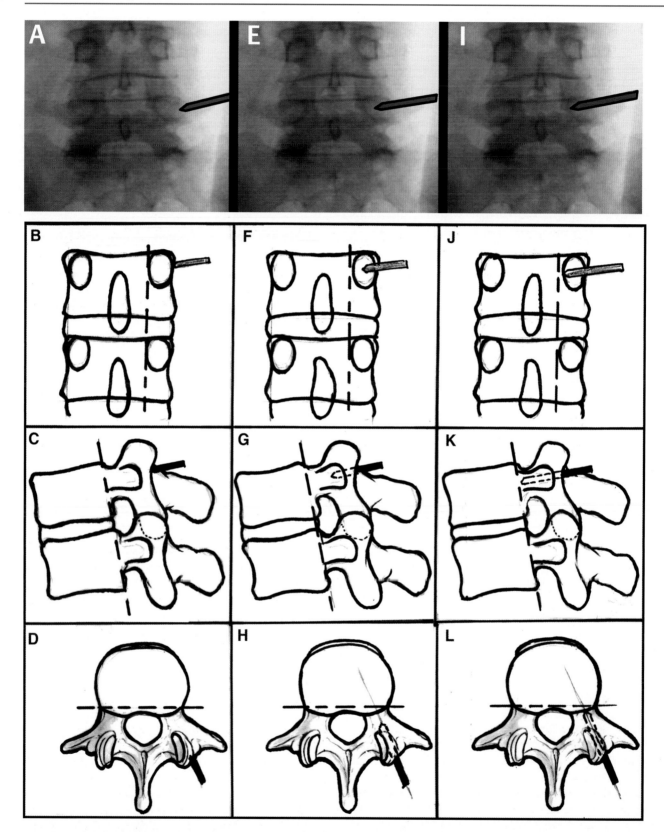

Fig. 29.5 The percutaneous pedicle screw placement illustration demonstrates the accurate starting point and controlled advancement of the Jamshidi needle across the pedicle to the posterior vertebral body without medial breach. **(A–D)** Initial docking point on anteroposterior x-ray, with corresponding anteroposterior, lateral, and axial illustrations. **(E–H)** The Jamshidi needle halfway across pedicle. **(I–L)** Position of the needle at the posterior aspect of the vertebral body after it has safely passed through the pedicle.

The lateral approach procedure offers some unique risks. The segmental vertebral vessels are at risk during this approach if the approach is away from the disc level. These vessels are generally encountered during corpectomies or from aberrant retractor pins placed into the midvertebral level. Immediate tamponade with long peanut elevators along with gentle electrocautery is usually sufficient to halt bleeding. Second, lateral approaches are associated with postoperative groin and/or thigh pain in ~30% of patients.

These symptoms are usually transient and generally do not last longer than a month.[35] Patients may also experience hip flexor weakness likely due to swelling of the psoas muscle itself. Patients should be counseled on this unique postoperative effect, which is usually mild and transient.

In all MIS fusion techniques, the use of fluoroscopy is imperative to remain anatomically oriented. Meticulous use of fluoroscopy begins as early as patient positioning and lasts through final implant insertion. Because of this,

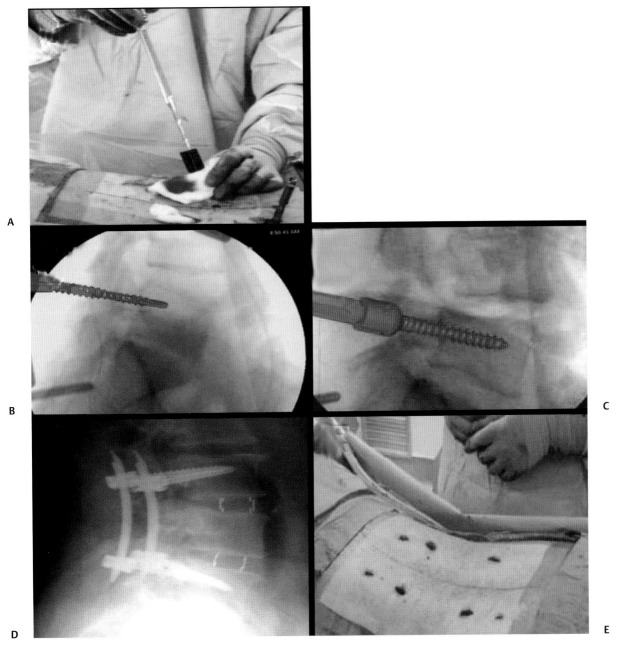

Fig. 29.6 Soft tissue dilation over a guide wire allows for cannulated tapping **(A)** and screw placement **(F)**. Computer navigation may be used to decrease radiation exposure during tapping **(B)** and pedicle **(C)** screw insertion. Percutaneous rod systems allow for segmental fixation **(D, G)** with only small stab incisions that minimize soft tissue trauma **(E)**.

(Continued on page 260)

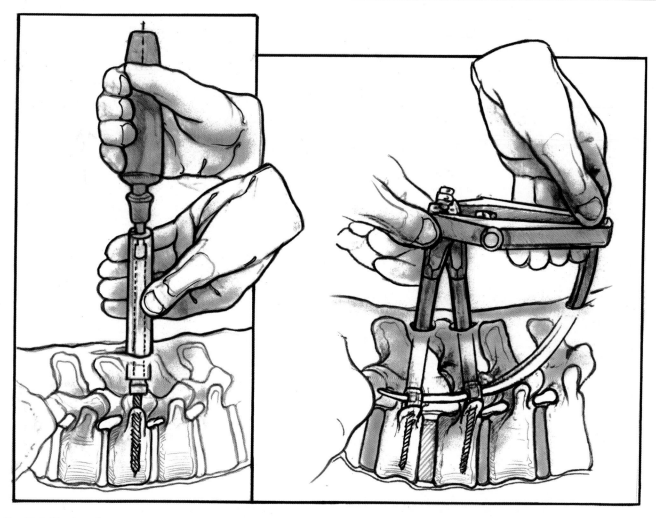

F   G

Fig. 29.6 (Continued)

the cumulative radiation exposure raises significant concerns. Recently, a study demonstrated that an average 3.3 minutes of fluoroscopic exposure was required per level instrumented.[36] Placement of pedicle screws with standard fluoroscopy has been shown to expose the spine surgeon to 10 to 12 times the ionizing radiation of nonspinal musculoskeletal procedures.[37,38]

Several options exist to lessen the radiation exposure. The two main categories are image guidance/navigation and robotics. Navigation systems permit "virtual" visualization of anatomy thus allowing immediate identification of anatomic landmarks in multiple planes (**Fig. 29.6C,D**). The use of navigation systems can dramatically decrease the cumulative radiation exposure to the entire surgical team.[39] Operating rooms of the future will likely be equipped with robotics. Studies of a miniature robotic guide have demonstrated accuracy to 1 mm of the planned placement.[40] Radiation exposure is minimal and the time for placement of

pedicle screws is about half as long when compared with standard fluoroscopy.[40]

■ Conclusion

As with all surgical procedures, spine surgery will evolve to become less invasive. This involves more than smaller incisions. MIS techniques strive to limit unnecessary injury to surrounding soft tissues; use intermuscular, internervous, and intervascular planes when possible; avoid elevated retractor pressures; and exploit the interbody compartment when fusions are necessary. Through MIS practices, there is decreased pain and quicker recovery. It is possible through soft tissue preservation that there will be long-term benefits. It is intriguing to postulate that long-term processes such as adjacent-level degeneration may be mitigated through the unhindered action of the paraspinal muscular complex. Similarly, the longevity of motion devices may be increased when the function of the paraspinal soft tissues is preserved. The indications and technologies for MIS are currently evolving. The technology to perform not only decompression but also fusion, deformity correction, and complex reconstruction are being developed. It is clear that there are significant conceptual differences between MIS and traditional open spine surgery. Working in confined spaces without landmarks fosters a dependence on fluoroscopy and consequently exposes the surgeon to potentially harmful ionizing radiation. These new challenges must be addressed to sustain meaningful progress in the field of minimally invasive spine surgery.

References

1. Kawaguchi Y, Matsui H, Tsuji H. Back muscle injury after posterior lumbar spine surgery: a histologic and enzymatic analysis. Spine 1996;21(8):941–944
2. Foley KT, Gupta SK, Justis JR, Sherman ME. Percutaneous pedicle screw fixation of the lumbar spine. Neurosurg Focus 2001;10(4):E10
3. Gejo R, Matsui H, Kawaguchi Y, Ishihara H, Tsuji H. Serial changes in trunk muscle performance after posterior lumbar surgery. Spine 1999;24(10):1023–1028
4. Mayer TG, Vanharanta H, Gatchel RJ, et al. Comparison of CT scan muscle measurements and isokinetic trunk strength in postoperative patients. Spine 1989;14(1):33–36
5. Rantanen J, Hurme M, Falck B, et al. The lumbar multifidus muscle five years after surgery for a lumbar intervertebral disc herniation. Spine 1993;18(5):568–574
6. Sihvonen T, Herno A, Paljarvi L, Airaksinen O, Partanen J, Tapaninaho A. Local denervation atrophy of paraspinal muscles in postoperative failed back syndrome. Spine 1993;18(5):575–581
7. Datta G, Gnanalingham KK, Peterson D, et al. Back pain and disability after lumbar laminectomy: is there a relationship to muscle retraction? Neurosurgery 2004;54(6):1413–1420
8. Styf JR, Willén J. The effects of external compression by three different retractors on pressure in the erector spine muscles during and after posterior lumbar spine surgery in humans. Spine 1998;23(3):354–358
9. Stevens KJ, Spenciner DB, Griffiths KL, et al. Comparison of minimally invasive and conventional open posterolateral lumbar fusion using magnetic resonance imaging and retraction pressure studies. J Spinal Disord Tech 2006;19(2):77–86
10. Kim KT, Lee SH, Suk KS, Bae SC. The quantitative analysis of tissue injury markers after mini-open lumbar fusion. Spine 2006;31(6):712–716
11. Hyun SJ, Kim YB, Kim YS, et al. Postoperative changes in paraspinal muscle volume: comparison between paramedian interfascial and midline approaches for lumbar fusion. J Korean Med Sci 2007;22(4):646–651
12. Watkins MB. Posterolateral fusion of the lumbar and lumbosacral spine. J Bone Joint Surg Am 1953;35(4):1014–1018
13. Moskovitz PA. Minimally invasive posterolateral lumbar arthrodesis. Orthop Clin North Am 1998;29(4):665–667
14. Lowe TG, Tahernia AD, O'Brien MF, Smith DA. Unilateral transforaminal posterior lumbar interbody fusion (TLIF): indications, technique, and 2-year results. J Spinal Disord Tech 2002;15(1):31–38
15. Ozgur BM, Hughes SA, Baird LC, Taylor WR. Minimally disruptive decompression and transforaminal lumbar interbody fusion. Spine J 2006;6(1):27–33
16. Holly LT, Schwender JD, Rouben DP, Foley KT. Minimally invasive transforaminal lumbar interbody fusion: indications, technique, and complications. Neurosurg Focus 2006;20(3):E6
17. Schwender JD, Holly LT, Rouben DP, Foley KT. Minimally invasive transforaminal lumbar interbody fusion (TLIF): technical feasibility and initial results. J Spinal Disord Tech 2005;18(Suppl):S1–S6
18. Capener N. Spondylolisthesis. Br J Surg 1932;19:374–386
19. Bums BH. An operation for spondylolisthesis. Lancet 1933;1:1233
20. Inamasu J, Guiot BH. Laparoscopic anterior lumbar interbody fusion: a review of outcome studies. Minim Invasive Neurosurg 2005;48(6):340–347
21. Escobar E, Transfeldt E, Garvey T, Ogilvie J, Graber J, Schultz L. Video-assisted versus open anterior lumbar spine fusion surgery: a comparison of four techniques and complications in 135 patients. Spine 2003;28(7):729–732
22. Mathews HH, Evans MT, Molligan HJ, Long BH. Laparoscopic discectomy with anterior lumbar interbody fusion: a preliminary review. Spine 1995;20(16):1797–1802
23. Zucherman JF, Zdeblick TA, Bailey SA, Mahvi D, Hsu KY, Kohrs D. Instrumented laparoscopic spinal fusion: preliminary results. Spine 1995;20(18):2029–2034
24. Zdeblick TA, David SM. A prospective comparison of surgical approach for anterior L4–L5 fusion: laparoscopic versus mini anterior lumbar interbody fusion. Spine 2000;25(20):2682–2687
25. Zdeblick TA. Laparoscopic spinal fusion. Orthop Clin North Am 1998;29(4):635–645
26. Flynn JC, Price CT. Sexual complications of anterior fusion of the lumbar spine. Spine 1984;9(5):489–492
27. Regan JJ, Yuan H, McAfee PC. Laparoscopic fusion of the lumbar spine: minimally invasive spine surgery: a prospective multicenter study evaluating open and laparoscopic lumbar fusion. Spine 1999;24(4):402–411
28. Liu JC, Ondra SL, Angelos P, Ganju A, Landers ML. Is laparoscopic anterior lumbar interbody fusion a useful minimally invasive procedure? Neurosurgery 2002; 51(5, Suppl):S155–S158
29. Saraph V, Lerch C, Walochnik N, Bach CM, Krismer M, Wimmer C. Comparison of conventional versus minimally invasive extraperitoneal approach for anterior lumbar interbody fusion. Eur Spine J 2004;13(5):425–431
30. Brau SA. Mini-open approach to the spine for anterior lumbar interbody fusion: description of the procedure, results and complications. Spine J 2002;2(3):216–223
31. Gaur DD. Laparoscopic operative retroperitoneoscopy: use of a new device. J Urol 1992;148(4):1137–1139

32. McDougall EM, Clayman RV, Fadden PT. Retroperitoneoscopy: the Washington University Medical School experience. Urology 1994; 43(4):446–452

33. McAfee PC, Regan JJ, Geis WP, Fedder IL. Minimally invasive anterior retroperitoneal approach to the lumbar spine: emphasis on the lateral BAK. Spine 1998;23(13):1476–1484

34. Ozgur BM, Aryan HE, Pimenta L, Taylor WR. Extreme lateral interbody fusion (XLIF): a novel surgical technique for anterior lumbar interbody fusion. Spine J 2006;6(4):435–443

35. Pimenta L, Vigna F, Bellera F, Schaffa T, Malcolm J, McAfee P. A new minimally invasive surgical technique for adult lumbar degenerative scoliosis. Paper presented at the 11th International Meeting on Advanced Spine Techniques (IMAST); July 2004; Southhampton, Bermuda

36. Mirza SK, Wiggins GC, Kuntz C IV, et al. Accuracy of thoracic vertebral body screw placement using standard fluoroscopy, fluoroscopic image guidance, and computed tomographic image guidance: a cadaver study. Spine 2003;28(4):402–413

37. Foley KT, Simon DA, Ampersand YR. Virtual fluoroscopy: computer-assisted fluoroscopic navigation. Spine 2001;26(4): 347–351

38. Theocharopoulos N, Perisinakis K, Damilakis J, Papadokostakis G, Hadjipavlou A, Gourtsoyiannis N. Occupational exposure from common fluoroscopic projections used in orthopaedic surgery. J Bone Joint Surg Am 2003;85-A(9):1698–1703

39. Kim CW, Lee YP, Taylor W, Oygar A, Kim WK. Use of navigation-assisted fluoroscopy to decrease radiation exposure during minimally invasive spine surgery. Spine J 2008;8(4):584–590

40. Togawa D, Kayanja MM, Reinhardt MK, et al. Bone-mounted miniature robotic guidance for pedicle screw and translaminar facet screw placement. Part 2. Evaluation of system accuracy. Neurosurgery 2007;60(2, Suppl 1)ONS129–ONS139.

30 Biologics for Spinal Fusion

Wellington K. Hsu and Jeffrey C. Wang

Spinal arthrodesis presents several obstacles to even the most experienced spine surgeon. Despite the use of internal fixation, pseudarthrosis still occurs in 10 to 15% of all spine fusion surgeries.[1-4] The significant rates of pseudarthroses and reports of operative morbidity from the harvest of autograft can limit the success rates of primary spine fusion in certain patients. In addition, the stringent biologic environment created from pseudarthrosis formation presents a complicated array of problems and unpredictable outcomes after further surgical intervention. Dense fibrous tissue, intervertebral disc, and muscle cells commonly encountered during revision procedures have been found to inhibit host bone repair.[5] Because the success rates of fusion in this poor osteoinductive environment are relatively low, recent studies have been directed toward the development of new bone graft substitutes to improve outcomes in both primary and revision procedures.

The arena of spinal biologics has expanded to include autogenous bone graft, allograft, autologous cells, demineralized bone matrix (DBM), recombinant growth factors, and tissue engineering therapies. Continued research has been conducted to identify the ideal bone graft substitutes for spine surgery, which should be osteogenic, biocompatible, user-friendly, and cost-effective, and should provide structural support.[6] In this chapter, we review the preclinical and clinical data regarding the use of biologics in the induction of spine fusion.

■ Autograft

Autogenous cancellous bone graft remains the gold standard material for the treatment of bone loss challenges because it alone offers three of the necessary components for bone repair: osteoinductive signals from associated growth factors, osteogenic cells, and an osteoconductive matrix. Several animal models have provided insight into the incorporation of cancellous grafts into host bone.[7] Histologic and biomechanical evidence indicates that autogenous cancellous graft offers incorporation into host bone in 6 to 12 months. Two distinct phases have been described in the incorporative process: an early phase characterized by active bone resorption and formation, and a late phase identified by creeping substitution.[8]

By 1 year after surgery, complete remodeling and incorporation of the graft are seen.[8]

Both autogenous cortical and cancellous bone grafts are currently used in spine fusion procedures. The majority of autografts harvested contain cancellous bone. Although without compressive strength, cancellous grafts have a large trabecular area, which encourages the consolidation of the fusion mass. The bone graft ultimately becomes denser than surrounding host bone.[9] Cortical grafts offer structural support for the spinal column and are used for a wide range of spinal defects (0.5 to 25 cm). This type of graft is incorporated slower with less efficiency than cancellous allograft. Furthermore, cortical grafts undergo resorption before host incorporation. Stress fractures have also been reported in longer grafts (12 to 25 cm).[10]

The use of autologous bone graft in the setting of spine fusion typically presents several concerns for the surgeon. The elderly patient population presents unique clinical problems such as osteoporosis, poor bone stock, and anesthetic risks of increased operative time. Studies have shown that the harvest of autogenous graft leads to clinically significant perioperative and postoperative morbidity.[11-14] Finally, the options for biologic supplementation in the setting of revision spine surgery are decreased when previous iliac crest bone graft was harvested.

■ Allograft

Allograft bone offers advantages over autogenous bone graft because there is an abundant supply of graft material and the morbidity associated with autograft harvest is avoided. By decreasing antigenicity and thus, the host immune response, the process of freeze-drying avoids a localized inflammatory response and possible rejection of the material. As a result, this leads to increased graft incorporation after implantation.[15,16] On the other hand, this modification also decreases osteogenic activity and hinders host vascular invasion. When compared with autografts, the loss of osteoinductive capabilities leads to a higher incidence of nonunion and delayed union.[7] The risk of disease transmission from musculoskeletal tissue donors exists from the use of allografts; however, this has been reported to be low.[17]

Cancellous allograft bone chips and cortical allografts have been used extensively in spinal fusions. Anterior femoral ring allografts have been shown to successfully induce spinal fusion (range 52% to 98%) when posterior instrumentation is used.[18–20] Clinical evidence has suggested that the use of tricortical allograft may offer comparable fusion rates and clinical outcomes to iliac crest autograft after revision anterior arthrodesis of the lumbar spine.[21] However, studies comparing outcomes between allograft and autograft in the posterolateral arthrodesis of the lumbar spine are more controversial. An et al[22] reported a prospective comparison of autograft and allograft preparations in the posterolateral arthrodesis of the lumbar spine and concluded that allograft was less efficacious in achieving radiographically evident spine fusion (80% versus 50% successful fusion, respectively).[22] Another prospective study concluded that ethylene oxide-treated allograft mixed with autogenous bone graft was significantly less reliable in inducing spinal fusion compared with iliac crest autograft alone.[23]

In studies involving the cervical spine, single-level anterior fusions comparing allograft and autograft bone have revealed higher fusion rates with the use of iliac crest autograft (78% versus 92%, respectively).[24–26] However, in these same studies, satisfactory fusion rates using allograft bone were reported (78 to 90% fusion). Evidence involving multilevel cervical fusion or corpectomies show a much higher fusion rate with the use of autograft versus allograft (83% versus 47%, respectively).[4,22,26,27]

■ Demineralized Bone Matrix

DBM is created through the acid extraction of the mineralized phase of bone. The preparation of DBM was originally characterized by Urist et al[28,29] and then modified by Reddi and Huggins.[30] Methods of processing follow the same initial steps; however, additives and refining techniques are different depending on the source and company involved. Commercial preparations also use different carriers such as glycerol, hyaluronic acid, gelatin, and calcium sulfate powder. This has led to wide biologic variability in terms of osteoinductive potential in vivo.[17,31,32]

DBMs have been found to have rich osteoconductive capabilities but questionable osteoinductive ability. DBMs have been shown to induce rapid revascularization, serving as an excellent osteoconductive scaffold.[33] However, osteoinductive capacity of DBM is dependent not only on the original donor, but also on the different commercial sterilization and handling methods. Sterilization by ethylene oxide and use of gamma irradiation, for example, have been found to significantly reduce osteoinductivity.[34,35]

Commercial preparations of DBMs also use different carriers that may impart unpredictable biologic effects. For example, a large number of DBMs have been combined with glycerol to help convert the allograft to a putty form. This carrier has been demonstrated to be lethally toxic to athymic rats in a dose-dependent manner.[36] Other studies have confirmed the renal toxicity of glycerol in large doses[37]; however, despite these findings, in more than 10 years of use of these DBMs in humans, there have been no reported cases of renal toxicity related to this carrier.

Despite their wide use and variable processing methods, DBMs have been tested in few animal models and laboratory studies. Recent studies have demonstrated the variability of these preparations in inducing osteogenic activity in an intramuscular animal model,[38] a rat femoral defect,[39] and a rat spine fusion model.[17] In a study using a rat spine fusion model, widely variable osteoinductive potential was demonstrated using different commercially available DBM preparations.[17] Histologic analysis of the spines 8 weeks after DBM implantation demonstrated variable rates of fusion, amount of new bone formation, and presence of residual DBM. This wide variability of biologic activity of DBMs is likely influenced by the associated donor the carrier, and the assorted demineralization and sterilization methods used.[17]

DBMs have been used successfully as bone graft extenders to promote spinal fusion and the healing of long bone nonunions.[6,40–42] Certain formulations have also induced successful spine arthrodesis when used alone or in conjunction with autograft, bone marrow, or ceramic carriers.[37,43–47] Additional studies have combined the use of autologous bone marrow and DBM in healing osseous defects.[48,49]

There is a need for further study of the influence of donor age and sex, processing, and success of DBMs.[50] Both the historic lack of Food and Drug Adminstration (FDA) oversight in the United States and the wide variety of donors to supply the graft contribute to the variability in outcome from the use of DBM. Furthermore, different preparations are combined with different carriers that impart variable osteoconductive and osteoinductive capabilities. However, it is important to note that DBMs should be used clinically solely as bone graft extenders and not substitutes. Because all DBMs do not have the same biologic potential, the optimal DBM for each clinical situation needs to be determined.

■ Autologous Cells

Bone marrow contains osteoprogenitor cells and growth factors that actively recruit host mesenchymal stem cells (MSCs) to undergo osteoblastic differentiation. Recent research has reported the ability of bone marrow to stimulate bone formation.[51] Autologous cells provide significant osteoinductive capabilities through osteogenic cells, however, when used alone, they lack localized structural support. For this reason, the combination of bone graft substitutes and autologous marrow has been assessed in tibial nonunions, bone cysts, and comminuted fractures associated with bone loss.[45,49,52,53]

MSCs in autogenous bone marrow are capable of developing into mature osteoblasts when exposed to the appropriate growth factors.[54-58] Furthermore, culture expansion of MSCs has been shown to amplify the number of osteoprogenitor cells in vitro.[58,59] In a preclinical critical-sized defect model in canines, culture-expanded MSCs exhibited superior healing rates when compared with bone marrow.[58] These results show promise for the use of MSC therapy in spinal fusion, particularly in the elderly patient population.

Bone marrow cells are readily accessible through aspiration from the posterior iliac wing, and a recent study has recommended the harvest of smaller volumes (2 mL) of bone marrow from any one location to obtain a higher concentration of osteoblast progenitor cells.[59] Muschler et al reported the efficacy of concentrating bone marrow-derived cells from bone marrow aspirates using a selective cell attachment technique in a canine posterior segmental spine fusion model.[60] Their results suggest that when used with a bone marrow clot, an enriched cellular composite graft of concentrated bone marrow cells induced a greater spine fusion mass volume in vivo than cancellous bone matrix alone.[60]

Together, the use of autologous cells with a carrier offers components for bone repair akin to that of autogenous bone graft. Complications are subsequently avoided, such as those associated with bone graft harvesting and the low risk of infection. However, there are concerns about the potential variability in human bone marrow cellularity as well as an age-related decline in progenitor cells.[61] Although the benefits are supported by a strong theoretical basis and success in animal models, further clinical studies into using autologous cells as a bone graft substitute in spine fusion are needed.

■ Bone Morphogenetic Proteins

The discovery of bone morphogenetic proteins (BMPs) by Urist in 1965[62] has led to a diverse area of research dedicated to the identification and characterization of osteoinductive growth factors. Members of the transforming growth factor-B (TGF-β) superfamily, BMPs have been proposed for several applications in orthopaedic surgery.[63] Although 14 different BMPs have been reported,[64] much of the recent study in the literature has focused on BMP-2, 6, 7, 9, and 14 (MP-52).

Recombinant BMP-2 (rhBMP-2) and BMP-7 (or osteogenic protein-1, rhOP-1) have been evaluated in numerous preclinical models, and successful healing in long bone defects has been reported.[63,65-67] Similar findings have been demonstrated in spinal arthrodesis models in animals.[68-71] In the United States, FDA approval has been granted for the use of rhBMP-2 to enhance anterior spinal fusion[72] and rhOP-1 to supplement posterior spine fusions for pseudarthrosis (under a humanitarian device exemption).[73]

Recombinant BMP-2 has been shown to reproducibly heal the lumbar spine in rodents and nonhuman primates.[65,71,74-82] Furthermore, rhOP-1 has also demonstrated consistent bone healing properties in rodent and sheep models.[76,83-86] Results from these studies suggest that the use of rhBMP results in similar if not superior fusion rates with biomechanically stronger fusion masses when compared with autogenous bone graft.[65,71,74-82]

Vaccaro and colleagues recently demonstrated the efficacy of rhOP-1 putty (3.5 mg rhOP-1 with 1 g type I collagen) in the enhancement of posterolateral lumbar arthrodesis.[87] In a randomized, prospective, multicenter study, 36 patients with degenerative spondylolisthesis were treated with either rhOP-1 or autogenous iliac crest bone graft in an uninstrumented posterolateral fusion following a decompressive laminectomy. At the one-year time point, 74% (14 of 19 patients) of the rhOP-1 and 60% (6 of 10 patients) in the autograft groups achieved a successful clinical and radiographic posterolateral arthrodesis using static and dynamic plain radiographs, which was not statistically significant.[87] These authors concluded that fusion in the absence of internal fixation with the use of rhOP-1 putty was safe and yielded comparable results to that of iliac crest bone graft.

Similarly, Boden et al reported the successful clinical use of rhBMP-2 in the healing of a posterolateral spine fusion both with and without instrumentation in a comparison study involving 25 patients.[88] Clinical improvement as defined by the mean Oswestry Disability Index score (6 weeks postoperatively) was greatest in the rhBMP-2 treatment only group. Interestingly, the authors concluded that the use of a higher dose of recombinant growth factor in nonhuman primates (1.5 to 2.0 mg/mL) than in rodents (0.2 to 0.4 mg/mL), was required in healing a posterolateral spine fusion.[89] To date, it remains unclear why concentrations of BMP a million times greater than that found in the human body are required to successfully induce a spinal arthrodesis.[90-92]

Follow-up studies utilizing rhBMP-2 have confirmed its successful use in inducing a posterolateral spinal fusion diagnosed by computed tomography (CT).[93,94] Glassman et al reported the use of a large INFUSE kit (12 mg rhBMP-2/ACS, Infuse Bone Graft, Medtronic Sofamor Danek) in the posterolateral fusion bed as equivalent fusion success to iliac crest bone graft (ICBG).[94] The authors concluded that INFUSE can effectively substitute for ICBG for both one- and two-level posterolateral instrumented fusions. Dimar and colleagues published 2-year radiographic results from an FDA interventional device exemption study comparing ICBG and rhBMP-2 combined with a compression-resistant matrix (CRM) carrier for single posterolateral fusions. The authors demonstrated that patients in the BMP/CRM group experienced significantly higher fusion rates yet had less surgical time and blood loss than the ICBG group (88% versus 73%; $P = 0.051$).[93]

The importance of associated carriers with BMP was elucidated when Barnes et al[95] reported the results of rhBMP-2 delivered on an absorbable collagen sponge wrapped around a bulking agent consisting of biphasic calcium phosphate and collagen in a posterolateral fusion model in rhesus monkeys. Results from this and other studies suggest that the required dosage of rhBMP-2 for spinal arthrodesis can be reduced by optimizing the delivery of growth factor by combining the strengths of different carriers.[96] On the other hand, carriers such as fibrin glue have been shown to inhibit bone formation induced from rhBMP and may provide protection from heterotopic ossification and diffusion of protein to undesirable adjacent areas.[97]

Because the treatment of spinal pseudarthrosis is fraught with relatively poor outcomes and potential complications, the interest in the utilization of rhBMP for these clinical challenges is on the rise. With the use of different preclinical pseudarthrosis models, recombinant growth factors may eventually prove to be a more appropriate bone graft option than other existing choices including ICBG. With the use of a nicotine-exposed rabbit lumbar pseudarthrosis model, OP-1 was found to increase the expression of crucial genes in bone repair such as angiogenin, vascular endothelial growth factor, and bone morphogenetic proteins.[98] In fact, these authors concluded that application of a single BMP in relatively high concentrations to a biologically stringent environment can induce angiogenic and osteogenic gene expression greater than that seen with autologous graft.

Despite the overwhelming evidence in support of the routine use of rhBMPs in the enhancement of spinal arthrodesis, several studies have suggested potential complications with its clinical use. Smucker et al[99] reported that 27.5% of 69 patients who underwent anterior cervical spine fusions using rhBMP-2 had a clinical significant neck swelling event compared with only 3.6% of patients in the non-rhBMP2 group. Other studies have confirmed the finding that the use of rhBMP-2 in the anterior cervical spine can be problematic.[100,101] Furthermore, the use of rhBMP-2 in transforaminal lumbar interbody fusion has been reported to lead to significant vertebral bone resorption in a total of 22 of 32 lumbar levels studied postoperatively with a CT scan.[102] These authors concluded that rhBMP-2 was the direct cause of resorption, which led to graft subsidence and prevented solid radiographic union in a significant number of cases.[102]

■ Tissue Engineering

Tissue engineering options are attractive as an adjunct to spine surgery because of their ability to closely approximate the biology of autologous bone graft. Furthermore, many of these treatment strategies offer a continuous delivery of recombinant protein, which may enhance spinal fusion rates in a compromised biologic environment. Protocols utilizing the combination of bone graft substitutes, recombinant proteins, and/or gene transfer systems could offer additional options for spine arthrodesis. Gene therapy involves the in vitro transfer of genetic material to cells to stimulate in vivo expression of a targeted protein. Gene therapy systems are composed of the DNA sequence, a vector, such as a virus, to mobilize the genetic material in question, and target cells to express the protein. Transduction of target cells can occur in several different ways. In vivo techniques involve the direct injection of the vector into the site of bony repair, whereas ex vivo systems require the harvest of responding cells and transduction with a virus in an in vitro setting. In general, ex vivo systems have been studied more extensively because of higher transduction efficiencies when compared with in vivo methods.

Early results using BMP gene transfer via an in vivo technique revealed successful fusion only in immunocompromised animals.[103–105] Since then, several immunocompetent animal studies have demonstrated the efficacy of gene therapy in the healing of long bone defects[106–108] and spinal fusion.[109,110] Wang et al reported the initial results with the use of ex vivo adenoviral gene transfer in a posterolateral spine fusion model in immunocompetent rats.[71] Histomorphometric analysis revealed that coarse trabecular bone had formed from cells generated by adenoviral gene transfer whereas thin, lace-like bone formed from that of recombinant BMP.[71] This finding has also been confirmed in a rat femoral critical-sized defect model.[107]

The success of gene therapy has also been reported in higher animal models.[105,111,112] In one study, harvested mesenchymal stem cells (MSCs) from pigs were used as targets for adenoviral-mediated transfer of the BMP-2 gene.[112] The transduced cells were then used to successfully heal the thoracic disc spaces of three pigs through an anterior thoracoscopic injection. Radiographic and histologic examination confirmed bridging bone in all six disc spaces treated with adenovirus; little bone formation was seen in the control injections.[112]

The utilization of growth factors other than BMP-2 with ex vivo gene therapy in bone formation has also been described. In addition to BMP-2 and BMP-7, recent reports have shown the successful use of other genes, such as BMP-4,[113] BMP-6,[114] and BMP-9.[115] Furthermore, Viggeswarapu et al[110] demonstrated solid posterolateral arthrodesis of the spine in a rabbit model from the adenoviral delivery of LIM mineralization protein-1 (LMP-1) into the fusion bed. LMP-1 is an intracellular protein that has been shown to function as an upstream regulator for several BMPs.

Although recombinant BMP homodimers such as BMP-2 and BMP-7 have been used successfully in animal models of spinal fusion, recent studies have suggested that the coexpression of multiple BMPs can lead to the formation of heterodimeric BMPs.[116–118] These studies also suggest that heterodimeric BMPs may have more potent osteoblastic potential than their homodimeric counterparts. Using a rat posterolateral spine fusion model, Zhu and colleagues[119] tested the in vivo and in vitro capacity of combination gene transfer using BMP-2 and BMP-7 in comparison to single BMP gene transfer. A549 cells were cotransfected with adenoviral vectors encoding for BMP-2 and BMP-7, and with each vector alone. The authors found that the animals treated with cotransfection of both BMP genes experienced a significantly greater number of mechanically stable spinal fusions with higher bone fusion mass assessed via CT scanning when compared with single gene transfer.[119] These findings suggest that the use of heterodimeric BMPs may possibly lead to lower required doses of recombinant protein and fewer responding cells in tissue engineering.

Further optimization to gene therapy protocols have been directed at the use of different cellular delivery vehicles. Although multiple types of target cells have been used to deliver growth factors for bone formation, bone marrow stromal cells have been the most widely used. However, studies demonstrate that bone marrow contains a relatively low percentage of MSCs that have the capability of differentiating into osteoblasts.[59] Moreover, this ratio is further diminished in elderly patients, those with metabolic diseases, and osteoporosis.[61]

Because of the inherent limitations of bone marrow stromal cells, several other gene delivery vehicles have been utilized. Buffy coat cells, which are a concentrate of white blood cells and platelets derived from either bone marrow or blood, have been used successfully to produce spine fusions in both rat and rabbit models after transduction with LMP-1.[110] Other target cells used successfully in gene transfer strategies include periosteal cells,[111] C2C12 myoblasts,[120] and muscle-derived stem cells.[121,122]

Recent interest has been directed toward human liposuction aspirates, obtained from human fat, which contain an abundance of pluripotent progenitor cells termed processed lipoaspirate cells. These cells can undergo purification steps to produce adipose-derived stem cells (ADSCs) that have demonstrated the ability to differentiate into cells of chondrogenic, osteogenic, myogenic, and adipogenic lineage. The prospect of using processed lipoaspirate cells is attractive because they offer a significantly higher yield of mesenchymal stem cells than bone marrow,[123] can be obtained through a minimally invasive procedure under local anesthesia, and are widely available among the patient population.[124]

Studies using adipose cells as gene delivery vehicles have reported initial success in the induction of bone formation in several different animal models.[125–127] One study from our laboratory has successfully described the use of ADSCs as cellular delivery vehicles in the induction of spine fusion in a rat posterolateral spine fusion model using an adenoviral vector.[126] Microcomputed tomographic and plain radiographic analysis of fusion masses revealed over twice as much bone formation in animals treated with ADSCs transduced with the adenoviral vector carrying the BMP-2 gene when compared with those from high-dose recombinant BMP-2.[126]

◾ Discussion and Conclusion

Spinal arthrodesis is complicated by challenges including osteoporotic bone, a stringent biologic environment, and poor local vascularity. Bone graft substitutes should provide for consistent arthrodesis without the morbidity associated with autogenous graft. As a whole, however, these substances vary widely in regard to available data, and careful evaluation is necessary to identify the appropriate use of various bone graft agents. In making these critical decisions, surgeons must assess the host biologic environment and must ensure that the four critical elements are present to promote bone repair: the presence of bioactive factors, responding cells, matrix, and an adequate vascular supply.

Currently established treatment options including the use of allograft, autograft, or DBM, may soon be regularly supplemented with recombinant growth factors or products from tissue engineering. Although its cost effectiveness must be assessed, use of these novel biologic substitutes may be used to enhance bone repair in more stringent biologic environments.

The body of evidence reporting the efficacy of recombinant BMP in clinical studies has grown considerably over the past 5 years. Since the first report of BMP-induced osteoinduction in a clinical trial,[72] additional studies have reported the superiority of rhBMP-2 to the use of autogenous bone graft.[72,83,89,93,128,129] Moreover, patients treated with rhBMP-2 alone have been found to show more rapid and significant clinical improvement after spine fusion.[89] Furthermore, multiple investigators have demonstrated the osteoinductive versatility of recombinant BMP using multiple approaches. Recent evidence has supported the efficacy of rhBMP in posterolateral, interbody, and transpedicular approaches in inducing radiographic and histologic spine fusion.[83,88,89,102,128,129]

However, despite excellent clinical results, many concerns still exist for the routine use of recombinant growth factors. Clinical studies, which confirm the safety from the use of rhBMP-2 in humans,[87,130] fall short in evaluating possible long-term effects. Several complications have also been associated with its use in both the cervical and lumbar spine.[99,101,102] Furthermore, the cost of recombinant BMPs currently precludes its routine use in spine arthrodesis; further study will be necessary to delineate the clear indications in which BMPs should be used.

Despite promising preclinical results from gene therapy, safety concerns have hindered the progress of tissue engineering in the clinical setting. Recent interest has been dedicated to characterizing the lifespan of transduced cells, duration of gene expression, and systemic effects on the host genome after the use of gene therapy. Additional studies in higher animal models are needed to assess the long-term effects of gene therapy before its clinical use in humans is widely accepted. With additional investigation into its safety profile in humans, the use of gene therapy may one day become a reality in the field of musculoskeletal surgery in the future.

Multiple avenues of research exist in the development of biologic substitutes for the enhancement of spine fusion. The continued laboratory and clinical characterization of spinal biologics will ultimately offer spine surgeons multiple options in the arena of spine fusion.

References

1. Bridwell KH, Sedgewick TA, O'Brien MF, Lenke LG, Baldus C. The role of fusion and instrumentation in the treatment of degenerative spondylolisthesis with spinal stenosis. J Spinal Disord 1993; 6(6):461–472
2. McGuire RA, Amundson GM. The use of primary internal fixation in spondylolisthesis. Spine 1993;18(12):1662–1672
3. West JL III, Bradford DS, Ogilvie JW. Results of spinal arthrodesis with pedicle screw-plate fixation. J Bone Joint Surg Am 1991; 73(8):1179–1184
4. Zdeblick TA. A prospective, randomized study of lumbar fusion: preliminary results. Spine 1993;18(8):983–991
5. Bae H, Kanim LEA, Zhao L, Wong P, Delamarter R. Cellular environments alter performance of rhBMP-2 and induce pseudarthrosis. Spine J 2004;4(5S):52S
6. Berven S, Tay BK, Kleinstueck FS, Bradford DS. Clinical applications of bone graft substitutes in spine surgery: consideration of mineralized and demineralized preparations and growth factor supplementation. Eur Spine J 2001;10(Suppl 2):S169–S177
7. Goldberg VM, Stevenson S. Natural history of autografts and allografts. Clin Orthop Relat Res 1987; (225):7–16
8. Urist MR. Bone transplants and implants. In: Fundamental and Clinical Bone Physiology. Philadelphia: JB Lippincott; 1980:331–368
9. Gupta MC, Maitra S. Bone grafts and bone morphogenetic proteins in spine fusion. Cell Tissue Bank 2002;3(4):255–267
10. Vaccaro AR, Chiba K, Heller JG, et al. North American Spine Society for Contemporary Concepts in Spine Care. Bone grafting alternatives in spinal surgery. Spine J 2002;2(3):206–215
11. Catinella FP, De Laria GA, De Wald RL. False aneurysm of the superior gluteal artery: a complication of iliac crest bone grafting. Spine 1990;15(12):1360–1362
12. Fernyhough JC, Schimandle JJ, Weigel MC, Edwards CC, Levine AM. Chronic donor site pain complicating bone graft harvesting from the posterior iliac crest for spinal fusion. Spine 1992;17(12): 1474–1480
13. Summers BN, Eisenstein SM. Donor site pain from the ilium: a complication of lumbar spine fusion. J Bone Joint Surg Br 1989; 71(4):677–680
14. Younger EM, Chapman MW. Morbidity at bone graft donor sites. J Orthop Trauma 1989;3(3):192–195
15. Bos GD, Goldberg VM, Zika JM, Heiple KG, Powell AE. Immune responses of rats to frozen bone allografts. J Bone Joint Surg Am 1983;65(2):239–246
16. Burwell RG. Studies in the transplantation of bone. V. The capacity of fresh and treated homografts of bone to evoke transplantation immunity. J Bone Joint Surg Br 1963;45-B:386–401
17. Peterson B, Whang PG, Iglesias R, Wang JC, Lieberman JR. Osteoinductivity of commercially available demineralized bone matrix: preparations in a spine fusion model. J Bone Joint Surg Am 2004;86-A(10):2243–2250
18. el-Masry MA, Katsochis A, Badawy WS, el-Hawary YK. Anterior lumbar interbody fusion using a hybrid graft. Acta Orthop Belg 2004;70(4):332–336
19. Holte DC, O'Brien JP, Renton P. Anterior lumbar fusion using a hybrid interbody graft: a preliminary radiographic report. Eur Spine J 1994;3(1):32–38
20. Sasso RC, Kitchel SH, Dawson EG. A prospective, randomized controlled clinical trial of anterior lumbar interbody fusion using a titanium cylindrical threaded fusion device. Spine 2004;29(2):113–122
21. Buttermann GR, Glazer PA, Hu SS, Bradford DS. Revision of failed lumbar fusions: a comparison of anterior autograft and allograft. Spine 1997;22(23):2748–2755
22. An HS, Lynch K, Toth J. Prospective comparison of autograft vs. allograft for adult posterolateral lumbar spine fusion: differences among freeze-dried, frozen, and mixed grafts. J Spinal Disord 1995;8(2):131–135
23. Jorgenson SS, Lowe TG, France J, Sabin J. A prospective analysis of autograft versus allograft in posterolateral lumbar fusion in the same patient: a minimum of 1-year follow-up in 144 patients. Spine 1994;19(18):2048–2053
24. Bishop RC, Moore KA, Hadley MN. Anterior cervical interbody fusion using autogeneic and allogeneic bone graft substrate: a prospective comparative analysis. J Neurosurg 1996;85(2):206–210
25. Martin GJ Jr, Haid RW Jr, MacMillan M, Rodts GE Jr, Berkman R. Anterior cervical discectomy with freeze-dried fibula allograft: overview of 317 cases and literature review. Spine 1999;24(9): 852–858
26. Zdeblick TA, Ducker TB. The use of freeze-dried allograft bone for anterior cervical fusions. Spine 1991;16(7):726–729
27. Zhang ZH, Yin H, Yang K, et al. Anterior intervertebral disc excision and bone grafting in cervical spondylotic myelopathy. Spine 1983;8(1):16–19
28. Urist MR, Dawson E. Intertransverse process fusion with the aid of chemosterilized autolyzed antigen-extracted allogeneic (AAA) bone. Clin Orthop Relat Res 1981; (154):97–113

29. Urist MR, Silverman BF, Buring K, Dubuc FL, Rosenberg JM. The bone induction principle. Clin Orthop Relat Res 1967;53:243–283

30. Reddi AH, Huggins C. Biochemical sequences in the transformation of normal fibroblasts in adolescent rats. Proc Natl Acad Sci U S A 1972;69(6):1601–1605

31. Lee YP, Jo M, Luna M, Chien B, Lieberman JR, Wang JC. The efficacy of different commercially available demineralized bone matrix substances in an athymic rat model. J Spinal Disord Tech 2005;18(5):439–444

32. Wang JC, Alanay A, Mark D, et al. A comparison of commercially available demineralized bone matrix for spinal fusion. Eur Spine J 2007;16(8):1233–1240

33. Finkemeier CG. Bone-grafting and bone-graft substitutes. J Bone Joint Surg Am 2002;84-A(3):454–464

34. Aspenberg P, Johnsson E, Thorngren KG. Dose-dependent reduction of bone inductive properties by ethylene oxide. J Bone Joint Surg Br 1990;72(6):1036–1037

35. Munting E, Wilmart JF, Wijne A, Hennebert P, Delloye C. Effect of sterilization on osteoinduction: comparison of five methods in demineralized rat bone. Acta Orthop Scand 1988;59(1):34–38

36. Wang JC, Kanim LE, Nagakawa IS, Yamane BH, Vinters HV, Dawson EG. Dose-dependent toxicity of a commercially available demineralized bone matrix material. Spine 2001;26(13):1429–1435

37. Bostrom MP, Yang X, Kennan M, Sandhu H, Dicarlo E, Lane JM. An unexpected outcome during testing of commercially available demineralized bone graft materials: how safe are the nonallograft components? Spine 2001;26(13):1425–1428

38. Schwartz Z, Mellonig JT, Carnes DL Jr, et al. Ability of commercial demineralized freeze-dried bone allograft to induce new bone formation. J Periodontol 1996;67(9):918–926

39. Oakes DA, Lee CC, Lieberman JR. An evaluation of human demineralized bone matrices in a rat femoral defect model. Clin Orthop Relat Res 2003; (413):281–290

40. Frenkel SR, Moskovich R, Spivak J, Zhang ZH, Prewett AB. Demineralized bone matrix. Enhancement of spinal fusion. Spine 1993;18(12):1634–1639

41. Johnson EE, Urist MR, Finerman GA. Resistant nonunions and partial or complete segmental defects of long bones: treatment with implants of a composite of human bone morphogenetic protein (BMP) and autolyzed, antigen-extracted, allogeneic (AAA) bone. Clin Orthop Relat Res 1992; (277):229–237

42. Kakiuchi M, Hosoya T, Takaoka K, Amitani K, Ono K. Human bone matrix gelatin as a clinical alloimplant: a retrospective review of 160 cases. Int Orthop 1985;9(3):181–188

43. Lindholm TS, Nilsson OS, Lindholm TC. Extraskeletal and intraskeletal new bone formation induced by demineralized bone matrix combined with bone marrow cells. Clin Orthop Relat Res 1982;171(171):251–255

44. Lindholm TS, Ragni P, Lindholm TC. Response of bone marrow stroma cells to demineralized cortical bone matrix in experimental spinal fusion in rabbits. Clin Orthop Relat Res 1988; (230):296–302

45. Lindholm TS, Urist MR. A quantitative analysis of new bone formation by induction in compositive grafts of bone marrow and bone matrix. Clin Orthop Relat Res 1980;(150):288–300

46. Morone MA, Boden SD. Experimental posterolateral lumbar spinal fusion with a demineralized bone matrix gel. Spine 1998;23(2):159–167

47. Ragni P, Lindholm TS. Interaction of allogeneic demineralized bone matrix and porous hydroxyapatite bioceramics in lumbar interbody fusion in rabbits. Clin Orthop Relat Res 1991;(272):292–299

48. Connolly JF. Injectable bone marrow preparations to stimulate osteogenic repair. Clin Orthop Relat Res 1995;(313):8–18

49. Tiedeman JJ, Garvin KL, Kile TA, Connolly JF. The role of a composite, demineralized bone matrix and bone marrow in the treatment of osseous defects. Orthopedics 1995;18(12):1153–1158

50. Greenwald AS, Boden SD, Goldberg VM, Khan Y, Laurencin CT, Rosier RN. Bone-graft substitutes: facts, fictions, and applications. J Bone Joint Surg Am 2001;83-A(Suppl 2 Pt 2):98–103

51. Whang PG. Clinical issues in the development of cellular systems for use as bone graft substitutes. In: Bone Graft Substitutes: A Multidisciplinary Approach. West Conshohocken, PA: American Society for Testing and Materials International; 2003:142–164

52. Connolly JF, Guse R, Tiedeman J, Dehne R. Autologous marrow injection as a substitute for operative grafting of tibial nonunions. Clin Orthop Relat Res 1991;(266):259–270

53. Ohgushi H, Goldberg VM, Caplan AI. Repair of bone defects with marrow cells and porous ceramic: experiments in rats. Acta Orthop Scand 1989;60(3):334–339

54. Cassiede P, Dennis JE, Ma F, Caplan AI. Osteochondrogenic potential of marrow mesenchymal progenitor cells exposed to TGF-beta 1 or PDGF-BB as assayed in vivo and in vitro. J Bone Miner Res 1996;11(9):1264–1273

55. Dennis JE, Haynesworth SE, Young RG, Caplan AI. Osteogenesis in marrow-derived mesenchymal cell porous ceramic composites transplanted subcutaneously: effect of fibronectin and laminin on cell retention and rate of osteogenic expression. Cell Transplant 1992;1(1):23–32

56. Grigoriadis AE, Heersche JN, Aubin JE. Differentiation of muscle, fat, cartilage, and bone from progenitor cells present in a bone-derived clonal cell population: effect of dexamethasone. J Cell Biol 1988;106(6):2139–2151

57. Jaiswal N, Haynesworth SE, Caplan AI, Bruder SP. Osteogenic differentiation of purified, culture-expanded human mesenchymal stem cells in vitro. J Cell Biochem 1997;64(2):295–312

58. Kadiyala S, Young RG, Thiede MA, Bruder SP. Culture expanded canine mesenchymal stem cells possess osteochondrogenic potential in vivo and in vitro. Cell Transplant 1997;6(2):125–134

59. Muschler GF, Boehm C, Easley K. Aspiration to obtain osteoblast progenitor cells from human bone marrow: the influence of aspiration volume. J Bone Joint Surg Am 1997;79(11):1699–1709

60. Muschler GF, Nitto H, Matsukura Y, et al. Spine fusion using cell matrix composites enriched in bone marrow-derived cells. Clin Orthop Relat Res 2003; (407):102–118

61. Muschler GF, Nitto H, Boehm CA, Easley KA. Age- and gender-related changes in the cellularity of human bone marrow and the prevalence of osteoblastic progenitors. J Orthop Res 2001;19(1):117–125

62. Urist MR. Bone: formation by autoinduction. Science 1965;150(698):893–899

63. Zabka AG, Pluhar GE, Edwards RB 3rd, et al. Histomorphometric description of allograft bone remodeling and union in a canine segmental femoral defect model: a comparison of rhBMP-2, cancellous bone graft, and absorbable collagen sponge. J Orthop Res 2001;19(2):318–327

64. Cheng H, Jiang W, Phillips FM, et al. Osteogenic activity of the fourteen types of human bone morphogenetic proteins (BMPs). J Bone Joint Surg Am 2003;85-A(8):1544–1552

65. Cook SD, Dalton JE, Tan EH, Whitecloud TS III, Rueger DC. In vivo evaluation of recombinant human osteogenic protein (rhOP-1) implants as a bone graft substitute for spinal fusions. Spine 1994; 19(15):1655–1663

66. Cook SD, Wolfe MW, Salkeld SL, Rueger DC. Effect of recombinant human osteogenic protein-1 on healing of segmental defects in non-human primates. J Bone Joint Surg Am 1995;77(5):734–750

67. Yasko AW, Lane JM, Fellinger EJ, Rosen V, Wozney JM, Wang EA. The healing of segmental bone defects, induced by recombinant human bone morphogenetic protein (rhBMP-2): a radiographic, histological, and biomechanical study in rats. J Bone Joint Surg Am 1992;74(5):659–670

68. Boden SD, Martin GJ Jr, Horton WC, Truss TL, Sandhu HS. Laparoscopic anterior spinal arthrodesis with rhBMP-2 in a titanium interbody threaded cage. J Spinal Disord 1998;11(2):95–101

69. Martin GJ Jr, Boden SD, Marone MA, Moskovitz PA. Posterolateral intertransverse process spinal arthrodesis with rhBMP-2 in a nonhuman primate: important lessons learned regarding dose, carrier, and safety. J Spinal Disord 1999;12(3):179–186

70. Sandhu HS, Kanim LE, Toth JM, et al. Experimental spinal fusion with recombinant human bone morphogenetic protein-2 without decortication of osseous elements. Spine 1997;22(11):1171–1180

71. Wang JC, Kanim LE, Yoo S, Campbell PA, Berk AJ, Lieberman JR. Effect of regional gene therapy with bone morphogenetic protein-2–producing bone marrow cells on spinal fusion in rats. J Bone Joint Surg Am 2003;85-A(5):905–911

72. Boden SD, Zdeblick TA, Sandhu HS, Heim SE. The use of rhBMP-2 in interbody fusion cages: definitive evidence of osteoinduction in humans. A preliminary report. Spine 2000;25(3):376–381

73. Food and Drug Administration. Device approval letter to Stryker. Available at: http://www.fda.gov/cdrh/pdf2/H020008a.pdf.

74. Boden SD, Martin GJ Jr, Morone M, Ugbo JL, Titus L, Hutton WC. The use of coralline hydroxyapatite with bone marrow, autogenous bone graft, or osteoinductive bone protein extract for posterolateral lumbar spine fusion. Spine 1999;24(4):320–327

75. Boden SD, Moskovitz PA, Morone MA, Toribitake Y. Video-assisted lateral intertransverse process arthrodesis: validation of a new minimally invasive lumbar spinal fusion technique in the rabbit and nonhuman primate (rhesus) models. Spine 1996;21(22):2689–2697

76. Grauer JN, Patel TC, Erulkar JS, Troiano NW, Panjabi MM, Friedlaender GE. 2000 Young Investigator Research Award Winner. Evaluation of OP-1 as a graft substitute for intertransverse process lumbar fusion. Spine 2001;26(2):127–133

77. Holliger EH, Trawick RH, Boden SD, Hutton WC. Morphology of the lumbar intertransverse process fusion mass in the rabbit model: a comparison between two bone graft materials–rhBMP-2 and autograft. J Spinal Disord 1996;9(2):125–128

78. Martin GJ Jr, Boden SD, Titus L. Recombinant human bone morphogenetic protein-2 overcomes the inhibitory effect of ketorolac, a nonsteroidal anti-inflammatory drug (NSAID), on posterolateral lumbar intertransverse process spine fusion. Spine 1999;24(21):2188–2193

79. Muschler GF, Hyodo A, Manning T, Kambic H, Easley K. Evaluation of human bone morphogenetic protein 2 in a canine spinal fusion model. Clin Orthop Relat Res 1994;(308):229–240

80. Sandhu HS, Kanim LE, Kabo JM, et al. Evaluation of rhBMP-2 with an OPLA carrier in a canine posterolateral (transverse process) spinal fusion model. Spine 1995;20(24):2669–2682

81. Schimandle JH, Boden SD, Hutton WC. Experimental spinal fusion with recombinant human bone morphogenetic protein-2. Spine 1995;20(12):1326–1337

82. Silcox DH III, Boden SD, Schimandle JH, Johnson P, Whitesides TE, Hutton WC. Reversing the inhibitory effect of nicotine on spinal fusion using an osteoinductive protein extract. Spine 1998;23(3):291–296

83. Blattert TR, Delling G, Dalal PS, Toth CA, Balling H, Weckbach A. Successful transpedicular lumbar interbody fusion by means of a composite of osteogenic protein-1 (rhBMP-7) and hydroxyapatite carrier: a comparison with autograft and hydroxyapatite in the sheep spine. Spine 2002;27(23):2697–2705

84. Kalodiki EP, Hoppensteadt DA, Nicolaides AN, et al. Deep venous thrombosis prophylaxis with low molecular weight heparin and elastic compression in patients having total hip replacement: a randomised controlled trial. Int Angiol 1996;15(2):162–168

85. Magin MN, Delling G. Improved lumbar vertebral interbody fusion using rhOP-1: a comparison of autogenous bone graft, bovine hydroxylapatite (Bio-Oss), and BMP-7 (rhOP-1) in sheep. Spine 2001;26(5):469–478

86. Masuda K, Takegami K, An H, et al. Recombinant osteogenic protein-1 upregulates extracellular matrix metabolism by rabbit annulus fibrosus and nucleus pulposus cells cultured in alginate beads. J Orthop Res 2003;21(5):922–930

87. Vaccaro AR, Patel T, Fischgrund J, et al. A pilot safety and efficacy study of OP-1 putty (rhBMP-7) as an adjunct to iliac crest autograft in posterolateral lumbar fusions. Eur Spine J 2003;12(5):495–500

88. Boden SD, Kang J, Sandhu H, Heller JG. 2002 Volvo Award Winner in Clinical Studies. Use of recombinant human bone morphogenetic protein-2 to achieve posterolateral lumbar spine fusion in humans: a prospective, randomized clinical pilot trial. Spine 2002;27(23):2662–2673

89. Suh DY, Boden SD, Louis-Ugbo J, et al. Delivery of recombinant human bone morphogenetic protein-2 using a compression-resistant matrix in posterolateral spine fusion in the rabbit and in the non-human primate. Spine 2002;27(4):353–360

90. Baltzer AW, Lieberman JR. Regional gene therapy to enhance bone repair. Gene Ther 2004;11(4):344–350

91. Hsu W, Sugiyama O, Feeley B, Liu N, Krenek L, An D, Chen I, Lieberman J. Lentiviral-mediated BMP-2 gene transfer enhances healing of segmental femoral defects in rats. Poster presented at American Society of Bone and Mineral Research 26th Annual Meeting; October 1–5, 2004; Seattle

92. Hsu WK, Sugiyama O, Park SH, et al. Lentiviral-mediated BMP-2 gene transfer enhances healing of segmental femoral defects in rats. Bone 2007;40(4):931–938

93. Dimar JR, Glassman SD, Burkus KJ, Carreon LY. Clinical outcomes and fusion success at 2 years of single-level instrumented posterolateral fusions with recombinant human bone morphogenetic protein-2/compression resistant matrix versus iliac crest bone graft. Spine 2006;31(22):2534–2539

94. Glassman SD, Carreon L, Djurasovic M, et al. Posterolateral lumbar spine fusion with INFUSE bone graft. Spine J 2007;7(1):44–49

95. Barnes B, Boden SD, Louis-Ugbo J, et al. Lower dose of rhBMP-2 achieves spine fusion when combined with an osteoconductive bulking agent in non-human primates. Spine 2005;30(10):1127–1133

96. Akamaru T, Suh D, Boden SD, Kim HS, Minamide A, Louis-Ugbo J. Simple carrier matrix modifications can enhance delivery of

recombinant human bone morphogenetic protein-2 for postero-lateral spine fusion. Spine 2003;28(5):429–434

97. Patel VV, Zhao L, Wong P, et al. Controlling bone morphogenetic protein diffusion and bone morphogenetic protein-stimulated bone growth using fibrin glue. Spine 2006;31(11):1201–1206

98. White AP, Maak TG, Prince D, et al. Osteogenic protein-1 induced gene expression: evaluation in a posterolateral spinal pseudarthrosis model. Spine 2006;31(22):2550–2555

99. Smucker JD, Rhee JM, Singh K, Yoon ST, Heller JG. Increased swelling complications associated with off-label usage of rhBMP-2 in the anterior cervical spine. Spine 2006;31(24):2813–2819

100. Perri B, Cooper M, Lauryssen C, Anand N. Adverse swelling associated with use of rh-BMP-2 in anterior cervical discectomy and fusion: a case study. Spine J 2007;7(2):235–239

101. Shields LB, Raque GH, Glassman SD, et al. Adverse effects associated with high-dose recombinant human bone morphogenetic protein-2 use in anterior cervical spine fusion. Spine 2006;31(5):542–547

102. McClellan JW, Mulconrey DS, Forbes RJ, Fullmer N. Vertebral bone resorption after transforaminal lumbar interbody fusion with bone morphogenetic protein (rhBMP-2). J Spinal Disord Tech 2006;19(7):483–486

103. Alden TD, Pittman DD, Beres EJ, et al. Percutaneous spinal fusion using bone morphogenetic protein-2 gene therapy. J Neurosurg 1999;90(1, Suppl):109–114

104. Helm GA, Alden TD, Beres EJ, et al. Use of bone morphogenetic protein-9 gene therapy to induce spinal arthrodesis in the rodent. J Neurosurg 2000;92(2, Suppl):191–196

105. Riew KD, Wright NM, Cheng S, Avioli LV, Lou J. Induction of bone formation using a recombinant adenoviral vector carrying the human BMP-2 gene in a rabbit spinal fusion model. Calcif Tissue Int 1998;63(4):357–360

106. Lee JY, Musgrave D, Pelinkovic D, et al. Effect of bone morphogenetic protein-2-expressing muscle-derived cells on healing of critical-sized bone defects in mice. J Bone Joint Surg Am 2001;83-A(7):1032–1039

107. Lieberman JR, Daluiski A, Stevenson S, et al. The effect of regional gene therapy with bone morphogenetic protein-2-producing bone-marrow cells on the repair of segmental femoral defects in rats. J Bone Joint Surg Am 1999;81(7):905–917

108. Lieberman JR, Le LQ, Wu L, et al. Regional gene therapy with a BMP-2-producing murine stromal cell line induces heterotopic and orthotopic bone formation in rodents. J Orthop Res 1998;16(3):330–339

109. Boden SD, Titus L, Hair G, et al. Lumbar spine fusion by local gene therapy with a cDNA encoding a novel osteoinductive protein (LMP-1). Spine 1998;23(23):2486–2492

110. Viggeswarapu M, et al. Adenoviral delivery of LIM mineralization protein-1 induces new-bone formation in vitro and in vivo. J Bone Joint Surg Am 2001;83-A(3):364–376

111. Breitbart AS, Grande DA, Mason JM, Barcia M, James T, Grant RT. Gene-enhanced tissue engineering: applications for bone healing using cultured periosteal cells transduced retrovirally with the BMP-7 gene. Ann Plast Surg 1999;42(5):488–495

112. Riew KD, Lou J, Wright NM, Cheng SL, Bae KT, Avioli LV. Thoracoscopic intradiscal spine fusion using a minimally invasive gene-therapy technique. J Bone Joint Surg Am 2003;85-A(5):866–871

113. Luk KD, Chen Y, Cheung KM, Kung HF, Lu WW, Leong JC. Adeno-associated virus-mediated bone morphogenetic protein-4 gene therapy for in vivo bone formation. Biochem Biophys Res Commun 2003;308(3):636–645

114. Laurent JJ, Webb KM, Beres EJ, et al. The use of bone morphogenetic protein-6 gene therapy for percutaneous spinal fusion in rabbits. J Neurosurg Spine 2004;1(1):90–94

115. Dumont RJ, Dayoub H, Li JZ, et al. Ex vivo bone morphogenetic protein-9 gene therapy using human mesenchymal stem cells induces spinal fusion in rodents. Neurosurgery 2002;51(5):1239–1244

116. Aono A, Hazama M, Notoya K, et al. Potent ectopic bone-inducing activity of bone morphogenetic protein-4/7 heterodimer. Biochem Biophys Res Commun 1995;210(3):670–677

117. Hazama M, Aono A, Ueno N, Fujisawa Y. Efficient expression of a heterodimer of bone morphogenetic protein subunits using a baculovirus expression system. Biochem Biophys Res Commun 1995;209(3):859–866

118. Israel DI, Nove J, Kerns KM, et al. Heterodimeric bone morphogenetic proteins show enhanced activity in vitro and in vivo. Growth Factors 1996;13(3–4):291–300

119. Zhu W, Rawlins BA, Boachie-Adjei O, et al. Combined bone morphogenetic protein-2 and -7 gene transfer enhances osteoblastic differentiation and spine fusion in a rodent model. J Bone Miner Res 2004;19(12):2021–2032

120. Okubo Y, Bessho K, Fujimura K, Iizuka T, Miyatake SI. In vitro and in vivo studies of a bone morphogenetic protein-2 expressing adenoviral vector. J Bone Joint Surg Am 2001;83-A(Suppl 1,(Pt 2):S99–S104

121. Musgrave DS, Pruchnic R, Bosch P, Ziran BH, Whalen J, Huard J. Human skeletal muscle cells in ex vivo gene therapy to deliver bone morphogenetic protein-2. J Bone Joint Surg Br 2002;84(1):120–127

122. Shen HC, Peng H, Usas A, Gearhart B, Fu FH, Huard J. Structural and functional healing of critical-size segmental bone defects by transduced muscle-derived cells expressing BMP4. J Gene Med 2004;6(9):984–991

123. Fraser JK, Wulur I, Alfonso Z, Hedrick MH. Fat tissue: an underappreciated source of stem cells for biotechnology. Trends Biotechnol 2006;24(4):150–154

124. Zuk PA, Zhu M, Mizuno H, et al. Multilineage cells from human adipose tissue: implications for cell-based therapies. Tissue Eng 2001;7(2):211–228

125. Dragoo JL, Choi JY, Lieberman JR, et al. Bone induction by BMP-2 transduced stem cells derived from human fat. J Orthop Res 2003;21(4):622–629

126. Hsu W, Wang J, Feeley B, et al. Gene therapy utilizing stem cells from human fat in a rat posterolateral spine fusion model. Spine J 2004;4(5S):51S

127. Peterson B, Zhang J, Iglesias R, et al. Healing of critically sized femoral defects, using genetically modified mesenchymal stem cells from human adipose tissue. Tissue Eng 2005;11(1–2):120–129

128. Burkus JK, Gornet MF, Dickman CA, Zdeblick TA. Anterior lumbar interbody fusion using rhBMP-2 with tapered interbody cages. J Spinal Disord Tech 2002;15(5):337–349

129. Vaccaro AR, Anderson DG, Patel T, et al. Comparison of OP-1 Putty (rhBMP-7) to iliac crest autograft for posterolateral lumbar arthrodesis: a minimum 2-year follow-up pilot study. Spine 2005;30(24):2709–2716

130. Valentin-Opran A, Wozney J, Csimma C, Lilly L, Riedel GE. Clinical evaluation of recombinant human bone morphogenetic protein-2. Clin Orthop Relat Res 2002;(395):110–120

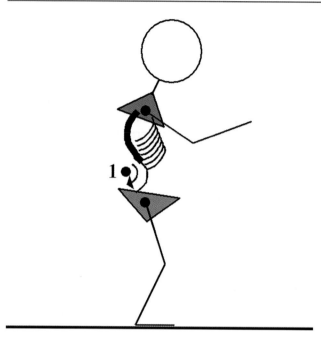

Fig. 31.2 A fixed thoracic hyperkyphotic deformity (bold) produces a compensatory lumbar hyperlordosis (1) in erect standing posture. Patients compensate for excess load on the posterior elements with hip and knee flexion.

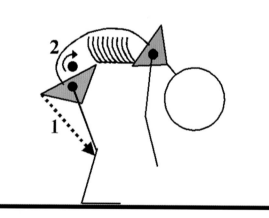

Fig. 31.3 Shortened hamstrings (1) prevent physiologic pelvic flexion over the hips during forward bending. This produces an excessive kyphotic force upon the lumbar spine (2). Patients compensate for hamstring tightness with knee flexion, increased thoracic kyphosis, and shoulder protraction when attempting to touch the floor.

Table 31.1 Patterns of Muscle Imbalance about the Pelvis and Trunk Affecting the Sagittal Balance of the Lumbar Spine[18]

Shortened Muscles	Weak Muscles
Hamstrings	Gluteus maximus
Rectus femoris	Rectus abdominis
Iliopsoas	
Erector spinae	

Muscles Exhibiting Tendency toward Shortening

Iliopsoas

The psoas portion of the iliopsoas complex originates from the transverse processes of T12 through L5 and crosses the pelvis and hip before attaching to the lesser trochanter of the femur (**Fig. 31.4**). Concentric contraction of the iliopsoas muscle is associated with increases in lumbar lordosis in experimental subjects[19] as well as hip flexion. The eccentric function of this muscle is to prevent uncontrolled hip extension. Shortening of this muscle mimics concentric contraction, and is associated with hyperlordosis (**Fig. 31.5**), secondarily causing increased mechanical force upon the posterior elements.[20-23]

Rectus Femoris

The rectus femoris originates from the anterior inferior iliac spine and crosses the hip before inserting into the patella via the common quadriceps tendon (**Fig. 31.6**). It is a "two joint muscle" and its effect on the hip and pelvis are realized

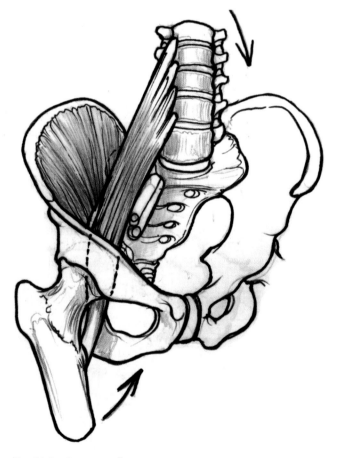

Fig. 31.4 Concentric iliopsoas contraction produces lumbar lordosis and hip flexion. Eccentric contraction controls hip extension.

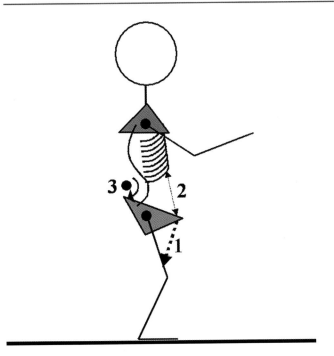

Fig. 31.5 Hyperlordosis of the lumbar spine (3) in erect standing posture may be caused by contracture of the hip flexors (1), weakness of the rectus abdominis (2), or both.

only with the knee in full extension, as in static standing. Concentric contraction of the rectus femoris produces hip flexion and knee extension. In static standing with the knee fully extended, shortening of this muscle produces flexion of the pelvis over the femoral heads, producing a secondarily exaggerated lumbar lordosis (**Fig. 31.5**) and again, increased mechanical force upon the posterior elements. The eccentric function of this muscle about the hip is to prevent uncontrolled hip extension, although this effect is diminished when the knee is flexed, as in the swing phase of gait.

Hamstrings

The hamstrings consist of the semimembranosus, semitendinosus, and biceps femoris long and short heads. Like the rectus femoris, this is a two joint muscle, and its effect on the hip and pelvis are realized only with the knee in full extension, as in static standing. The hamstrings originate from a common tendon off the ischial tuberosity and insert into the medial proximal tibia and posterior capsule of the knee (**Fig. 31.7**). Concentric contraction of the hamstrings produces hip extension and knee flexion. In static standing with the foot planted and knee fully extended, shortening of this muscle produces extension of the pelvis over the femoral heads, limiting hip flexion during bending at the waist, producing a secondarily exaggerated

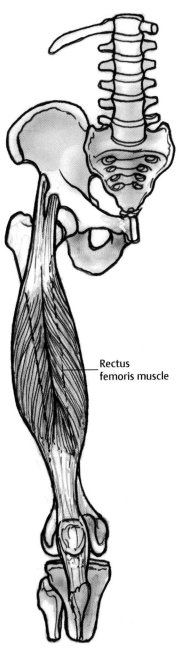

Rectus femoris muscle

Fig. 31.6 Rectus femoris concentric contraction produces hip flexion and knee extension. Its eccentric function about the hip and pelvis is limited by a short lever arm and maximized with the knee in full extension.

lumbar kyphosis (**Fig. 31.3**). This kyphotic force places increased mechanical force upon the anterior column of the spine, including the disc.[24] This is one of the reasons that it is recommended to bend at the knees when picking objects off the floor. The eccentric function of this muscle about the hip is to prevent uncontrolled hip flexion,[25] but this effect is markedly diminished when the knee is flexed, as in the swing phase of gait.

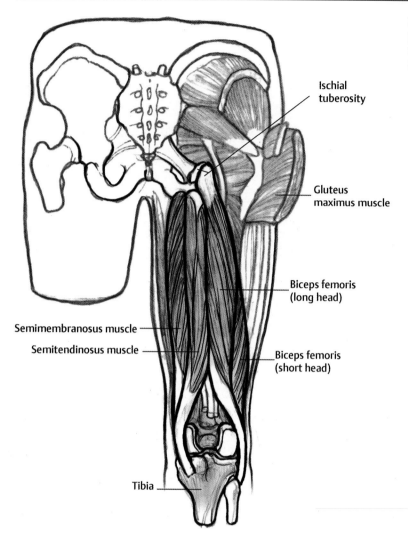

Fig. 31.7 Concentric contraction of the hamstrings produces hip extension and knee flexion. Its eccentric role about the hip in erect posture is to guard against uncontrolled pelvic flexion over the hips.

Ischial tuberosity

Gluteus maximus muscle

Biceps femoris (long head)

Semimembranosus muscle

Semitendinosus muscle

Biceps femoris (short head)

Tibia

Muscles Exhibiting Tendency toward Weakness

Rectus Abdominis

The rectus abdominis originates from the anterior ribs and traverses the anterior abdominal wall, attaching into the symphysis pubis (**Fig. 31.8**). Concentric contraction of the rectus muscle produces lumbar flexion, reducing lordosis. The eccentric function of this muscle is to prevent uncontrolled lumbar extension.[26,27] Eccentric weakness of this muscle produces hyperlordosis by allowing flexion of the pelvis over the hips in erect posture (**Fig. 31.5**), secondarily causing increased mechanical force upon the posterior elements.

Gluteus Maximus

The gluteus maximus originates from posterior iliac crests and thoracolumbar fascia and inserts into the greater trochanter and iliotibial band (**Fig. 31.9**). Concentric contraction of the gluteus maximus muscle produces hip

extension, and it is the most powerful of the hip extensors. The eccentric function of this muscle is to prevent uncontrolled hip flexion.[28] Eccentric weakness of this muscle (and the hamstrings) during dynamic forward flexion causes the secondary activation of the erector spine[29] and other paraspinals to prevent hyperflexion of the trunk. As the paraspinal muscles have significantly less contractile strength than the gluteus, the paraspinals are subject to failure, leading to muscle sprain or injury to the anterior column structures, including the disc.

Thoracolumbar Fascia

The thoracolumbar fascia controls lumbar lordosis by its attachment to the lumbar spinous processes (**Fig. 31.10**). Tension of the thoracolumbar fascia is provided by the pull of the transversus abdominis and latissimus dorsi on the edges of the fascia,[30] and maintains normal lordosis by tending to align the spinous processes in the plane of the

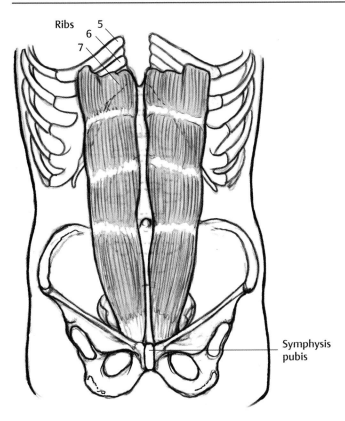

Fig. 31.8 The rectus abdominis produces trunk flexion with concentric contraction. Eccentric contraction protects against uncontrolled lumbar extension.

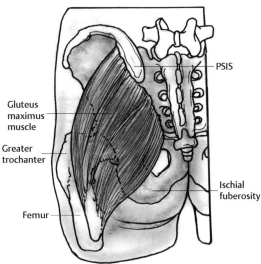

Fig. 31.9 The gluteus maximus is a powerful hip extensor in its concentric mode. Eccentrically, it prevents uncontrolled pelvic flexion. PSIS, posterosuperior iliac spine.

fascia. Weakness of the attached muscles allows hyperlordosis due to laxity of the thoracolumbar fascia.

Segmental Anatomy and Biomechanics

Spine biomechanics may also be examined from the viewpoint of the motion segment, consisting of two adjacent vertebrae and involving three joints. The three-joint complex consists of the intervertebral joint, spaced by the disc, and two posterolateral synovial facet joints (**Fig. 31.11**).[31]

Passive Stabilizers of Segmental Motion

The intervertebral disc is constructed of a multilayered anulus fibrosus surrounding a viscous proteoglycan and water-laden nucleus pulposus.[32] Annular fibers are aligned at 30 degrees from the horizontal[33] and resist intervertebral rotation (**Fig. 31.12**).[34] Repeated microtears of the anulus may result in a loss of structural integrity, allowing the nucleus pulposus to herniate.[31] Internal disc pressure is greatest in lumbar flexion,[24] and the normal intervertebral joint bears ~72% of body weight in static standing.[23]

The facet joints are true synovial joints and are oriented vertically, allowing segmental flexion and extension, but

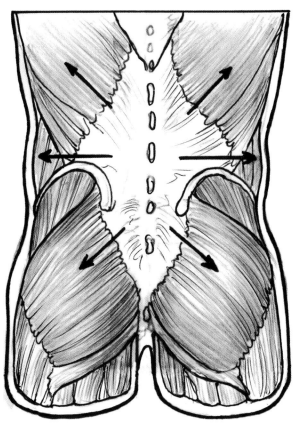

Fig. 31.10 Tension of the thoracolumbar fascia tends to control lumbar lordosis by way of its attachment to the lumbar spinous processes. The transversus abdominis muscle attaches deep to the fascia and latissimus dorsi superiorly to maintain tension. The inferior portion of the fascia serves as an attachment site of the gluteus maximus.

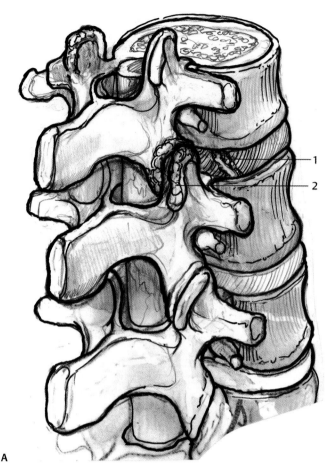
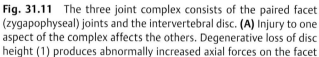
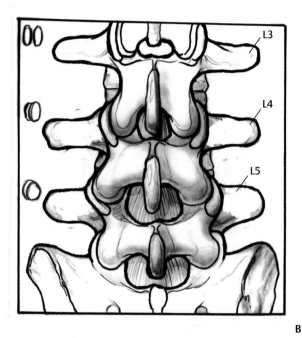

Fig. 31.11 The three joint complex consists of the paired facet (zygapophyseal) joints and the intervertebral disc. **(A)** Injury to one aspect of the complex affects the others. Degenerative loss of disc height (1) produces abnormally increased axial forces on the facet joints, leading to premature proliferative arthritic changes (2). **(B)** The facet orientation limits lateral bending and axial rotation of the motion segment.

limiting lateral bending and rotation (**Fig. 31.11**).[35] Normal joints bear ~28% of body weight in static standing, but lumbar extension increases the facet load by more than twice over neutral standing,[23] and the presence of disc space narrowing can increase facet loading to 70% of body weight.[36] The pars interarticularis is likewise susceptible to high loads with lumbar extension.

The static stabilizers of lumbar flexion are the posterior longitudinal ligament, ligamentum flavum, facet capsules, interspinous ligament, supraspinous ligament, and anterior disc compression. These stabilizers become important only upon full flaccid lumbar flexion.[29,37]

Active Stabilizers of Segmental Motion

The deep paraspinal muscle layer, including the rotatores, multifidi, and intertransversarii, appears to control intersegmental postural alignment.[38] Electromyographic activity of the deep muscle layer is associated with increased intradiscal pressure.[39] Knowledge of the dynamic muscular stabilizers of segmental rotation is unclear, but the erector spinae[38] and abdominal oblique muscles may play a role. The anulus appears to be the primary stabilizer.[35]

■ Rehabilitation Principles

Therapeutic exercise programs follow a standard progression. The initial goal of rehabilitation is to control inflammation either pharmacologically or with modalities such as ice.[40] The next step is to correct ROM restrictions of structures adjacent to the painful or injured area. This is accomplished with stretching or related techniques such as muscle energy, strain-counterstrain, etc. Stretching and lengthening of muscles may be aided by preheating with superficial or deep heating modalities.[41] Once ROM and inflammation are controlled, the focus is on strengthening the dynamic stabilizers of the injured area. Concentric exercise may be better tolerated in the early stages of the exercise program as this mode

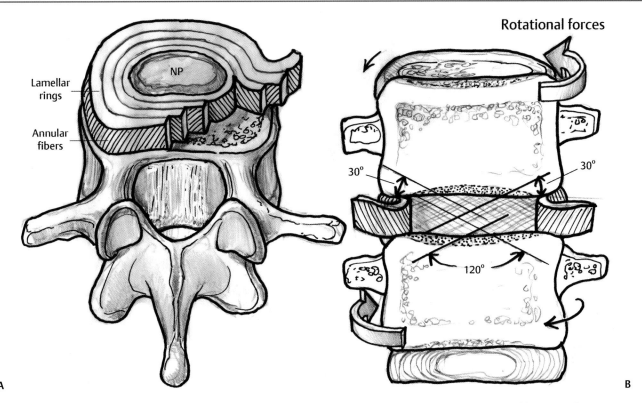

Fig. 31.12 Anulus fibrosus. The lamellated structure **(A)** and the oblique, crossed arrangement **(B)** of annular fibers provide resistance to lumbar segmental rotation. NP, nucleus pulposus.

of strengthening produces lower muscle tension for a given load.[42] Eccentric muscle strength training of the protective muscle is essential to protect against future injury. As it produces high muscle tension,[42] however, eccentric strengthening across the injured or postoperative region should be avoided until pain is under good control. Endurance training in the form of aerobic exercise is interwoven with the above program to diminish fatigability of the dynamic stabilizers. Proprioceptive training reinforces neuromuscular engrams that prevent injury.[5]

One cannot overemphasize the importance of active exercise. Modalities should be used spaningly to facilitate successful active participation in the exercise program, and overdependence on passive modalities should be avoided. The patient must come to understand that a lifetime of active exercise is often necessary for long-term control of spinal symptoms. This often requires a behavioral change that many patients will find difficult, and they may require significant encouragement and counseling.

Rehabilitation Program for Discectomy Patients

The biomechanical milieu of the postoperative region in discectomy patients is substantially different from the normal anatomy. There is disruption of the anulus from herniation and operative intervention, decreasing the disc's capacity to control rotational forces.[43,44] Facetectomy may produce sagittal or rotational instability of the motion segment.[45–47] Wide laminectomy with resection of the spinous process and interspinous ligaments increases flexion–extension travel of the motion segment, decreases rotational stability,[48] and removes muscle attachment sites. Operative injury to the paraspinal muscles reduces intersegmental balance and stability of the operated segment. Generally speaking a theme of *instability* of the operated segment is noted. Epidural fibrosis is a result of granulation tissue about the operative site and may mature in as few as 5 weeks or remain immature indefinitely.[49]

The goal of the therapeutic exercise program is to protect the disc and surrounding structures to allow healing and prevent reinjury. Specifically, it is desirable to promote controlled and avoid uncontrolled flexion and rotation moments over the operated spinal segment. In forward bending, restricted flexion of the pelvis over the hips from tight hamstrings puts excessive flexion moment on the lumbar segments. It is recommended that hamstrings be lengthened to allow 90 degrees of hip flexion with a straight knee. Control of dynamic trunk flexion is encouraged by eccentric strengthening of the gluteus maximus, erector spinae, and particularly, the hamstrings. Control of dynamic axial rotation is encouraged by eccentrically strengthening the abdominal oblique, erector spinae, and hip rotator muscles. As paraspinal spasm increases intradiscal pressure, therapeutic massage or lengthening of these muscles with muscle energy techniques is indicated. Therapeutic philosophies such as neutral spinal stabilization[50] and the McKenzie[51] methods focus on protection of injured discs. Therapeutic exercise is initially performed avoiding lumbar flexion, but as pain decreases, exercises are gradually performed in the full range of spinal motion. Protective reflexes are promoted in muscles by the challenge of hip and trunk stabilizers under controlled conditions. Aerobic conditioning and endurance training are indicated to prevent muscle fatigue during prolonged activities. Neuromobilization techniques as described by Butler may be helpful to reduce the symptoms of epidural scarring.[52]

Rehabilitation Goals for Fusion Patients

In distinction to the discectomy situation when introduction of *instability* is the major biomechanical challenge, fusion patients have a biomechanical milieu characterized by nonphysiologic *rigidity* of the surgical segments. Although the concept of adjacent segment dysfunction is under debate,[53–55] it is clear that the spinal segments above and below the fusion site are subject to supranormal forces.[56–59] Although there are varying opinions,[60] recent studies indicate that adjacent segment forces may also cause the sacroiliac joint to become painful when fusions incorporate the sacrum.[61,62] Paraspinal muscle disruption is more extensive in standard posterior fusion approaches compared with routine discectomy but is minimized in anterior and minimally invasive approaches.

Once the surgical site has achieved solid bony fusion, a postoperative exercise program is recommended to protect adjacent structures minimize the effect of scar tissue, and promote aerobic reconditioning. The role of oral antiinflammatory medication postfusion is controversial as these medications may retard bony union.[63] As we have discussed already,[17] humans have a predisposition to certain patterns of muscle shortening and weakness affecting erect posture, and these alterations place undue forces on the spine. In patients who have undergone a lumbar fusion, the rehabilitation goals are to maximize the flexibility of the surrounding structures and provide controlled eccentric contraction for protection of the adjacent segments. As in discectomy patients, minimization of epidural fibrosis-related symptoms is of importance.

Specific rehabilitation goals in postfusion patients include stretching muscles prone to shortening to above-average lengths. Hamstrings should optimally lengthen to achieve 90 degrees of hip flexion with the knee fully extended without diminishing physiologic lumbar lordosis during the stretch. Iliopsoas stretching should achieve hip extension to at least neutral and preferably 5 to 10 degrees of hip extension without producing lumbar hyperlordosis. The rectus femoris should be lengthened to allow contact of the heel to the gluteal muscles in prone lying, controlling for lumbar hyperlordosis. Paraspinal muscle tension should be reduced over the proximal and distal segments adjacent to the fusion to avoid increased intradiscal pressure.[39] This is accomplished with muscle energy techniques, massage, or manual medicine. Muscles prone to weakness must be strengthened in both their concentric and eccentric functions. Targets include the rectus abdominis, the gluteal muscles, and the muscles controlling the thoracolumbar fascia, namely the transverses abdominis and latissimus dorsi. Protective reflexes are promoted in muscles by challenge of hip and trunk stabilizers under controlled conditions. Aerobic conditioning and endurance training are indicated to prevent muscle fatigue during prolonged activities. As in discectomy patients, neuromobilization techniques as described by Butler may be helpful to reduce the symptoms of epidural scarring.[52]

■ Conclusion

In this chapter, we have formulated biomechanically based rehabilitation programs for discectomy and fusion patients. The medical literature is fraught with studies measuring the outcomes of "one size fits all" rehabilitation programs with widely varying results. Individually tailored, biomechanically based rehabilitation programs make intuitive sense, but require further substantiation with outcome studies.

References

1. Abenhaim L, Rossignol M, Valat JP, et al. The role of activity in the therapeutic management of low back pain: report on the International Paris Task Force on Back Pain. Spine 2000;25(4 suppl)1S–33S
2. Bigos S, Bowyer O, Braen G, et al. Acute Low Back Problems in Adults: Clinical Practice Guidelines (Quick Reference Guide No. 14). Rockville, MD: US Department of Health and Human Services, Agency for Health Care Policy and Research; 1994
3. Practitioners RCoG. Clinical Guidelines for the Management of Acute Low Back Pain. London: Royal College of General Practitioners; 1999
4. Long A, Donelson R, Fung T. Does it matter which exercise? A randomized control trial of exercise for low back pain. Spine 2004;29(23):2593–2602
5. Kjellby-Wendt G, Styf J. Early active training after lumbar discectomy: a prospective randomized and controlled study. Spine 1998;23(21):2345–2351
6. Millisdotter M, Strömqvist B. Early neuromuscular customized training after surgery for lumbar disc herniation: a prospective controlled study. Eur Spine J 2007;16(1):19–26

7. Dolan P, Greenfield K, Nelson RJ, Nelson IW. Can exercise therapy improve the outcome of microdiscectomy? Spine 2000;25(12): 1523–1532

8. Filiz M, Cakmak A, Ozcan E. The effectiveness of exercise programmes after lumbar disc surgery: a randomized controlled study. Clin Rehabil 2005;19(1):4–11

9. Ostelo RW, de Vet HC, Waddell G, Kerckhoffs MR, Leffers P, van Tulder M. Rehabilitation following first-time lumbar disc surgery: a systematic review within the framework of the Cochrane Collaboration. Spine 2003;28(3):209–218

10. Christensen FB, Laurberg I, Bünger CE. Importance of the back-café concept to rehabilitation after lumbar spinal fusion: a randomized clinical study with a 2-year follow-up. Spine 2003;28(23): 2561–2569

11. Soegaard R, Christensen FB, Lauerberg I, Bünger CE. Lumbar spinal fusion patients' demands to the primary health sector: evaluation of three rehabilitation protocols: a prospective randomized study. Eur Spine J 2006;15(5):648–656

12. Watt D, Jones GM. On the functional role of the myotactic reflex in man. Proc Can Fed Biol Soc 1966;9:13

13. Carlsöö S, Johansson O. Stabilization of and load on the elbow joint in some protective movements: an experimental study. Acta Anat (Basel) 1962;48:224–231

14. Basmajian JV, DeLuca CJ. Muscles Alive: Their Functions Revealed by Electromyography. Baltimore: Williams and Wilkins; 1985:367–388

15. Pavone E, Moffat M. Isometric torque of the quadriceps femoris after concentric, eccentric, and isometric training. Arch Phys Med Rehabil 1985;66:168–170

16. Gregersen GG, Lucas DB. An in vitro study of the axial rotation of the human thoracolumbar spine. J Bone Joint Surg Am 1967;49: 247–262

17. Janda V. Muscles and motor control in low back pain: assessment and management. In: Twomey L, ed. Physical Therapy of the Low Back. New York: Churchill Livingstone; 1987:253–278

18. Janda V. Comparison of spastic syndromes of cerebral origin with the distribution of muscular tightness in postural defects. Paper presented at Reha-biliticia Supplementum 14-15: the 5th International Symposium of Rehabilitation in Neurology; 1977

19. Basmajian JV, DeLuca CJ. Muscles Alive: Their Functions Revealed by Electromyography. Baltimore: Williams and Wilkins, 1985.

20. Hakim NS, King AI. Static and dynamic facet loads. In: Proceedings of the 20th Stapp Car Crash Conference. Warrendale, PA: Society of Automotive Engineers; 1976:607–639

21. Lin HS, Liu YK, Adams KH. Mechanical response of the lumbar intervertebral joint under physiological (complex) loading. J Bone Joint Surg Am 1978;60:41–54

22. Markolf KL. Deformation of the thoracolumbar intervertebral joints in response to external loads. J Bone Joint Surg Am 1972;54:511–533

23. Lorenz M, Patwardhan A, Vanderby R. Load bearing characteristics of lumbar facets in normal and surgically altered spinal segments. Spine 1983;8:122–130

24. Nachemson A. The load on lumbar disks in different positions of the body. Clin Orthop Relat Res 1966;45:107–122

25. Carlsoeoe S. Influence of frontal and dorsal loads on muscle activity and on the weight distribution in the feet. Acta Orthop Scand 1964;34:299–309

26. Partridge MJ, Walters CE. Participation of the abdominal muscles in various movement of the trunk in man: an electromyographic study. Phys Ther Rev 1959;39:791–800

27. Ono K. Electromyographic studies of the abdominal wall muscles in visceroptosis: I. Analysis of patterns of activity of the abdominal wall muscles in normal adults. Tokohu J Exp Med 1958;68:347–354

28. Karlsson E, Jonsson B. Function of the gluteus maximus muscle: an electromyographic study. Acta Morphol Neerl Scand 1965;6:161–169

29. Floyd WF, Silver PHS. Function of erectores spinae muscles in certain movements and postures in man. J Physiol 1955;129:184–203

30. Gracovetsky S, Farfan HF, Lamy C. The mechanism of the lumbar spine. Spine 1981;6:249–262

31. Kirkaldy-Willis WH. Pathology and pathogenesis of low back pain. In: Kirkaldy-Willis WH, Burton CV, eds. Managing Low Back Pain. New York: Churchill Livingstone; 1992

32. Lipson SJ, Muir H. Proteoglycans in experimental intervertebral disc degeneration. Spine 1981;6:194–210

33. White A, Panjabi M. Clinical Biomechanics of the Spine. 2nd ed. Philadelphia: JB Lippincott; 1990:38–79

34. Farfan HF, Cosette JW, Robertson GH, et al. The effects of torsion on the lumbar intervertebral joints: the role torsion in the production of disc degeneration. J Bone Joint Surg Am 1970;52:468–497

35. Haher TR, Felmly W, Devlin V, et al. The contribution of the three columns of the spine to rotational stability: a biomechanical model. Spine 1989;14:663–669

36. Adams MA, Hutton WC. The mechanical function of the lumbar apophyseal joints. Spine 1983;8:327–330

37. Allen CE. Muscle action potentials used in the study of dynamic anatomy. Br J Phys Med. 1948;11:66–73

38. Donisch EW, Basmajian JV. Electromyography of deep muscles in man. Am J Anat 1972;133:25–36

39. Andersson BJ, Örtengren R, Nachemson A, et al. The sitting posture: an electromyographic and discometric study. Orthop Clin North Am 1975;6:105–120

40. Grant AE. Massage with ice (cryokinetics) in the treatment of painful conditions of the musculoskeletal system. Arch Phys Med Rehabil 1964;45:233–238

41. Lehmann JF, Masock AJ, Warren CG, et al. Effect of therapeutic temperatures on tendon extensibility. Arch Phys Med Rehabil 1970; 51:481–487

42. Guyton AC. Textbook of Medical Physiology. 8th ed. Philadelphia: WB Saunders; 1991

43. Goel VK, Nishiyama K, Weinstein JN, Liu YK. Mechanical properties of lumbar spinal motion segments as affected by partial disc removal. Spine 1986;11(10):1008–1012

44. Natarajan RN, Andersson GB, Patwardhan AG, Verma S. Effect of annular incision type on the change in biomechanical properties in a herniated lumbar intervertebral disc. J Biomech Eng 2002;124(2): 229–236

45. Lee KK, Teo EC, Qiu TX, Eng M, Yang K. Effect of facetectomy on lumbar spinal stability under sagittal plane loadings. Spine 2004;29(15): 1624–1631

46. Natarajan RN, Andersson GBJ, Patwardhan AG, et al. Study on effect of graded facetectomy on change in lumbar motion segment torsion flexibility using three-dimensional continuum contact representation for facet joints. J Biomech Eng 1999;121:215–221

47. Abumi K, Panjabi MM, Kramer KM, et al. Biomechanical evaluation of lumbar spine stability after graded facetectomies. Spine 1990; 15:1142–1147

48. Zander T, Rohlmann A, Bergmann G. Analysis of simulated single ligament transection on the mechanical behaviour of a lumbar functional spinal unit. Biomed Tech (Berl) 2004;49(1–2):27–32

49. Bundschuh CV, Stein L, Slusser JH, et al. Distinguishing between scar and recurrent herniated disc in postoperative patients: value of contrast enhanced CT and MR imaging. AJNR Am J Neuroradiol 1990;11:949–958

50. Saal JA. Dynamic muscular stabilization in the nonoperative treatment of lumbar pain syndromes. Orthop Rev 1990;19(8):691–700

51. McKenzie RA. The Lumbar Spine: Mechanical Diagnosis and Therapy. Waikanae, New Zealand: Spinal Publications; 1981

52. Butler DS. Mobilisation of the Nervous System. Melbourne, Australia: Churchill Livingstone; 1991

53. Penta M, Sandhu A, Fraser RD. Magnetic resonance imaging assessment of disc degeneration 10 years after anterior lumbar interbody fusion. Spine 1995;20(6):743–747

54. Dekutoski MB, Schendel MJ, Ogilvie JW, et al. Comparison of in vivo and in vitro adjacent segment motion after lumbar fusion. Spine 1994;19(15):1745–1751

55. Chou WY, Hsu CJ, Chang WN, Wong Cy. Adjacent segment degeneration after lumbar spinal posterolateral fusion with instrumentation in elderly patients. Arch Orthop Trauma Surg 2002;122(1):39–43

56. Axelsson P, Johnsson R, Stromqvist B. The spondylolytic vertebra and its adjacent segment: mobility measured before and after posterolateral fusion. Spine 1997;22(4):414–417

57. Weinhoffer SL, Guyer RD, Herbert M, Griffith SL. Intradiscal pressure measurements above an instrumented fusion: a cadaveric study. Spine 1995;20(5):526–531

58. Chow DH, Luk KD, Evans JH, Leong JC. Effects of short anterior lumbar interbody fusion on biomechanics of neighboring unfused segments. Spine 1996;21(5):549–555

59. Frymoyer JW, Hanley EN Jr, Howe J, et al. A comparison of radiographic findings in fusion and nonfusion patients ten or more years following lumbar disc surgery. Spine 1979;4(5):435–440

60. Frymoyer JW, Howe J, Kuhlmann D. The long-term effects of spinal fusion on the sacroiliac joints and ilium. Clin Orthop Relat Res 1978;(134):196–201

61. Katz V, Schofferman J, Reynolds J. The sacroiliac joint: a potential cause of pain after lumbar fusion to the sacrum. J Spinal Disord Tech 2003;16(1):96–99

62. Maigne JY, Planchon CA. Sacroiliac joint pain after lumbar fusion: a study with anesthetic blocks. Eur Spine J 2005;14(7):654–658

63. Dahners LE, Mullis BH. Effects of nonsteroidal anti-inflammatory drugs on bone formation and soft-tissue healing. J Am Acad Orthop Surg 2004;12(3):139–143

32 Surgical Treatment of Degenerative Lumbar Disc Disease: A Critical Review

Stewart M. Kerr, Andrew P. White, and Todd J. Albert

Surgery rates for degenerative lumbar conditions vary regionally within the United States.[1] There also is a dramatic difference seen when comparing U.S. trends to other developed nations.[2] The volume of spinal surgery has also been increasing over time; investigators have reported a 200% increase in the number of lumbar spinal fusions performed in the United States annually since the late 1980s.[3,4] This epidemiologic information, considered alongside lay press editorials and conflicting medical opinions, has raised questions regarding the appropriateness of surgery for degenerative lumbar conditions.

Although it is widely accepted that some degenerative lumbar pathology such as neurocompressive conditions that result in progressive lower extremity motor deficit or cauda equina syndrome should be managed operatively, surgical indications for many other degenerative lumbar processes are not as clear. Most humans will experience back pain at some point in their life and most often an identifiable cause cannot be determined.

The contemporary literature is replete with reports describing operative treatments for various lumbar degenerative conditions. Collectively determining which patients will likely benefit from spinal surgical procedures is not well described, and unfortunately many current reports lack sufficient power or have inherent methodologic flaws hindering management consensus. Indeed, even high-quality level 1 studies often show fairly equivocal results when evaluated with "intent-to-treat" principles. These results are understandably perplexing to clinicians, patients, policymakers, and the health insurance industry.

The extent of surgical intervention, if any, for many of the degenerative processes in the lumbar spine remains controversial from an evidence-based medicine standpoint. Society is relying on the sound judgment of health care professionals to "do the right thing" with limited fiscal resources. The need for evidence to guide our surgical actions will likely grow in importance as budgets experience the costly reality of an aging population.

■ Decision Making about Treatment

In the absence of tumor or infection, the etiology of lumbar pain is poorly understood. Even in relatively straightforward clinical scenarios such as nerve root compression caused by a herniated nucleus pulposus, it is clearly possible for a wide variety of symptoms or even no correlation with the extent of abnormality seen on radiographs or magnetic resonance imaging (MRI).[5–10]

Resolution of the painful motion segment often requires (1) decompression of symptomatic neural elements that are persistently refractory to nonoperative management, (2) fusion of unstable motion segments while restoring anatomic lordosis, and (3) pain generator ablation. If possible, this would be performed without disruption of nonpathologic physiologic structures such as the paraspinal musculature.

Determining the pain generators for less obvious findings or selecting which region or segment is problematic within the lumbar spine is not always possible. Of those patients with back pain, only a small proportion go on to have chronic symptoms. A much smaller percentage will eventually undergo surgery.

Locating pain etiology begins with careful clinical evaluation and, in addition to various imaging studies such as MRI (**Fig. 32.1**), may include invasive procedures such as provocative discography (**Fig. 32.2**), epidural steroid injections, facet injections, and selective nerve root blocks. Psychological evaluation is also warranted to identify depression,

The views expressed in this chapter are those of the authors and do not necessarily reflect the official policy or position of the Department of the Navy, Department of Defense, or the United States Government.

Table 32.2 Comparison of Treatment Interventions for Chronic Back Pain Randomized Trials

	Study		
	Fritzell et al (2002)	**Brox et al (2003, 2006)**	**Fairbank et al (2005)**
Intervention in the treatment group (lumbar fusion)	(1) PLF using iliac crest autograft without fixation	—	Spinal stabilization using any technique, devices, and graft material at the discretion of the surgeon
	(2) PLF using pedicle screws and iliac crest autograft (3) ALIF or PLIF using bone blocks cut from the iliac crest	PLF using pedicle screws (VSP) and iliac crest autograft —	— —
Therapy in the control group (no surgery)	The treatment could vary within the broad but commonly used limits reflecting the nonsurgical treatment policy in the society	Cognitive intervention and exercises in a supervised treatment period of 25 hours per week at first, followed by 2 weeks at home, then another period of 2 weeks, and follow-up consultations at 3 and 6 months	A daily outpatient program of education and exercise running on 5 days per week for 3 weeks continuously averaging 75 hours, with 1 day of follow-up sessions at 1, 3, 6, or 12 months after treatment

Source: Mirza SK, Deyo RA. Systematic review of randomized trials comparing lumbar fusion surgery to nonoperative care for treatment of chronic back pain. Spine 2007:32(7):816–823; reprinted with permission.

Abbreviations: ALIF, anterior lumbar interbody fusion; PLF, posterolateral fusion; PLIF, posterior lumbar interbody fusion; VSP, variable screw placement.

One significant limitation of this study was the high degree of crossover between assigned patient groups; many patients ultimately received treatment that they were not originally randomized to receive which limited the power of the intention to treat analysis. Therefore, "as treated" analysis was used, which devalued the report.

The Swedish Lumbar Spine Study also reported the results of three spinal fusion techniques for treatment of degenerative, disabling low back pain.[16] Patients were randomized to groups for posterolateral fusion (PLF) without internal fixation, PLF with variable screw placement (VSP), and interbody fusion (anterior or posterior, per surgeon preference). Fusion rates were 91%, 87%, and 72% for interbody, PLF with VSP, and PLF without screw fixation, respectively. Even with this difference in fusion rates, however, patient outcomes did not significantly differ; all groups experienced decreased pain and disability at 2 years of postoperative follow-up.

Brox and colleagues attempted to repeat the Swedish Lumbar Spine Study in 2003 and 2006. They compared PLF with VSP to nonoperative treatment in an effort to address the shortfalls related to high crossover rates and a heterogeneous nonoperative cohort. Cognitive rehabilitation and therapy that stressed core strengthening were emphasized. The primary outcome measure (Oswestry Disability Index; ODI) showed no significant difference between the treatment cohorts. Understandably, the nonsurgical experienced significantly higher fear-avoidance scores compared with those surgically managed. The power of each of these studies has been criticized due to the number of participants was small (61 in 2003 and 57 in 2006).[12,13]

In 2005, Fairbank and colleagues published a related randomized prospective study of 349 patients comparing fusion to nonsurgical treatment. The nonoperative group followed an intensive rehabilitation program that emphasized endurance, stretching, and stabilization exercises along with cognitive therapy. Improvement in the ODI was only marginal; it was concluded that even though such an intense rehab program was unlikely to be available to the average patient, it was effective at reducing both low back pain and the inherent complications that arose in almost 11% of the surgical cohort.[15] In summary, all four studies report modest advantages of surgery compared with nonoperative treatment for lumbar pain secondary to spondylosis. Mirza and Deyo suggest that the large differences seen in nonsurgical improvement may be important for further investigation.[11]

The Spine Patient Outcomes Research Trial (SPORT) reports the results of two large studies representing level 1 evidence on the treatment of common spinal disorders. Eleven centers across the United States were used to compare clinical outcomes for surgical versus nonsurgical

Table 32.3 Comparison of Oswestry Disability Index (ODI) Results from Randomized Trials Comparing Nonoperative Care to Surgery for Chronic Back Pain

	Study			
	Fritzell et al (2002)	Brox et al (2003)	Fairbank et al (2005)	Brox et al (2006)
Final follow-up interval	2 year	1 year	2 year	1 year
Follow-up rate	98%	97%	82%	97%
Surgery Group	$n = 201$	$n = 35$	$n = 176$	$n = 29$
Baseline ODI*	47.3 (11.4)	42.0 (11.0)	46.5 (14.6)	47.0 (9.4)
Final ODI*	35.7 (18.0)	26.4 (16.4)	34.0 (21.1)	38.1 (20.1)
Charge (final-baseline)	−11.6	−15.6	−12.5	−8.9
Percent improvement[†]	24.5%	37.1%	26.9%	18.9%
Nonoperative group	$n = 63$	$n = 26$	$n = 173$	$n = 31$
Baseline ODI*	48.4 (11.9)	43.0 (13.0)	44.8 (14.8)	45.1 (9.1)
Final ODI*	45.6 (16.1)	29.7 (19.6)	36.1 (20.6)	32.3 (19.1)
Change (final − baseline)	−2.8	−13.3	−8.7	−12.8
Percent improvement[†]	5.8%	30.1%	19.4%	28.4%
Differential improvement across treatments (Δsurgery − Δnonoperative)				
Change in ODI[‡]	8.8	2.3	3.8	(−3.9)
Percent benefit with surgery[¶]	18.7%	7.0%	7.5%	(−9.5%)[#]

Source: Mirza SK, Deyo RA. Systematic review of randomized trials comparing lumbar fusion surgery to nonoperative care for treatment of chronic back pain. Spine 2007:32(7):816–823; reprinted with permission.

*Mean (SD).

[†]Change in ODI expresses as a percentage of the baseline value.

[‡]Difference of the differences: final-to-baseline ODI change in surgery group − final-to-baseline ODI change in nonsurgery group.

[¶]Difference in improvement over baseline score for surgery group − percent improvement over baseline score in nonsurgery group.

[#]Results favor nonoperative treatment.

treatment for several diagnoses at various follow-up times. The study examining lumbar disc herniation enrolled 743 patients. All had symptoms and confirmatory signs of lumbar radiculopathy with a corresponding disc herniation validated by imaging. Five-hundred twenty-eight of these received surgical treatment of a standard open discectomy with decompression of the nerve root if needed; 191 received nonsurgical treatment (i.e., therapy, education, home exercises, nonsteroidal antiinflammatory drugs). At 3 months of follow-up as defined by the SF-36 Pain Survey, the surgical group experienced significantly better bodily pain measures compared with the nonsurgical group (40.9 versus 26.0). The ODI scores also favored the operative group at 3 months (mean change, −36.1 versus −20.9). This significant margin reduced at 2 years; the nonsurgical group showed steady pain reduction to a score of 32.4. Bodily pain reported by the surgical group showed only

moderate continued improvement to 42.6. Likewise, the ODI scores also followed this trend at 2 years with the nonoperative group (−24.2) gaining more ground than the surgical group (−37.6).[17,18] The authors concluded that although both treatments helped to resolve back pain and sciatica at 2 years of follow-up, those who received surgery experienced more immediate pain relief and greater initial improvement.

For patients with spondylolisthesis, more favorable results are likewise experienced with surgery. Recently, Weinstein and colleagues reported their outcomes for 303 observational and 304 patients randomized to surgical versus nonsurgical management for degenerative spondylolisthesis as part of the SPORT.[19]

The study highlighted some of the difficulties associated with randomized trials. Approximately 40% of patients crossed over between randomized cohorts thereby

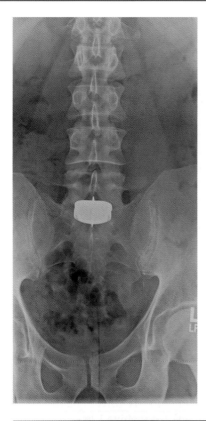

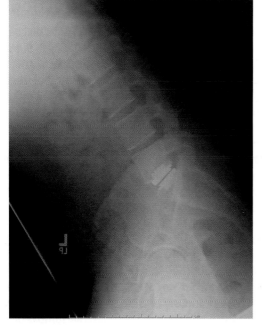

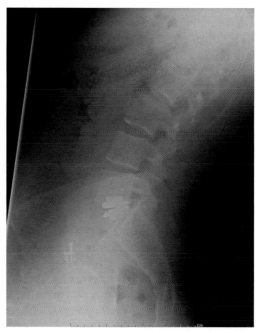

Fig. 32.4   Anteroposterior **(A)**, lateral flexion **(B)**, and extension **(C)** radiographs demonstrating satisfactory implant placement and motion at the L5–S1 intervertebral motion segment.

The gross majority of the modern literature still lacks scientific rigor. Methodologic issues limit the usefulness of the data, further confounding the question of which patients are best indicated for surgical management and if so, what procedures are necessary to accomplish the goal of a cost-effective, acceptable outcome that allows for return to work and leisure without disabling symptoms. The myriad underlying categories of degenerative lumbar spondylosis or degenerative disc disease presents additional challenges to investigators as many patients exhibit numerous symptomatic findings that include components of both back and lower extremity discomfort. To date, there remains a need for more rigorous study design that includes careful description of the degenerative process to answer these difficult questions.

References

1. Weinstein JN, Lurie JD, Olson PR, Bronner KK, Fisher ES. United States' trends and regional variations in lumbar spine surgery: 1992–2003. Spine 2006;31:2707–2714

2. Cherkin DC, Deyo RA, Loeser JD, Bush T, Waddell G. An international comparison of back surgery rates. Spine 1994;19:1201–1206

3. Deyo RA, Gray DT, Kreuter W, Mirza S, Martin BI. United States trends in lumbar fusion surgery for degenerative conditions. Spine 2005;30:1441–1445 discussion 1446–1447

4. Deyo RA. Back surgery–who needs it? N Engl J Med 2007;356: 2239–2243

5. Boden SD, Davis DO, Dina TS, Patronas NJ, Wiesel SW. Abnormal magnetic-resonance scans of the lumbar spine in asymptomatic subjects: a prospective investigation. J Bone Joint Surg Am 1990; 72:403–408

6. Boden SD, McCowin PR, Davis DO, Dina TS, Mark AS, Wiesel S. Abnormal magnetic resonance scans of the cervical spine in asymptomatic subjects: a prospective investigation. J Bone Joint Surg Am 1990;72:1178–1184

7. Jensen MC, Brant-Zawadzki MN, Obuchowski N, Modic MT, Malkasian D, Ross JS. Magnetic resonance imaging of the lumbar spine in people without back pain. N Engl J Med 1994;331:69–73

8. Boos N, Rieder R, Schade V, Spratt KF, Semmer N, Aebi M. 1995 Volvo Award in Clinical Sciences. The diagnostic accuracy of magnetic resonance imaging, work perception, and psychosocial factors in identifying symptomatic disc herniations. Spine 1995;20: 2613–2625

9. Borenstein DG, O'Mara JW Jr, Boden SD, et al. The value of magnetic resonance imaging of the lumbar spine to predict low-back pain in asymptomatic subjects: a seven-year follow-up study. J Bone Joint Surg Am 2001;83-A:1306–1311

10. Carragee EJ, Tanner CM, Yang B, Brito JL, Truong T. False-positive findings on lumbar discography: reliability of subjective concordance assessment during provocative disc injection. Spine 1999; 24:2542–2547

11. Mirza SK, Deyo RA. Systematic review of randomized trials comparing lumbar fusion surgery to nonoperative care for treatment of chronic back pain. Spine 2007;32:816–823

12. Brox JI, Sorensen R, Friis A, et al. Randomized clinical trial of lumbar instrumented fusion and cognitive intervention and exercises in patients with chronic low back pain and disc degeneration. Spine 2003;28:1913–1921

13. Brox JI, Reikeras O, Nygaard O, et al. Lumbar instrumented fusion compared with cognitive intervention and exercises in patients with chronic back pain after previous surgery for disc herniation: a prospective randomized controlled study. Pain 2006;122: 145–155

14. Fritzell P, Hagg O, Wessberg P, Nordwall A, Swedish Lumbar Spine Study Group. 2001 Volvo Award Winner in Clinical Studies. Lumbar fusion versus nonsurgical treatment for chronic low back pain: a multicenter randomized controlled trial from the Swedish Lumbar Spine Study Group. Spine 2001;26:2521–2532

15. Fairbank J, Frost H, Wilson-MacDonald J, et al. Randomised controlled trial to compare surgical stabilisation of the lumbar spine with an intensive rehabilitation programme for patients with chronic low back pain: the MRC spine stabilisation trial. BMJ 2005;330:1233

16. Fritzell P, Hagg O, Wessberg P, Nordwall A, Swedish Lumbar Spine Study Group. Chronic low back pain and fusion: a comparison of three surgical techniques: a prospective multicenter randomized study from the Swedish Lumbar Spine Study Group. Spine 2002; 27:1131–1141

17. Weinstein JN, Lurie JD, Tosteson TD, et al. Surgical vs nonoperative treatment for lumbar disk herniation: the spine patient outcomes research trial (SPORT) observational cohort. JAMA 2006;296: 2451–2459

18. Weinstein JN, Tosteson TD, Lurie JD, et al. Surgical vs nonoperative treatment for lumbar disk herniation: the spine patient outcomes research trial (SPORT): a randomized trial. JAMA 2006;296:2441–2450

19. Weinstein JN, Lurie JD, Tosteson TD, et al. Surgical versus nonsurgical treatment for lumbar degenerative spondylolisthesis. N Engl J Med 2007;356:2257–2270

20. Gibson JN, Grant IC, Waddell G. The Cochrane Review of surgery for lumbar disc prolapse and degenerative lumbar spondylosis. Spine 1999;24:1820–1832

21. Gibson JN, Waddell G. Surgery for degenerative lumbar spondylosis: updated Cochrane Review. Spine 2005;30:2312–2320

22. Gibson JN, Waddell G. Surgical interventions for lumbar disc prolapse. Cochrane Database Syst Rev 2007;(2):CD001350

23. Weatherley CR, Prickett CF, O'Brien JP. Discogenic pain persisting despite solid posterior fusion. J Bone Joint Surg Br 1986;68:142–143

24. Slosar PJ, Reynolds JB, Schofferman J, Goldthwaite N, White AH, Keaney D. Patient satisfaction after circumferential lumbar fusion. Spine 2000;25:722–726

25. Videbaek TS, Christensen FB, Soegaard R, et al. Circumferential fusion improves outcome in comparison with instrumented posterolateral fusion: long-term results of a randomized clinical trial. Spine 2006; 31:2875–2880

26. Christensen FB, Hansen ES, Eiskjaer SP, et al. Circumferential lumbar spinal fusion with Brantigan cage versus posterolateral fusion with titanium Cotrel-Dubousset instrumentation: a prospective, randomized clinical study of 146 patients. Spine 2002;27:2674–2683

27. Linson MA, Williams H. Anterior and combined anteroposterior fusion for lumbar disc pain: a preliminary study. Spine 1991;16: 143–145

28. O'Brien JP, Dawson MH, Heard CW, Momberger G, Speck G, Weatherly CR. Simultaneous combined anterior and posterior fusion: a surgical solution for failed spinal surgery with a brief review of the first 150 patients. Clin Orthop Relat Res 1986;(203):191–195

29. Anderson DG, Risbud MV, Shapiro IM, Vaccaro AR, Albert TJ. Cell-based therapy for disc repair. Spine J 2005;5:297S–303S

30. Bridwell KH, Anderson PA, Boden SD, Vaccaro AR, Wang JC. What's new in spine surgery. J Bone Joint Surg Am 2006;88:1897–1907